Linda Gallo
personal copy
Rm 538
X3521

NUTRITION and HEART DISEASE

CONTEMPORARY ISSUES IN CLINICAL NUTRITION

VOLUME 6

SERIES EDITOR
Richard S. Rivlin M.D.

EDITORIAL ADVISORY BOARD
Myron Brin, Ph.D

Leon Ellenbogen, Ph.D.

Elaine B. Feldman, M.D.

Sami A. Hashim, M.D.

Sheldon Konigsberg, M.D.

NUTRITION and HEART DISEASE

Edited by

Elaine B. Feldman, M.D.

Professor of Medicine
Chief, Section of Nutrition
Director, Clinical Nutrition Research Unit
and Georgia Institute of Human Nutrition
Medical College of Georgia
Augusta, Georgia

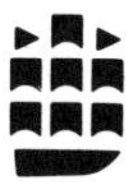

Churchill Livingstone
New York, Edinburgh, London, and Melbourne
1983

First published 1983
Printed in USA

ISBN 0-443-08243-X

9 8 7 6 5 4 3 2 1

Library of Congress Cataloging in Publication Data
Main entry under title:

Nutrition and heart disease.
    (Contemporary issues in clinical nutrition; v. 6)
    Bibliography: p.
    Includes index.
    1. Heart—Diseases—Nutritional aspects—Addresses,
essays, lectures.—I. Feldman, Elaine B.
II. Series. [DNLM: 1. Heart diseases—Etiology. 2. Heart
diseases—Prevention and control. 3. Diet. 4. Diet,
Atherogenic. 5. Nutrition. W1 CO769MQH v.6 / WG 200
N976]
RC682.N86   1983   616.1'2071   83-15354
ISBN 0-443-08243-X

Contributors

Robert E. Burch, M.D.
Price-Goldsmith Professor of Clinical Nutrition
Tulane University School of Medicine
Associate Chief of Staff for Research
Veterans Administration Medical Center
New Orleans, Louisiana

Arlene W. Caggiula, Ph.D.
Associate Professor of Nutrition
Department of Epidemiology
Graduate School of Public Health
University of Pittsburgh
Pittsburgh, Pennsylvania

William E. Connor, M.D.
Professor of Medicine
Section of Clinical Nutrition and Lipid Metabolism
Director, Lipid-Atherosclerosis Research Laboratory
Co-Director, Lipid Disorders Clinic
The Oregon Health Sciences University
Portland, Oregon

Elaine B. Feldman, M.D.
Professor of Medicine
Chief, Section of Nutrition
Director, Clinical Nutrition Research Unit
    and Georgia Institute of Human Nutrition
Medical College of Georgia
Augusta, Georgia

John P. Foreyt, M.D.
Associate Professor of Medicine
Department of Medicine
Baylor College of Medicine—The Methodist Hospital
Houston, Texas

Howard S. Friedman, M.D.
Associate Professor of Medicine
Downstate Medical Center
State University of New York
Chief, Section of Cardiology
The Brooklyn Hospital
Brooklyn, New York

Linda L. Gallo, Ph.D.
Associate Professor of Biochemistry
The George Washington University Medical Center
Washington, D.C.

Scott H. Goodnight, Jr., M.D.
Professor of Medicine
Head, Hematology and Medical Oncology
Director, Hemostasis and Thrombosis Research Laboratory
Department of Medicine
The Oregon Health Sciences University
Portland, Oregon

Antonio M. Gotto, Jr., M.D.
Chairman, Department of Medicine
Baylor College of Medicine
Chief, Active Staff Services
The Methodist Hospital
Houston, Texas

Henry K.J. Hahn, Ph.D.
Associate Professor of Medicine and Biochemistry
Tulane University School of Medicine
Research Chemist
Veterans Administration Medical Center
New Orleans, Louisiana

William S. Harris, Ph.D.
Research Fellow
Section of Clinical Nutrition and Lipid Metabolism
Department of Medicine
The Oregon Health Sciences University
Portland, Oregon

David Kritchevsky, M.D.
Professor of Biochemistry in Surgery
University of Pennsylvania
Associate Director
The Wistar Institute of Anatomy and Biology
Philadelphia, Pennsylvania

Lewis H. Kuller, M.D., Dr.P.H.
Professor and Chairman
Department of Epidemiology
Graduate School of Public Health
University of Pittsburgh
Pittsburgh, Pennsylvania

Terrence T. Kuske, M.D.
Professor of Medicine
Associate Dean for Curriculum
Associate Director, Georgia Institute of Human Nutrition
Medical College of Georgia
Augusta, Georgia

Charles S. Lieber, M.D.
Professor of Medicine and Pathology
Mt. Sinai School of Medicine
Director, Alcohol Research and Treatment Center
Veterans Administration Medical Center
Bronx, New York

Trevor J. Orchard, M.B.B.Ch., M.Med.Sci.
Assistant Professor
Department of Epidemiology
Graduate School of Public Health
University of Pittsburgh
Pittsburgh, Pennsylvania

Lynn W. Scott, M.D.
Assistant Professor of Medicine
Department of Medicine
Baylor College of Medicine—The Methodist Hospital
Houston, Texas

R. Joe Teague, M.D.
Assistant Professor of Medicine
Section of Nutrition
Medical College of Georgia
Augusta, Georgia

Foreword

In the decade since 1970 it has been recognized that regular, vigorous exercise can raise the plasma level of the high-density lipoproteins in human plasma, and that such lipids protect the arteries from formation of plaques rich in triglyceride and cholesterol. For a century it has been known that coronary disease is rarely found in the bodies of poor people dying in city hospitals, although it is a common cause of death in doctors, lawyers, businessmen, and persons in easy circumstances due to inheritance. This greater incidence of coronary disease was proved to be largely a consequence of diets rich in dairy products, eggs, and meat with a high fat content. In 1970, the experiments of Zelis and colleagues* showed conclusively that the arterial lesions could be prevented and even reversed by diets and drugs that limited triglyceride and cholesterol absorption.

When persons are on a high caloric intake, due to alcohol or refined carbohydrate, the liver can swiftly produce triglyceride and cholesterol to form the precursor of low-density lipoprotein. Reduction in caloric intake and increase in physical activity, as well as a change from saturated to polyunsaturated fatty acids in the diet, is the key to good coronary health. Exercise does not merely burn up the calories that should have been avoided, it causes increased production of lipoproteins rich in protein and phosphorus and, hence, lipoproteins of high density (atomic weight P = 31, H = 1, C = 12, N = 14). These protect the arteries.

Since exercise also causes restructuring of bones and prevents osteoporosis, we should be grateful to parents who taught us the joy of walking in the hills. Patients should not take seriously the advice of overweight physicians, who are not likely to give sound advice or stimulate them to lead normal, healthy lives. The authors of this volume bring us up to date on the relation between our nutrition, our habits, and our health.

William Dock, M.D.
Paris

---

* Mason DT, Spann JF Jr, Zelis R, and Amsterdam EA: Comparison of the cardiac contractile state in patients with idiopathic myocardial disease and in ventricular hypertrophy secondary to prolonged systolic pressure overloading. J Clin Invest 38:196A, 1970.

Preface

A variety of nutritional factors are implicated in the etiology and pathogenesis of coronary heart disease, hypertension, cardiomyopathy and specific deficiency diseases affecting the heart.

This volume brings together primarily new information acquired in the past decade implicating components of the diet, in addition to lipids, which influence levels of serum lipids, lipoprotein composition and atherosclerosis.

The contributing authors, experienced investigators in nutrition research, not only review critically the scientific data relating various nutrients to the clinical, physiological, biochemical and pathologic manifestations of cardiac disorders but also provide practical information to use in preventing or treating heart disease and counseling patients. This volume is therefore informative to nutrition researchers and educators and medical practitioners, especially in primary care.

I would like to thank all the contributors, my colleagues in the Nutrition Section at MCG who helped in the review process, my patient and efficient secretaries, Sue Wetherington and Barbara Trill, and my husband "Dr. Dan" who is all of the above.

Elaine B. Feldman, M.D.

Contents

NUTRITION and HEART DISEASE

1 Epidemiologic Studies of Nutrition and Heart Disease

Arlene W. Caggiula
Trevor J. Orchard
Lewis H. Kuller

THE MEASUREMENT OF NUTRITIONAL FACTORS

The ability to establish a relationship between nutritional factors and cardiovascular disease has been hampered to a large extent by limitations in the methodology used. Many studies have employed methods that were either inappropriate or inadequate for measuring the relationships in question. Additionally, some studies that have used valid methods have suffered from misinterpretation or inappropriate application of their results. Our knowledge of methods is also seriously limited because many of the studies that evaluated them were done before the availability of computerized data bases and, therefore, involved relatively small samples. Applying the conclusions from these earlier studies to contemporary large-scale epidemiologic studies and clinical trials clearly involves some risk.

Basically, there are two approaches for measuring nutritional factors or patterns: direct and indirect. Methods employing the direct approach include the collection of phantom food samples and observation of foods or meals eaten. While both of these methods should provide data with the highest validity, they have a number of disadvantages, especially for studies with large samples. To utilize phantom food samples (duplicate portions of all foods eaten within a prescribed period of time), the study population must be highly motivated and compliant. Since it is expensive to analyze these samples even for a relatively small number of nutrients, sample size is limited. Finally, the validity of the data may be decreased if the collection of the sample results in changes in food intake (reactivity) or if the subject fails to collect the duplicate portion correctly. This latter disadvantage can be overcome by utilizing trained nutrition personnel to collect the sample. However, this would substantially add to the cost of collecting the data[1] and might also affect the usual pattern of dietary intake.

The major disadvantage of the alternative direct approach, the observation method, is that its application is largely confined to populations that are institutionalized or who are fed from a cafeteria or meal service. It also requires the use of trained observers to record the data. The validity of the data would also be decreased if subjects had access to foods from other sources, such as snack bars, that were not under observation.

While neither of these methods would be appropriate for large-scale studies of free-living populations, they might be utilized in small subsamples to provide a measure of internal validity for the indirect method(s) actually employed.[2]

The methods most commonly used in large-scale studies are indirect ones, that is, they rely on the subjects' ability to record or recall foods or meals eaten over a specified period of time. These include the diet history (Burke type), the food or diet record, the dietary recall, and the food frequency questionnaire. Each method differs from the others with respect to its strengths and weaknesses, and the selection of the appropriate method should be made after consideration of the factors discussed below.

Measurement of Group Differences

In many epidemiologic studies the objective is to characterize the relationship between an individual's intake of a specific nutrient or food pattern and an outcome measure such as serum cholesterol or blood pressure, or an endpoint measure such as rate of fatal and/or nonfatal coronary heart disease (CHD). However, when the study design includes an intervention component for one or more randomized subgroups, it would be important to measure the differences between the groups in question. In general it is easier to characterize the dietary intake of groups than it is to accurately characterize the intake of individuals, and a smaller amount of data needs to be collected for each subject. Two methods, the 24-hour recall and the food record are appropriate when considering only differences between groups. The 24-hour recall method is only reliable for groups of greater than 50 people, but can be used instead of a 7-day food record if errors of 10 percent between methods for some nutrients can be tolerated.[3] The 24-hour recall should be conducted by a trained interviewer in a standardized fashion using open-ended probing questions and food models to estimate portion sizes.

Similarly, a 1-day food record (the subject's recorded food intake for the day in question) can be substituted for a 24-hour recall. The major advantage of the record is that it does not rely on the subject's memory. However, to improve validity the subject must be instructed in the procedures for keeping the record, and the resulting data should be documented by a trained nutritionist working with the subject. If greater precision is required in the estimate of mean intake, it is more efficient to increase the sample size than to increase the number of days recorded by each subject. A major disadvantage is that the record-keeping procedure may produce changes in the subject's eating behavior so that the validity of the data, as an estimate of usual intake, is reduced.

Collection of data by either of these methods is not particularly time consuming for the subject or for the nutrition personnel. A thorough 24-hour recall interview for the average subject should take 20 minutes, and the total time needed for patient instruction and documentation of a 1-day record usually would not exceed the time required for the recall. While there does not appear to be a consistent variability in dietary intake by "day of the week" for most population groups, a potential bias can be avoided by randomly assigning days to be recorded, or by scheduling recalls so that equal amounts of data are collected for each day of the week.[4]

Measurement of Individuals

As already mentioned, it is fairly difficult to accurately characterize the dietary intake of individuals, primarily because of the large degree of daily variability. The degree of variability among individuals is related both to the nutrient(s) and the population group to be investigated. For example Keys[1] reported that in dietary surveys of men from the islands of Crete and Corfu, the intra-individual variance for protein and fat was not significantly smaller than the inter-individual variance, while Liu and colleagues[5] reported that for three populations studied, the ratios of intra- to inter-individual variance for dietary cholesterol were greater than one. In fact, for two of these populations the estimated ratios were >3. Balogh and colleagues[6] also reported much larger coefficients of variation (standard deviation between days divided by mean intake of nutrient) for nutrients such as cholesterol and linoleic acid than for calories and total carbohydrate. In rural populations or in populations that subsist on diets containing a limited number of food items, the daily variability for most nutrients would likely be smaller than in highly industrialized groups with access to a large variety of foods and food products.

Any of the four indirect methods previously identified can be used to measure the dietary intake of individuals. However, it should be noted that the results from any one of these methods do not predict the results of another to a very high degree, so that they cannot be used interchangeably within the same study.[7] While the Burke-type diet history frequently results in higher levels for the nutrients in question than either the food record or recall, there is no evidence that the data from the food history is a more valid measure than the others. The validity and choice of method will depend on other design characteristics, such as the nutritional factors or variables of interest, availability of trained personnel and time for data collection, availability of valid food-table values, and method of data analyses.

Retrospective/Prospective Design Implications

For prospective studies, a choice of methods can be made from those previously mentioned. However, the choice is severely limited in retrospective studies. Two methods, the Burke-type diet history and the food frequency questionnaire, can be utilized, but the validity of the data from both will decrease as the retrospective period increases in duration. The Burke-type diet history has usually represented dietary intake for periods of less than 1 year, and it is questionable whether subjects can accurately remember more than whether selected food items were consumed on frequent versus occasional or never basis if the time period of interest is more than 1 or 2 years in the past. Therefore, a food frequency questionnaire is probably the method of choice for retrospective studies of periods of greater than 1 year.

Dietary Factors of Interest

Young and Trulson[7] state, "Each investigator in epidemiological studies must decide which method appears to give the most valid index of what it is about dietary intake that he is trying to correlate with various aspects of a disease." In fact, the specific indexes selected to represent the nutritional factors under investigation have the greatest influence on the selection of an appropriate method for data collection. There are several indexes that have been used in epidemiologic studies as measures, and they vary in terms of their quantitative and descriptive nature. The most quantitative indexes provide data on the quantity of specific nutrients, such as calories, protein, saturated fat, or individual vitamins and minerals such as sodium or potassium, consumed by an individual or group for a specified period of time. The data can also be expressed as food groups, that is, as percentages of calories from high-fat foods, high-sodium foods, high-fiber foods, or high–β-carotene foods. This latter approach is particularly useful when the quantity of the nutrient in question is clearly differentiated by food group, in other words, the values are not continuous across all food groups. For example, high β-carotene–containing foods are primarily fruits and vegetables, thus, expressing the data in that way provides a clear indication that it represents a measure of fruit and vegetable intake. Further, data of this type is particularly useful when describing the effects of an intervention program on food choices. In this case, the investigator is primarily concerned with the behavioral effects obtained, and is less interested in actual nutrient values.

To obtain either of these indexes, data must be collected by the 24-hour recall, food record, or Burke-type diet history. Since the 24-hour recall and food record represent limited food intake periods, they must be collected on a repeated basis (preferably over an extended period of time) if a valid estimate of individual intake is to be obtained. The number of samples or days to be collected will vary according to the nutritional factors and population under investigation, however, a *minimum* of 6 days is probably required in order to accurately estimate intake of most nutrients. For nutrients such as cholesterol and vitamin A that have very high intra-individual variability, 10 days or more are necessary.

A third approach is to describe food patterns or habits. For example, salting habits have been used to differentiate levels of sodium intake, while alternative dietary patterns such as vegetarian or lactovegetarian have denoted quantitative differences in the consumption of animal fat or protein. These indexes will only provide data that will allow a population or individual to be loosely characterized or scaled in relation to the intake of the nutritional factors in question. In fact, the major disadvantage of this approach is that it may not provide enough data to adequately differentiate levels of intake either between or among individuals or groups. For example, Sacks and colleagues[8] studied lipoprotein patterns in two groups of young adults and found levels of total cholesterol, LDL cholesterol, and triglycerides in the vegetarian group living in a commune that were significantly lower than those levels in the free-living group eating the "usual" American diet. However, except for Dahl's study,[9] studies by other investigators have been unable to find a relationship between salting habits (as a measure of sodium intake) and blood pressure.

These examples illustrate how the nature of the population and the nutritional factors to be studied influence the choice of appropriate method and indexes. In a free-living population, sodium intake cannot be characterized simply by salting habits. This is particularly true now, since many foods that are commonly eaten are precooked, convenience, or fast foods that contain large amounts of salt. In a sense, sodium has been ubiquitous in the normal food environment of industrialized countries; to adequately assess intake levels, consumption of all foods must be measured. However, in the Sack's study[8] dietary intake within the commune group was fairly homogeneous and represented a significantly different food pattern than that of the matched controls. Because of this high degree of homogeneity, it was not necessary to measure the nutrient intake of each individual to characterize the group. Instead, a simple description of the food pattern and the frequency of consumption for animal-protein foods was adequate.

Finally, intake can be expressed simply by the frequency of consumption of specific foods. As is true of the food grouping approach, this index is most useful and valid when a few foods characteristically represent the major portion of intake for the nutrient(s) in question. For example, since eggs have been the primary source of dietary cholesterol in westernized diets, egg consumption patterns provide a rough index for total intake of cholesterol. Similarly, the consumption patterns of bananas and citrus fruits and juices provides an index of total potassium intake. These indexes clearly grow less useful and less accurate as diversification of dietary intake increases, since the chance of misclassifying an individual's intake is greater. There is also the danger that, because of changing patterns of consumption within a population, the food or foods chosen as the index no longer represent total intake. Twenty years ago total intake of dietary cholesterol was very much defined by egg consumption patterns. Since egg consumption has decreased markedly, it no longer represents a valid index of dietary cholesterol intake, and other foods that represent the primary sources will have to be used.

Resources for Data Analyses

In addition to the design implications discussed above, the availability of certain resources for data analyses also has a decided influence on the methods and indexes chosen to measure nutritional factors. As discussed before, lack of computerized data bases and analyses has limited sample size in many studies. Even today, however, in studies with relatively small samples, computer analyses should be utilized, because they provide a higher level of accuracy and consistency than hand calculation.

Valid and reliable food table values are available for most of the major nutrients but are not yet available for trace minerals or micronutrients. Therefore, if the objective is to measure the intake of nutrients such as zinc or selenium, the only appropriate methods would be those based on direct analyses of phantom or duplicate food samples.

There are also problems associated with the construction of valid food tables (data bases) even for major nutrients. First, it is not clear whether variability in nutrient content is introduced by the effect of growing area or by techniques used in food processing. Secondly, it is difficult to obtain and maintain accurate information on commercially manufactured foods, which make up an increasing proportion of the westernized diet. While food companies usually provide data on a selected group of major nutrients, this group may not include the ones of greatest interest to a study. This information is critical, however, since content of nutrients such as sodium may vary so much by brand that existing values in the food table cannot be considered accurate estimates. For example, there is a three-fold difference in the sodium content between several brands of salted potato chips, and this difference can be as high as 10 mEq or 230 mg.

Error is also introduced when ingredients such as added fat, alcohol, or sodium are used in the preparation of foods and are not accounted for in the analysis. This source of error can be minimized, however, if the food intake data is collected and/or documented carefully by trained nutrition personnel. The time and availability of these personnel should also be considered a resource, if not a critical one. Even in studies utilizing self-reporting or self-administered questionnaires, the design of instruments and a review for additional documentation and completeness by nutritionists are important.

It is clear that estimating dietary intake is difficult, particularly for individuals within highly industrialized populations. However, applying appropriate methods with well-trained personnel can greatly improve the accuracy of the estimate and the potential for establishing a relationship between nutritional factors and cardiovascular disease.

THE MEASUREMENT OF CARDIOVASCULAR DISEASE IN THE COMMUNITY

The Problem of Changing Fashions

Like many areas of epidemiologic study, cardiovascular disease epidemiology is hampered by both imprecise and variable measures of the disease endpoints of interest. The use of stringent criteria that are universally accepted and that remain constant over time is a vital requisite for investigators interested in trying to interpret geographic differences and temporal changes. For example, it is likely that the epidemic of heart disease in the early and middle parts of this century may be attributable, in part, to changing fashions in signing death certificates. This is suggested by the decline in deaths ascribed to nonischemic heart disease that occurred between 1950 and 1968, and the concomitant rise in ischemic heart disease deaths. Conversely, "other" forms of heart disease rose by 47 percent between 1968 and 1976 in the United States, while ischemic, rheumatic, and hypertensive heart disease fell by over 20 percent.[10] How much of these changes can be ascribed to changing fashions in signing death certificates is difficult to assess, and this is further complicated by the changes in the International Classification of Disease codes, which occur every 10 years.

In order to permit monitoring of cardiovascular disease and to overcome some of these difficulties in terms of disease endpoint definition and criteria, a number of surveillance studies have been developed within the United States[11,12] and, through the World Health Organization (WHO), throughout the world.[13] The latest study within the United States is beginning its pilot phases as of this writing, and is called the Community Cardiovascular Surveillance Project. A major problem in studies such as these is arriving at a standard set of criteria for each cardiovascular event, particularly when the clinical and laboratory data available vary from hospital to hospital, from doctor to doctor, from area to area, and over time.

These studies, it is hoped, will enable the investigators to examine geographic and temporal changes, particularly with regard to whether these are a result of changes in incidence (that is, a change in the amount of disease occurring in the community) or of changes in case fatality (that is, the mortality experience of those with the disease).

The Problem of Disease Manifestation

Another aspect of the difficulties in documenting cardiovascular disease is the fact that there is no single reliable and valid test to ascertain whether a person actually has the *underlying* disease. For coronary or ischemic heart disease, the underlying disease would be atherosclerotic-thrombotic occlusive disease of the coronary arteries. In terms of cerebral vascular disease, the situation is further complicated by the importance of hypertension and embolic disease. The one possible exception to this lack of a definitive test (apart from pathologic studies) might be arteriography, which can be performed both on coronary and cerebral vessels. However, this test is far from an epidemiologic tool, since it is expensive, carries a moderate risk (approximately 0.1 percent mortality), is difficult to perform and is unpleasant for the participant, who may suffer considerable morbidity.[14]

Consequently, because we do not have a measure of the disease process, we are obliged to use as our measure the *effects* of the arterial disease and not the arterial disease itself. This, then, raises considerable problems because, like any biologic factor, the expression of coronary artery disease (for example, in terms of heart disease events) is very variable. The events that are documented in epidemiologic studies range from various fatal events, such as fatal myocardial infarction and sudden death, to morbid events. These include asymptomatic myocardial infarction (detectable by regular ECG recording); definite, probable, or possible acute myocardial infarction; angina (determined in a variety of ways, including questionnaire and physician diagnosis); and a range of other conditions, including acute coronary insufficiency, atypical angina, and the intermediate coronary syndrome. The variability in the criteria used in different studies for these endpoints makes the epidemiologic data very difficult to interpret.

The Problem of Different Etiologies

As already indicated, the etiologic point of interest in ischemic heart disease is the process in the arteries that leads to the impairment of the blood supply to the heart muscle (myocardium). However, there are many theories that have been proposed to account for this atherosclerotic-thrombotic disease process.[15] These include (1) the lipid infiltration hypothesis, (2) an hypothesis that the primary lesion comprises a proliferation of smooth muscle cells, and (3) an hypothesis that suggests that the major lesion is one of thrombosis or blood clotting and that the other atherosclerotic features represent subsequent developments stemming from this abnormality.[15] While it is quite feasible that all of these and other elements are involved, the atherothrombotic process remains a major unknown in the investigation of cardiovascular etiology for the measures of disease endpoints we are using may relate to these different hypotheses to varying degrees in different people. The major emphasis in the United States appears to have been on the atherosclerotic or lipid hypotheses while less attention has been paid in epidemiologic studies to the hemostatic factors. This is partly the result of a deficiency of suitable tests, although it is interesting to note that in a prospective study in England, hemostatic factors including Factors VII, VIII, and fibrinogen have been shown to be equally predictive, if not more predictive, compared with cholesterol, in the development of ischemic heart disease in a middle-aged, community-based population.[16]

Thus, not only do we use variably defined endpoints as our measures of the disease process(es), we also use the same endpoints in all patients, although it would seem likely that different patients would have different mixtures of the etiologic processes outlined above. Another example of this difficulty is the recent description of coronary artery spasm[17] as a disease process that can lead to both variant angina and, conceivably, to fatal coronary heart disease. A further example is the possibility of a primary arrhythmic process resulting in fatal heart disease, which may be entirely independent of the atherothrombotic processes (yet still may be similarly classified along with disease endpoints resulting from atherothrombosis) as shown by reports of ventricular fibrillation occurring without any evidence of myocardial infarction or severe atherosclerosis.[18]

The Problem of Other Factors Affecting Mortality

Another aspect of this problem of measuring cardiovascular disease in the community lies in the fact that different factors affect the mortality of people who develop the various forms of cardiovascular disease. Thus, if one is using deaths from various types of heart disease as a measure of the amount of heart disease in a community over a time period, the deaths that are counted reflect not only the frequency of disease, but also the medical care that the patients receive and the severity of any primary nonfatal disease that the patients have developed. For example, the number of patients who suffer first myocardial infarctions and die rapidly may be a fair measure of the incidence of fatal myocardial infarction. However, for patients who do not die, the prognosis then is a result of other factors. Among these are the extent of the myocardial damage, the degree of pump failure that may have developed, the precise part of the myocardium that is affected, and whether there is an irritable zone causing dysrhythmias. Consequently, a measure of cardiovascular mortality involving a high proportion of secondary cases, that is, deaths occurring to people who already have the disease, is a more imprecise measure of the incidence of that disease, and is a composite of the manisfestations of the disease and the care received. Clearly, if the proportions of primary and secondary deaths is different in a community over time or between communities, then comparisons of disease death rates in those two communities or time periods will be difficult to interpret.

In summary, it would seem that in the realm of cardiovascular epidemiology we use relatively imprecise disease endpoints to measure a disease process that is likely to be multifactorial, perhaps even a process that involves a number of completely different processes, but which are collectively measured by these imprecise disease endpoints. Our measures are further weakened by the fact that nonetiologic factors, including medical care, are involved in the manifestation of the various fatal disease endpoints that are commonly used. Thus, despite the many advances that have been made in cardiovascular epidemiology, there is much work still to do if we are to understand the pathogenetic processes that underlie the cardiovascular diseases.

ECOLOGICAL STUDIES

The original studies of the relationship between nutrition and coronary heart disease (CHD) were classical ecological analyses. Estimated nutritional intake in the population was provided by data related to food production, consumption of available nutrients, and estimated nutritional intake from household or individual surveys. The mortality rate for the same population was determined and compared with its estimated nutrient intake.[19] This ecological approach has been used very successfully in the investigation of other nutritional disorders, such as Goldberger's classical description of pellagra in the southeastern United States.[20]

These early ecological studies described a strong relationship between dietary intake of cholesterol and saturated fat and CHD mortality on a community basis. Similar studies have also noted an association between the intake of sodium or salt in the diet and hypertension. Ecological studies, however, have important limitations. Conclusions drawn from such studies alone can be criticized legitimately because other factors that may differ among communities and that are correlated with nutrient intake may be the primary determinants of the disease. The relationship between nutritional intake and disease may be spurious because of a common correlation of specific nutrient intake, disease, and other factors that may be the true etiologic factors; for example, behavioral characteristics, social organization, stress, or genetic differences may correlate with nutritional factors and may play parts in the etiology of the disease as well.

The ecologic analyses also do not make it possible to compare the relationships among nutritional intake, biochemical measurements, and disease for any specific individual. From individual to individual within a population, the relationship between nutrition and disease may be very different from that among populations. However, if atherosclerosis is an example of a so-called common-source epidemic (the common source being the amount or percent of calories consumed that include cholesterol or saturated fat), comparing overall measurements of exposure obtained from populations that differ widely in their fat intake may be more useful than comparing measurements from individuals within a homogeneous population in which a large segment has similar exposure. For example, if consumption of greater than 10 percent of total calories as saturated fat is considered the common-source risk for atherosclerotic disease, then probably the entire United States population (except certain religious groups, vegetarians, and those on therapeutic diets) would be considered exposed to the common source, and thus would be considered at risk. The variation and frequency of disease within the population in which all are exposed would then be a function of other factors, for example, genetic response to the common source, smoking, hypertension, exercise, behavior, and the like.[22] There may still be a gradation in risk in relation to the dose of the common source, that is, the amount of saturated fat or cholesterol in the diet.[23] However, it is possible that increased consumption of fat or cholesterol above our "threshold" point would make relatively little difference, compared with the other factors. Nevertheless, fat or cholesterol intake above threshold would still be *sine qua non* for the disease.

Measurements of Serum Lipoproteins

Unfortunately, measuring differences among individuals in diet, especially over time, is extremely difficult because of the marked "within," as compared with "between," individual variations.[24] This problem has made it practically impossible to test a relationship between dose of nutrient and risk of disease.[25] Lipoprotein levels in the blood have therefore been used as a surrogate for estimating dietary intake in many individual-based studies. There is clearly a strong relationship between plasma cholesterol, or LDL cholesterol, and the risk of heart attack, and probably also between the degree of atherosclerosis, especially in younger individuals (those below the age of 50 years).[26] There is, however, little proof of a strong relationship between dietary intake of cholesterol and saturated fat, or any other known nutrient, and an individual's specific plasma cholesterol levels. The use of lipoprotein levels in the blood may, therefore, be a relatively inaccurate measure of the relationship between dietary intake and atherosclerosis. Clinical trials in humans have focused primarily on changes in diet in an intervention group, compared with a control group, and have related the resulting changes in plasma cholesterol or other lipoprotein subfractions to the subsequent risk of disease. Animal experimental studies probably offer the best approach to determine any specific relationship between differences in dietary intake for a single animal and the extent of atherosclerosis.[27] Unfortunately, most such experiments have either used very large doses of "fat" or "cholesterol" or hyperresponding animals to measure effects on plasma cholesterol. It is also difficult to extrapolate from animal studies to humans. For example, a rapid change in dietary intake over one or two generations in an experimental animal may not be an appropriate model for the more gradual and long-term changes in diet that humans have experienced.

Special Populations

The ecological studies have been extended in recent years. The observations of either a very low or high rate of coronary heart disease in a population have suggested possible specific determinants of risk. For example, because of the very low rates of ischemic heart disease in Greenland Eskimos, a major focus is now placed on their dietary pattern in which fish provides the major portion of animal protein (see Chapter 4). The effects of eating fish oils high in eicosapentaenoic acid on platelet behavior and plasma cholesterol concentrations has been studied. There is a decrease in low density lipoprotein (LDL) and an increase in high density lipoprotein (HDL) cholesterol, a change in platelet aggregation, and a possible reduction in platelet-vessel wall interaction.[28]

Studies of Seventh Day Adventists who are predominantly lactoovovegetarians have also demonstrated lower CHD mortality (especially for men) compared with other populations living in the same area. Further, detailed comparisons of more representative comparison groups within the Seventh Day Adventist populations have substantiated these observations.[29] For example, it has been possible within the Seventh Day Adventist population to classify individuals by dose of "meat intake" per week, controlling for other risk factors and then demonstrating a positive dose relationship between "meat intake" and risk of heart disease. This relationship is obviously not an example of a randomized trial of the diet hypothesis. Individuals who eat meat within the Seventh Day Adventist religion may also not participate in other specific observations, such as abstinence from cigarettes or alcohol, although these have been controlled in some of the analyses.

There are very marked geographic variations in coronary heart disease mortality within the United States.[30] There have been few studies that have compared dietary intake in various areas of the United States with the coronary heart disease mortality rates. Studies relating plasma cholesterol levels in the United States population and CHD death rates have generally not been able to determine any relationship between diet and heart attack.[31] The relative homogeneity of the United States diet, except for certain subgroups such as the Seventh Day Adventist, may preclude attempts to relate diet to either lipoprotein levels or coronary heart disease mortality among the different areas of the United States.

Several investigators have also explored the marked inverse relationship between social class and coronary heart disease mortality in the United States, and at least one study suggested that serum cholesterol levels may be higher in the low-income groups, and may contribute to higher mortality in the lower-income groups.[32] Again, however, there are marked differences in blood pressure, smoking, physical activity, and other characteristics, which may account along with diet for the marked social-class variations in mortality.

Several investigators have been particularly interested in the possible relation between deficiency of trace elements (such as selenium) in the diet and the risk of heart disease (see Chapter 9).[33] The classical ecologic approach has been to compare the soil concentration of selenium or other trace metals to the coronary heart disease incidence or mortality. The presumption is that in areas in which the soil is low in selenium, the dietary intake will also be low. The use of commercially prepared foods, supermarket shopping, and the frequency with which meals are eaten at restaurants all weaken this hypothesis except in selected rural areas of the United States. A recent study in Finland, however, has evaluated the relationship between selenium intake, coronary heart disease deaths, and myocardial infarction. The coronary heart disease death rates in East Finland are some of the highest in the world, and the soil in Finland as well as the diet of the Finns are very low in selenium.[33] Serum samples were available at baseline for a random sample of the population in two areas of East Finland surveyed in 1972. The mean concentration of serum selenium was 51.8 μg/L with a standard deviation of 13.8 for all coronary heart disease cases, and 55.3 μg/L with a standard deviation of 14.7 for all controls—a significant difference. The relative risk of coronary disease was very high (6.9 percent) for those with low serum selenium ($\leq$34 μg/L), in comparison with the risk for those whose levels were greater than 45 μg/L. The results are very interesting, but must be interpreted cautiously. It is very possible that the selenium levels may be correlated with another factor that is related to the risk of coronary heart disease mortality. Further, it was not possible within the homogeneous population to describe the relationship between dietary intake of selenium, serum selenium levels, and the risk of disease.

Lipids and Other Diseases

The incidence or mortality of other diseases have been related to the consumption of cholesterol or fat and/or serum cholesterol concentrations. Carcinoma of the colon [34] and breast [35] have both been correlated with the population's consumption of dietary fat and cholesterol, as has coronary heart disease. Several studies, however, have demonstrated that the plasma cholesterol levels are lower in individuals who subsequently die of colon cancer than in controls.[36] It has been suggested that cholesterol or bile acid metabolism in the colon may result in the formation of carcinogens. Increasing dietary intake of cholesterol may be related to both atherosclerosis and colon cancer.[37] The development of atherosclerosis may primarily depend on the plasma cholesterol response, especially LDL cholesterol, to the dietary intake, while the risk of colon cancer may relate to the amount of cholesterol or bile acid secreted or the poor absorption of cholesterol in the gastrointestinal tract. No clinical data are available describing the change in plasma cholesterol in relationship to dietary cholesterol intake among individuals destined to develop colon cancer, as compared with coronary heart disease or other controls. This type of study, which would have to be done in a metabolic unit after the development of disease such as cancer or heart disease, may be flawed because of any specific effect of the disease itself on cholesterol absorption and metabolism. Two recent observations, however, may be pertinent. First, a report from the New Orleans pathology studies suggested a relationship between the extent of coronary atherosclerosis and the presence of colonic polyps at postmortem examination;

and, second, the observations in two studies suggested an association between cholecystectomy and right-sided colon cancer. It is also important to note that in populations in which the plasma cholesterol (especially the LDL cholesterol) is low and the dietary intake of cholesterol and saturated fat is low, such as among native Japanese and lactoovovegetarian Seventh Day Adventists,[39] the risk of both colon cancer and coronary artery disease is low. The possible relationship between plasma cholesterol and colon cancer may be limited, therefore, to those populations in which the intake of cholesterol or fat in the diet is high. The important question within these populations is whether the individuals who have a low plasma cholesterol and a possible increased risk of colon cancer also have high or low dietary intakes of cholesterol and saturated fat compared with controls or individuals who develop coronary artery disease.

Studies of Migrants

Studies of migrants represent another approach. The studies of the Japanese migrants to Hawaii and California have generated the greatest interest in the United States.[40] It is clear that within a short period of time there is a substantial increase in the cholesterol levels and subsequent CHD mortality among migrants from Japan to either Hawaii and California, and that this increase is associated with marked changes in the diet. Baseline nutritional patterns (assessed by 24-hour recall) indicated group mean intakes of total fat, saturated fat, and animal protein were very much lower in Japanese men than in Japanese-American men, while group mean intakes of total carbohydrates, complex carbohydrates, alcohol, and salt were higher in the Japanese. However, there has been some concern that other factors related to Japanese life-style, especially the loss of the traditional family structure, may be related to coronary disease, independent of the change in dietary intake. Further, within these populations (that is, in Hawaii or California), the relationship between dietary intake and the plasma cholesterol levels, or between dietary intake and risk of disease, is not as clear as the association among populations. Dietary changes and changes in blood pressure and smoking do not explain all of the increased disease experienced by migrants. Thus, although the studies of migrants strengthen the association between population intake of cholesterol or saturated fat and risk of heart disease, they do not resolve the question of any possible independent, linear relationship between dietary intake of cholesterol and saturated fat and the risk of heart disease, nor the important question about whether there is a threshold effect associated with a common source epidemic.

DIETARY INTAKE AND INDIVIDUAL RISK

Observational Studies

While ecological studies have found a strong relationship between nutritional factors, serum cholesterol, and disease, these relationships in general have not been confirmed by individually based observational studies. Dietary studies have been conducted in populations from several large, prospective, epidemiologic studies. These studies differ considerably in their sample size and characteristics, in their methods for collecting dietary data, and the nutritional variables tested.

In the first Framingham Diet Study, data on nutritional factors were collected using the Burke-type diet history in a subsample of 1,049 participants (503 males, 546 females) drawn from the total cohort.[41] Approximately 300, or 55 percent, of the female sample were not randomly selected but were the wives of men selected for the study. Almost no associations were found between reported dietary intake variables and serum cholesterol levels in either sex, except for a very weak negative association between caloric intake and serum cholesterol in men. Further, no relationship was found between dietary variables and the subsequent development of CHD in the study group, although serum cholesterol levels of the cases of CHD were 30 percent higher than in the age-adjusted population (part of this difference may be due to sampling).

The dietary habits of 4,057 adult participants of the Tecumseh Study[42] were estimated from the frequency of consumption of 110 different food items. Individual average weekly consumption of foods high in fat, sugar, starch, and alcohol were calculated and correlated with cholesterol and triglyceride (nonfasting) values. No positive correlations were found between these variables; however, they did find a significant association between serum lipids and a measure of adiposity (an index based on height, weight, and two measures of skinfold thickness).

The largest study was conducted on 8,829 middle-aged Israeli males sampled from six birth groups.[43] While mean values for serum cholesterol differed significantly between birth groups, the range of 23 mg (194 to 219 mg) between groups was relatively small and less than the standard deviation within groups.[39–41] Dietary intake was estimated from a short questionnaire administered by trained nurses. While mean values for each of nine dietary variables differed very little between groups, standard deviations within groups reflected substantial inter-individual variability. No significant associations between these dietary variables and serum cholesterol were found and correlation coefficients were all less than 0.15.

The smallest group studied was a subgroup of 26 age-matched, male pairs (each pair consisting of one subject with a high serum cholesterol level and one with a low level) randomly selected from the population in Evans County, Georgia.[44] Dietary data were collected by a nutritionist using a method similar to the Burke-type diet history. The data represent two interviews conducted 6 months apart (fall and spring). While group means for each nutrient differ by season, lack of data on individual variability make this effect difficult to interpret. None of the correlations between the 14 dietary variables and serum cholesterol were significant, either singly or when part of a multiple regression model. However, exercise (stratified on three levels—high, middle, and low) was found to have a significant negative relationship with serum cholesterol. When the effect of exercise was removed in a covariate analysis, the relationship between dietary variables and cholesterol was not improved.

Morris and colleagues[45] measured dietary intake in 337 middle-aged British males using 7 day weighed food records, and related intake variables to lipid levels and incidence of CHD (up to 20 years follow-up). No significant correlations were found (all below 0.2) between dietary variables and either total serum cholesterol or various lipoprotein fractions. They did, however, find that high energy intake and high intakes of cereal fiber were related to lower rates of CHD, even after adjusting for age, occupation, and length of follow-up. Further, they reported an inverse (although not significant) relationship between the ratio of polyunsaturated fatty acids to saturated fatty acids (P-S ratio) and incidence of CHD. The rate for men with low P-S ratios (.09–15) was almost three times greater than in men with the highest P-S ratios (.16–.28).

The only prospective intrapopulation study to demonstrate a relationship between dietary fat components (as expressed by the Keys or Hegsted diet score [see Chapters 3 and 5]) and serum cholesterol levels at baseline, change in diet score and change in serum cholesterol, as well as association between baseline diet score and risk of CHD, has recently been published by Shekelle and colleagues.[46] The study group was composed of 1,900 middle-aged men who were randomly selected from a utility company of Chicago, Illinois. Dietary data was collected by nutritionists using the Burke-type diet history, first at the initial examination and again at the second examination 1 year later. Diet scores for individuals were calculated using the values obtained for the percentage of calories from saturated and polyunsaturated fat and milligrams of dietary cholesterol per day in the predictive equations derived by Keys and colleagues and Hegsted and colleagues. The correlation between score values obtained by each equation was 0.984, and both were found to have a significant positive relationship to serum cholesterol at baseline. When the dietary variables were entered directly (not part of the score), serum cholesterol varied positively with dietary saturated fat and cholesterol, and less strongly but inversely with polyunsaturated fatty acids. Further, change in both scores as well as in saturated fatty acids and dietary cholesterol intake (from the first to the second examination) were positively related to a change in serum cholesterol level. There was a nonsignificant negative association for polyunsaturated fatty acids.

Finally, risk of CHD death during the ensuing 19-year period was positively related to baseline levels of both dietary scores and dietary cholesterol, and was inversely related to polyunsaturated fatty acid intake (after adjustment for a variety of other variables related to CHD risk).

Two other studies demonstrating intra-population relationships between dietary factors, serum cholesterol, and incidence of CHD are the Ni-Ho-San study[47] and the Puerto Rico Heart Health Program.[48] Nutritional data in both studies were collected using the same method, the 24-hour recall, administered by trained nutritionists. Kato and colleagues[47] found significant regression coefficients between a number of nutritional indexes and serum cholesterol in the Japanese and Hawaiian subgroups, with fewer significant associations noted in the San Francisco cohort, probably due to its much smaller sample size. Positive coefficients were found for dietary cholesterol, animal protein, and saturated fat, as well as for percentage of calories from total protein and animal protein, total fat, and saturated fat. Negative associations (all significant for Japanese and Hawaiian) were found for calories/weight and absolute intake of complex carbohydrate, as well as for percentage of calories from both complex and total carbohydrate. Interestingly, mean intake of complex carbohydrate was almost twice as high in the Japanese subgroup (278 gm) compared to the San Francisco cohort of Japanese American men (155 gm).

In the Puerto Rico Heart Study,[48] pronounced differences were found between the nutrient intake of the rural population (N = 2,426) and urban subgroup (N = 5,828). Rural men had higher intakes of total carbohydrate, starch, and lower intakes of saturated fatty acids than urban men. While serum cholesterol was associated with relative weight in the subgroups from both areas, dietary variables only showed significant relationships in the urban men. In this group, serum cholesterol was associated with percentage of calories from total and saturated fat, total carbohydrate, percentage of carbohydrate from starch, and dietary cholesterol intake (mg/day).

A recent paper by Gordon and colleagues[25] has investigated the incidence of CHD endpoints (MI, angina pectoris, or death) and dietary intake in the Honolulu (Hawaii) cohort of the Ni-Ho-San study, the cohort from the Puerto Rico Heart Study, and a subgroup (N = 859) of the Framingham Study. The nutritional data for the latter subgroup was collected in a second survey during the years 1966 to 1969 in 859 men using the 24-hour recall to insure consistency of data collection methods across all three studies. None of the dietary fat variables were found to be related to CHD; however, starch consumption for the Honolulu and Puerto Rico study groups was inversely related. Men who consumed more alcohol were less likely to develop CHD, but more likely to die of other causes, particularly in the Honolulu study. Calorie intake (either absolute or per kilogram of body weight) was negatively related to CHD, while men with greater body weight were more likely to develop CHD.

It should be noted that nutrient intake varied considerably among the three population groups, as did the rate of CHD, and these findings support the hypothesis that populations consuming a lower proportion of their calories in the form of fat and saturated fat tend to have a lower incidence of CHD. Intake of total fat and saturated fat was highest in the Framingham population, which also had the highest rate of CHD. Conversely, men in the Puerto Rico and Honolulu study groups consumed about 50 percent more starch than Framingham men, a difference which is even greater when expressed as percentage of calories.

While the results of these studies do not provide consistant evidence for the relationship of dietary variables of serum cholesterol and CHD for individuals, they do reaffirm the group or population relationships shown in the ecological data. Possible explanations for the failure to find significant associations on an individual basis are detailed below.

First of all, it is clear that diet is only one of many factors that influence serum cholesterol and the development of CHD. Serum cholesterol levels are also controlled by heredity, exercise or physical activity, weight, and/or adiposity, as well as weight change. In the Puerto Rico study,[48] the investigators found that diet and relative weight only accounted for 6 percent of the variability in serum cholesterol, with at most 2.5 percent of the variability due to diet alone.

Similarly, many factors such as family history, blood pressure, and cigarette smoking contribute to the development of atherosclerosis and CHD. When studies were partially controlled for some of these characteristics, significant relationships between intake of starch, cereal fiber, calorie intake,[25,45] and dietary fat components[46] were observed.

An additional limitation is that in all of these studies except one, total serum cholesterol was the primary lipid measured. It is now known that nutritional variables have differential effects on each lipoprotein fraction (see Chapter 3). For example, fat and dietary cholesterol components would have the most impact on LDL cholesterol, while calorie intake, adiposity and physical activity would influence very low density lipoprotein (VLDL) and HDL cholesterol more specifically. By using only total cholesterol, the potential for measuring an association is weakened. For example, if an individual is overweight, it is possible that his total blood cholesterol is controlled more by his triglyceride and VLDL cholesterol levels than the qualitative nature of his dietary fat intake.

A parallel problem is that people eat a whole diet or pattern but analyses are usually designed to measure the strength of the relationship between one nutrient or food and the endpoint in question. This approach also weakens the ability to obtain significant correlation. A better approach may be the one suggested by Shekelle and colleagues.[46] In their study, a score was derived that expressed the combined effect of the three major dietary fat components; saturated fatty acids, polyunsaturated fatty acid, and dietary cholesterol. The advantage of the method can be seen when reviewing some of the population data, particularly that from the Puerto Rico Study.[48] The investigations found that urban men had a higher intake of saturated fat than rural men. However, the effect of differences in saturated fat intake between the two groups of serum cholesterol may very well have been diminished, since it was also observed that urban men had considerably higher mean intakes of polyunsaturated fat (about 50 percent greater) than rural men. If a diet score had been calculated to represent intake of both saturated and polyunsaturated fat as well as dietary cholesterol, this would have controlled for all three variables simultaneously and perhaps would have resulted in a stronger association with blood cholesterol and/or CHD. This argument is also strengthened by the more consistent findings that starch or a predominant carbohydrate is more frequently found to have significant relationships with either blood cholesterol or CHD (see Chapter 6). The association has been found more frequently in populations with less westernized diets in which carbohydrate, predominantly starch, represents the major portion of calories.

The last and probably the most important limitation in all of these studies is the validity of the dietary data or the degree to which it represents the "usual" intake of the individual. Even in studies that use the Burke-type diet history, which is supposed to provide a more valid measure of intake over some period of time, one or even two interviews may be inadequate to characterize individuals. Stamler and his group[5] have suggested recently that this in fact is the case, and that it is necessary to collect a good deal more data for each person if individual relationships are to be measured accurately. However, the need for large amounts of data should not discourage investigators from doing this type of research. We now have vastly improved computerized data handling and analyses, which greatly facilitate the process.

Clinical Trials

Two generations of clinical trials, those done in the 1950s and 1960s and those conducted in the 1970s, clearly demonstrated that changing dietary intake resulted in mean decreases in serum cholesterol. This effect was seen in every study, despite great disparity in populations and type of intervention employed. However, due largely to small sample size or other design limitations, most of these trials failed to provide consistent and unequivocal evidence that lowering serum cholesterol had a beneficial effect on the incidence of CHD.

Two of these earlier studies, the Los Angeles Veterans Administration Study[49] and the Finnish Mental Hospital Study[50] were both conducted with institutionalized populations and utilized essentially a passive intervention design. Participants were fed from cafeterias or from other food service facilities, a condition which would conceivably improve compliance. However, since neither population was stable over the course of the trials, consistent levels of compliance were not achieved for all participants. Compliance was also reduced since the population had access to foods from snack bars and family members. Dietary modification for experimental groups consisted of reducing dietary cholesterol consumption, primarily through a reduction in egg consumption, and a substantial substitution of polyunsaturated fat for animal fat accomplished through the use of filled milk and other products and margarine instead of butter. Levels of total fat (40 percent of calories) and dietary cholesterol (365 mg/day) were quite high, but were less than that consumed by the general population at that time. Correspondingly, the levels of polyunsaturated fat in both studies was also quite high, approximately 20 percent of total calories. These dietary modifications produced cholesterol responses ranging from 12 to 18 percent (Table 1-1). In the Finnish trial, CHD mortality rates were consistently lower in those Finns residing in the experimental hospital, compared with the controls—53 percent for men and 34 percent for women. The trends for death rates for all cardiovascular disease were similar but smaller than for CHD. The difference in total mortality (at least for men) was favorable but not significantly different between the groups.

The results of the V.A. trial also showed benefit for hard artherosclerotic endpoints, particularly in subgroups that were free of disease, younger (less than age 66 years), and hypercholesteremic. However, no difference in all-cause mortality was observed due to excess neoplastic and accidental death in the experimental group. At the time this study was first published, there was a suspicion that the high levels of polyunsaturated fat in the diet may have been related to the excess of neoplastic disease (particularly of the GI tract) in the experimental group. Subsequent analysis of compliance data for this subgroup did not confirm the hypothesis[51]; however, since the level of polyunsaturates used in this trial was four times higher than usual population intakes, it probably represents an unusual eating pattern. All subsequent trials have utilized much lower levels of polyunsaturates, usually no more than 10 percent of total calories.

Two other trials, the Coronary Prevention Evaluation Program (CPEP) and the New York Anti-coronary Club, also done during the first generation period, are particularly interesting. While interpretation of CHD endpoints is difficult because

Table 1-1. Cholesterol Response in Clinical Trials

Study	Number E	Number C	Duration	Diet Specifications	Cholesterol Response Experimental Group BL	Final	Diff	mg% Δ	C–E MG	Diff %
V.A. Trial	422	424	Up to 8 years	40% Fat—Substitution of 2/3 of animal fat by poly fat reduced cholesterol in E group = 365 mg/day	232					12.7
Finnish Mental Hospital Study	Hospital N 390	Hospital K 286	6 years on each diet	31–33% Total Fat Polyunsaturate levels tripled Saturated fat reduced by 50% P-S ratio = 1.48 Cholesterol <350 mg/day	Hospital N 267 Hospital K 268	216 236	51 32	19 11.9		
N.Y. Anti-coronary Club	478	420	5 years	30–33% Fat—Approximately equal quantities of sat., mono., and polys. P-S ratio = 1.25–1.50 400 mg cholesterol/day	260	225	35	13.5	30	11.5
CPEP	516		Up to 9 years	30% Fat—<10% of Cal from sat. fat 7% of Cal from poly fat <300 mg/day cholesterol	270	239	31	11.4		
Diet-Heart Study	Diet B 332		1 year	Diet B <9% saturated fat, 30% fat, 15% or more poly P-S ratio = 1.5 350–450 mg cholesterol/day	221	206	25	11		

E = experimental, C = control, BL = baseline, Diff = difference neither study had randomized control groups, they were the first trials to demonstrate that significant cholesterol reductions could be obtained utilizing active intervention programs with free-living individuals. Dietary specifications included approximately 30 percent of calories from total fat, 10 percent from saturated fat, and between 7 and 10 percent of calories from polyunsaturated fat. Dietary cholesterol was reduced to 400 mg/day in the New York trial,[52] and to less than 300 mg/day in the CPEP.[53] Absolute reductions in serum cholesterol for both intervention groups were very similar, 31 mg (11.4 percent) and 35 mg (13.5 percent). These long-term reductions are impressive, considering the difficulties inherent in maintaining high levels of compliance in free-living individuals. Both studies produced favorable but not conclusive endpoint data, in part because of their small sample sizes.

The most sophisticated study demonstrating the relationship between diet and change in serum cholesterol levels in open populations was the Diet-Heart Study.[54] Conceived originally as the basis for a large-scale national study, it compared the cholesterol response between several groups placed on different diets. The active intervention program was unique in that both the nutritionists and participants were blinded with respect to the actual diet condition. Nutrient differences between conditions were achieved by the use of specially modified foods made available to participants through food distribution centers. Cholesterol response even in these open populations was related to the specifications of each dietary condition. Diet B (Table 1-1) produced a 25 mg, or 11 percent, reduction in serum cholesterol over a 1-year period of time, and group response was shown to be highly related to levels of dietary compliance. This study not only demonstrated the relationship between dietary patterns and changes in serum cholesterol but added greatly to our knowledge of intervention methodology and compliance measurement. It was not, however, designed to measure or compare CHD endpoints between groups.

The conclusions that can be drawn from these trials are that free-living individuals can be recruited, and that serum cholesterol levels of groups can be manipulated by changes in dietary patterns, specifically the reduction of saturated fat and dietary cholesterol and the concomitant increase in polyunsaturated fat. The latter three trials also demonstrated that this effect is not confined to institutionalized populations but can be produced in free-living individuals from a variety of geographic centers and ethnic groups.

While a single diet-heart study has not been and probably will not be conducted, large multirisk trials in both the United States and Europe that incorporated dietary modifications to lower blood cholesterol levels have recently been completed. Two of these studies, the Multiple Risk Factor Intervention Trial (MRFIT)[55] and the Oslo Study,[57] have endpoint data available. While both were multirisk studies, they differ substantially from each other in overall design, sample size, population characteristics, and intervention approaches.

The MRFIT[55] was designed to intervene simultaneously on three major risk factors, serum cholesterol, blood pressure, and cigarette smoking in middle-aged men (35 to 54 years of age) in the upper 10 to 15 percent of risk for CHD. A sample of 12,866 individuals were recruited from 22 centers across the United States and randomized into two groups, Usual Care (UC, seen once a year for an examination)

Table 1-2.   Mean Serum Cholesterol at First Screen and 72 Months for MRFIT Usual Care and Special Intervention Participants by First Screen Cholesterol mg%

First Screen	72 Mo.		Difference First Screen to 72 Mo.		
Cholesterol	SI	UC	SI	UC	SI—UC
<220	199	202	0.3	−3.5	3.8
220–239	221	224	9.0	6.2	2.7
240–259	233	237	16.1	12.6	3.5
260–279	247	252	21.8	16.8	5.0
280–299	258	267	30.7	22.7	8.0
≥300	272	284	44.1	33.6	10.6
Total	236	240	18.3	13.0	5.2

SI = Special Intervention; UC = Usual Care

and Special Intervention (SI). This latter group entered into an extensive intervention program, implemented for the first 4 months through a group format and carried on over a 6 year period primarily through individual counseling provided by a variety of health professionals. The intervention approach was unique in that risk factor reduction was attempted simultaneously; in other words, treatment for high blood pressure was initiated along with smoking cessation efforts and/or eating pattern changes to reduce blood cholesterol.

Through the course of the trial several eating patterns reflecting different levels of saturated fat, polyunsaturated fat, and dietary cholesterol were utilized in order to maintain and improve blood cholesterol response.[56] It became apparent after the initial intervention that simultaneous intervention on blood pressure and smoking produced interactions that diminished the overall cholesterol response in the SI group. Additionally, nutrient intake data obtained at baseline indicated that the overall population entered the study consuming less saturated fat and dietary cholesterol and more polyunsaturated fat than had been anticipated, so that the potential for cholesterol lowering using the original eating pattern was reduced.

Serum cholesterol reduction in the overall SI group was equal to 7.2 percent, at the end of 6 years (Table 1-2). However, the best responses were seen in men who had the highest levels at baseline, in those who were not on antihypertensive therapy or were not smoking, in those who lost weight (≥5 lbs) and in those who adhered to the Progressive Eating Pattern (<5 percent of calories from saturated fat, 10 percent of calories from polyunsaturated fat, and ≤100 mg cholesterol per day). Some of these relationships are illustrated in Table 1-3, which represents the mean change in cholesterol from years 1 to 3 by hypertensive and smoking status at baseline and weight change. Since MRFIT was a multifactor trial and simultaneous reduction of other risk factors essentially interfered with the potential for cholesterol lowering, the results cannot be perceived as a pure demonstration of the relationship of diet change and cholesterol responses. However, the compliance data even for the overall group (Table 1-4) clearly show that a strong relationship does exist.

Significant reductions in the other two risk factors were also observed over the course of the trial. At the end of 6 years, diastolic blood pressure had decreased by

Table 1-3.   Change in Serum Cholesterol from Baseline (S_1) to Years 1–4, According to Weight Change and to Smoking and Blood Pressure Category in MRFIT SI Participants[a]

Weight change:	Loss ≥10 lb	Loss 5–9 lb	Little change	Gain ≥5 lb	All participants
Number of participants	1,391	922	1,899	1,096	5,308
Mean change in serum cholesterol (%)					
Non hypertensive[b]					
Nonsmokers	−14.6	−10.2	−7.3	−4.7	−10.2
Smokers who quit	−12.0	−8.1	−7.0	−5.7	−7.4
Smokers	−8.4	−7.0	−6.0	−3.6	−6.2
Hypertensive					
Nonsmokers	−10.1	−9.0	−7.2	−5.7	−8.4
Smokers who quit	−7.7	−5.5	−3.9	−2.5	−4.4
Smokers	−4.8	−4.4	−3.2	−1.3	−3.5
All participants	−9.6	−7.5	−5.8	−3.9	−6.7
Mean S_1 serum cholesterol (mg/dl)					
Nonhypertensive					
Nonsmokers	273.0	270.7	274.3	265.5	272.1
Smokers who quit	257.1	257.0	258.3	253.8	256.3
Smokers	260.0	256.2	255.1	252.1	255.7
Hypertensive					
Nonsmokers	264.3	264.5	263.2	265.0	264.1
Smokers who quit	243.8	243.4	240.8	237.0	240.6
Smokers	239.2	239.0	234.2	232.8	236.0
All participants	258.0	256.0	253.0	248.8	254.0

[a]In this table, the data represent all participants for whom complete serum cholesterol and lipoprotein information was available at years 1–4; the cholesterol response is the change from baseline to the mean of years 1–4; weight change is from baseline to year 4; smoking status is at year 4.

[b]Nonhypertensive status is defined as DBP < 90 mm Hg and not on antihypertensive therapy at baseline. DBP = diastolic blood pressure.

Caggiula AW, Christakis G, Farrand M, Hulley SB, Johnson R, Lasser NL, Stamler J, Widdowson G: The multiple risk factor intervention trail (MRFIT), IV, Intervention on blood lipids. Prev Med 10:443–475, 1981.

10.6 mm Hg from baseline (the average of screen 2 and 3 blood pressures) in the total SI group, and the reported quit rate for smokers was 45 percent.

Unfortunately, despite impressive risk-factor reduction in the SI group, no significant reduction in CHD mortality between the SI and UC groups was observed. A more detailed analysis of the CHD mortality data and their interpretation has recently been published.[55] This report also provides information on risk-factor reduction in the UC group, which was largely unanticipated at the beginning of the trial. There is also evidence from other subgroup analyses that cholesterol response was related to outcome. In Table 1-5, survivors in both the SI and UC groups are

Table 1-4. Mean Serum Cholesterol Change,[a] SI Participants, Baseline Through Year 6, by FRR Adherence Category at Followup Prior to 6th Annual Exam

| | FRR | | |
| | $\leqslant 3$ | 4–9 | $\geqslant 10$ |
	(PEP)	(Basic)	(Other)
All SI	11.1	8.3	6.8
NHNS[b]	16.4	11.3	12.2

[a]Mean Percent Change: $\dfrac{\text{Baseline}^{c} - \text{6th Annual}}{\text{Baseline}^{c}} \times 100$

[b]Nonhypertensive, nonsmoker. [c]Baseline represents screen 1 serum value. FRR = food record rating; PEP = progressive eating pattern

Data presented at the 65th Annual Meeting of the American Dietetic Association, San Antonio, October, 1982.

shown to have a greater decrease in serum cholesterol than participants who died from CHD.

While the results with respect to overall CHD mortality are inconclusive in the MRFIT study, the results from the Oslo study are not.[57] This trial included 1,200 high-risk men (upper 15 to 20 percent) based on serum cholesterol and cigarette smoking, and did not include individuals with elevated blood pressure at baseline. For the 604 men randomized to the intervention group, advice on risk factors, diet, and smoking was provided primarily through several individual counseling sessions at the beginning of the trial. Follow-up visits were semiannual for intervention subjects and annual for controls. While exact dietary specifications have not been published, intervention participants with high cholesterol levels were encouraged to reduce saturated fat intake and slightly increase their intake of polyunsaturates. Weight reduction and reduced intake of simple sugars and alcohol was also recommended for those with high triglyceride levels.

At the end of 5 years there was a 13 percent difference in serum cholesterol between the intervention and control group (based on the mean of the three prerandomization values and the mean of the yearly values), and the quit rate for smokers was 25 percent in the intervention group, versus 17 percent in the control group.

Further, these intervention results were associated with a significantly lower incidence ($p = 0.028$) of myocardial infarction (fatal and nonfatal) and sudden death in the intervention group, compared with the control group. Changes in serum cholesterol accounted for about 60 percent of the reduction in CHD incidence, while smoking cessation only accounted for about 25 percent.

In comparing the intervention results with those from MRFIT, one may con-

Table 1-5. Mean Change in Serum Cholesterol (Screen 1–12 Months) for CHD Deaths and Survivors for MRFIT SI and UC Participants

| | SI | | UC | |
	CHD Deaths	Survivors	CHD Deaths	Survivors
Number	96	6,001	105	5,958
Δ Cholesterol	10.6	15.6	3.6	7.0

Deaths during the first year as well as surviving participants who did not attend the 12-month visit are excluded. Includes deaths after 12 months from causes other than CHD.

clude that the serum cholesterol response was much greater in this trial while the quit rate for smoking was much lower. In actuality, the cholesterol response was somewhat greater, but the difference is not as large if one compares the response in the MRFIT cohort that most closely resembled the study population in Oslo. Because the Oslo Study did not include hypertensives, this population had much higher cholesterol levels (lst serum mean = 325 mg%) than the overall MRFIT cohort (lst serum mean = 254 mg%). The cholesterol response in the MRFIT SI subgroup with first screen cholesterol ⩾300 ($\bar{x}$ = 316 mg%) was 14 percent, which was very similar to the serum levels in the Oslo intervention subgroup. However, in the latter study almost no change in cholesterol levels were observed in the control group, while in MRFIT the control subgroup with the highest baseline levels (⩾300 mg%) experienced an 11 percent decrease in serum cholesterol from first screen to 72 months. Therefore, the difference between SI and UC responses for this subgroup was only 3 percent (Table 1-2), compared with 13 percent in the Oslo Study group. Since the frequency of follow-up contact (yearly examination) for the control groups is similar for both studies, some other factor or factors must be responsible for the considerable reduction seen in the serum cholesterol levels of the MRFIT UC (control) participants, particularly those with the highest baseline levels.

The results from these clinical trials have not provided unequivocal evidence that lowering blood cholesterol levels is related to decreased incidence of CHD. However, they do provide consistent support for serum cholesterol as a risk factor for CHD as well as a clear demonstration that changing dietary patterns in both free-living and institionalized populations results in decreases in blood cholesterol levels. While the definitive diet-heart study will not be done, it is apparent that the United States population has changed their eating pattern in the direction of lower intakes of saturated fat and cholesterol and increased intakes of polyunsaturated fat. There has also been a substantial decline in the mean cholesterol levels and in CHD death rates. These associated events do not provide definitive proof but are certainly suggestive of a relationship between nutritional factors and cardiovascular disease.

REFERENCES

1. Keys A: Dietary survey methods. In Levy R, Rifkind B, Dennis B, Ernst N, eds. Nutrition, Lipids, and Coronary Heart Disease. New York, Raven Press, 1979.
2. Madden JP, Goodman SJ, Guthrie HA: Validity of the 24-hr. recall. J Am Diet Assn 68(2):143–147, 1976.
3. Young CH, Hagan GC, Tucker RE, Foster WD: A comparison of dietary study methods: Dietary history vs. seven-day record vs. 24-hr recall. J Am Diet Assn 28(3):218–221, 1952.
4. Chalmers FW, Clayton MM, Gates LO, Tucker RE, Wertz AW, Young CM, Foster WD: The dietary record—how many and which days? J Am Diet Assn 28(8):711–717, 1952.
5. Liu K, Stamler J, Dyer A, McKeever J, McKeever P: Statistical methods to assess and minimize the role of intra-individual variability in obscuring the relationship between dietary lipids and serum cholesterol. J Chron Dis 31:399–418, 1978.

6. Balogh M, Kahn HA, Medalie JH: Random repeat 24-hour dietary recalls. Am J Clin Nutr 24:304–310, 1971.
7. Young CH, Trulson MF: Methodology for dietary studies in epidemiological surveys: II. Strengths and weaknesses of existing methods. Am J P H 50:803–814, 1960.
8. Sacks FM, Castelli WP, Donner A, Kass EH. Plasma lipids and lipoproteins in vegetarians and controls. N Engl J Med 292:1148–1151, 1975.
9. Dahl LK: Salt and hypertension. Am J Clin Nutr 25:231–244, 1972.
10. Havlik RJ, Feinheit M: Proceedings of the Conference on the Decline in Coronary Heart Disease Mortality. NIH Pub No 79-1610, May 1979.
11. Gillum RF, Prineas RV, Luepper RV: The decline in coronary deaths: A search for explanations: The Minnesota mortality and morbidity surveillance program. Minn Med 65(4):235–8, 1982.
12. Fortmann SP: The community health survey of the Stanford five city project: Community epidemiologic surveillance for cardiovascular diseases: Manual of operations, 2nd ed. Board of Trustees of the Leland Stanford Junior University, 1981.
13. WHO Proposal for the multination monitoring of trends and determinants in cardiovascular disease and provisional protocol. Geneva Pub WHO CVD 81.2, 1981.
14. Editorial: Risk of coronary arteriography. Brit Med J 281:627–628, 1980.
15. Steinberg D: Research related to underlying mechanisms in artherosclerosis. Circulation 60:7, 1979.
16. Meade TW, Chakrabarti R, Haines AP, North WRS, Stirling Y, Thompson SG: Haemostatic function and cardiovascular death—early results of a prospective study. Lancet (i): 1050–1053, 1980.
17. Kirshenbaum HD, Ockene IS, Alpert JS: The spectrum of coronary artery spasm. JAMA 246:4, 354–9, 1981.
18. Mackintosh AF, Crabb ME, Granger R, Williams JH, Chamberlain DA: The Brighton resuscitation ambulances: review of 40 consecutive survivors of out-of-hospital cardiac arrest. Brit Med J 1:1115–1118, 1978.
19. Keys A: Seven countries, a multivariate analysis of death and coronary heart disease. Cambridge, MA, and London A Commonwealth Fund Book, Harvard University Press, 1980.
20. Milton T (ed): Goldberger on Pellagra. Baton Rouge, Louisiana State University Press, 1964.
21. Marmot MG, Syme SL, Sacks ST, Kwok LW: Japanese culture and coronary heart disease. In Orimo H, Shimada K, Iriki M, Maeda D (eds): Recent Advances in Gerontology. Proceedings of the XI International Congress of Gerontology, Tokyo 2025: 476–479, Aug 1978, 1979.
22. Knuiman, Jan T: Serum total and high density lipoprotein cholesterol concentrations and body mass index in adult men from 13 countries. Am J Epidemiol 116:631–642, 1982.
23. Shekelle, Richard B, et al: Original contributors, dietary lipids and serum cholesterol level, change in diet confounds the cross-sectional association. Am J Epidemiol 115: 506–514, 1982.
24. Jacobs DR Jr, Anderson JT, Blackburn H: Diet and serum cholesterol, do zero correlations negate the relationship? Am J Epidemiol 110:77–87, 1979.
25. Gordon T, et al: Diet and its relation to coronary heart disease and death in three populations. Circulation 63:500–515, 1981.
26. Vlietstra E, et al: Risk factors and angiographic coronary artery disease. A Report from the Coronary Artery Surgery Study (CASS). Circulation 62:254–261, 1980.
27. Gotto M Jr, Smith LC, Allen B (eds): Atherosclerosis V. Proceedings of the Fifth International Symposium. New York, Heidelberg, Berlin, Springer-Verlag, 1980.

28. Hay CRM, Durber AP, Saynor R: Effect of fish oil on platelet kinetics in patients with ischaemic heart disease. Lancet:1269–1272, 1982.
29. Kuller L, Neaton J, Caggiula A, Falvo-Gerard L: Primary prevention of heart attacks. The multiple risk factor intervention trial. Am J Epidemiol 112:185–199, 1980.
30. Levy RI, Moskowitz J: Cardiovascular research. Decades of progress, a decade of promise. Science 217:121–129, 1982.
31. Stolley PD, Kuller LF, Nefzger MD, Tonascia S, Lilienfeld AM, Miller GD, Diamond EL: Three-area epidemiological study of geographic differences in stroke mortality, II results. Stroke 8:551–557, 1977.
32. Kraus JF, Borhani NO, Franti CE: Socioeconomic status, ethnicity, and risk of coronary heart disease. Am J Epidemiol 111:407–414, 1980.
33. Salonen JT, et al: Association between cardiovascular death and myocardial infarction and serum selenium in a matched-pair longitudinal study. Lancet 2:175–179, 1982.
34. Graham S, Mettlin C.: Reviews and commentary, diet and colon cancer. Am J Epidemiol (formerly Am J Hygiene) 109:1–20, 1979.
35. Reddy BS, Cohen LA, McCoy GD, Hill PW, John H, Wynder EL: Nutrition and its relationship to cancer. Advances in Cancer Research 32:237–345, 1980.
36. Salonen JT: Risk of cancer and death in relation to serum cholesterol, A longitudinal study in an eastern Finnish population with high overall cholesterol level. Am J Epidemiol 116:622–630, 1982.
37. Committee on Diet, Nutrition, and Cancer; Assembly of Life Sciences, National Research Council: Diet, Nutrition, and Cancer, 1982. Washington, National Academy Press, 1982.
38. Correa PS, Strong JP, Johnson WD, Pizzolato P, Haensel W: Atherosclerosis and polyps of the colon quantification of precursors of coronary heart disease and colon cancer. J Chron Dis 35:313:320, 1982.
39. Philips RL, Garfinkel L, Kuzma JW, Beeson WL, Lotz T, Brin B: Mortality among California Seventh-Day Adventists for selected cancer sites. J Natl Cancer Inst 65: 1097–1107, 1980.
40. Hirotsugu U, et al: Dietary intake and serum total cholesterol level, their relationship to different lifestyles in several Japanese populations. Circulation 66:519–526, 1982.
41. Gordon T: The Framingham Diet Study. Diet and the regulation of serum cholesterol. The Framingham Study—An Epidemiol Invest Cardiovascular Dis. Section 24. Washington, United States Department of Health, Education and Welfare, 1970.
42. Nichols AB, Ravenscroft C, Lamphiear DE, Ostrander LD: Independence of serum lipid levels and dietary habits. The Tecumseh Study. JAMA 236, 17:1948–1953, 1976.
43. Kahn HA, Medalie JH, Neufeld HN, Riss E, Balogh M, Groen JJ: Serum cholesterol: Its distribution and association with dietary and other variables in a survey of 10,000 men. Israel J Med Sci 5(6):1117–1127, 1969.
44. Stulb SC, McDonough JR, Greenberg BG, Hames CG: The relationship of nutrient intake and exercise to serum cholesterol levels in white males in Evans County, Georgia. Am J Clin Nutr 16:238–242, 1965.
45. Morris JN, Marr JW, Clayton DG: Diet and heart: a postscript. Brit Med J 2:1307–1314, 1977.
46. Shekelle RB, Shryock AM, Oglesby P, Lepper M, Stamler J, Shguey L, Raynor WJ Jr: Diet, serum cholesterol, and death from coronary heart disease. Engl J Med 304(2): 65–70, 1981.
47. Kato H, Tillotson J, Nichaman MZ, Rhoads GG, Hamilton HB: Epidemiologic studies of coronary heart disease and stroke in Japanese men living in Japan, Hawaii and California. Am J Epidemiol 97, 6:372–385, 1973.

48. Garcia-Palmieri MR, Tillotson J, Cordero E, Costas R Jr, Sorlie P, Gordon T, Kannel WB, Colon AA: Nutrient intake and serum lipids in urban and rural Puerto Rican men. Am J Clin Nutr 30:2092–2100, 1977.

49. Dayton S, Pearce ML, Hashimoto S, Dixon WJ, Tomiyasu U: A controlled clinical trial of a diet high in unsaturated fat. In preventing complications of Atherosclerosis. Am Heart Assoc 25:II-I-II-63, 1969.

50. Turpeinen O, Karvonen MJ, Pekkarinen M, Miettinen M, Elosuo R, Paavilainen F: Dietary prevention of coronary heart disease: The Finnish Mental Hospital Study. Int J Epidemiol 8(2):99–118, 1979.

51. Ederer F, Leren P, Turpeinen O, Frantz ID Jr: Cancer among men on cholesterol lowering diets. Lancet 203–206, 1971.

52. Christakis G, Rinzler SH Archer M, Winslow G, Jampel S, Stephenson J, Friedman G, Fein H, Kraus A, James G: The Anti-coronary Club: a dietary approach to the prevention of coronary heart disease—a seven year report. Am J Pub Health 56:299, 1966.

53. Stamler J: Prevention of atherosclerotic coronary heart disease. In Morgan Jones A (ed): Modern Trends in Cardiology, 2nd ed. London, Butterworths, 1968.

54. National Diet Heart Study Final Report, National Diet Heart Study Research Group 37(suppl 1):1–419, 1968.

55. Multiple Risk Factor Intervention Trial Research Group: Multiple risk factor intervention trial. JAMA 248:1465–1477, 1982.

56. Caggiula AW, Christakis G, Farrand M, Hulley SB, Johnson R, Lasser NL, Stamler J, Widdowson G: The multiple risk factor intervention trail (MRFIT), IV, Intervention on blood lipids. Prev Med 10:443–475, 1981.

57. Hjermann I, Holm I, Byre KV, Leren P: Effect of diet and smoking intervention on the incidence of coronary heart disease. Report from the Oslo Study Group of a randomized trial in healthy men. Lancet 1303–1310, 1981.

2 | Nutritional Theories of Atherogenesis*

David Kritchevsky

There is a statistically significant relationship between elevated levels of serum cholesterol and the risk of coronary disease.[1] Cholesterolemia is one of the major risk factors of coronary heart disease,[2] together with elevated blood pressure and cigarette smoking. Strasser[3] identified as many as 30 risk factors and Hopkins and Williams[4] have identified 246 factors that impinge on atherosclerosis, many of which are diet related. They classified the risk factors as initiators, promoters, potentiators, and precipitators. Under general classifications, 16 factors were listed as constitutional and demographic; 5, as environmental; 54, under habits, lifestyle, and psychosocial; 16, as physical or biochemical measurements; 44, as serum or blood measurements; 16, as platelet and coagulation tests; 45, under medical conditions; 21, under dietary excess and positive association; 23, as dietary deficiencies and inverse association; and 6, under drug liabilities. Because cholesterolemia is a risk factor in coronary heart disease (CHD) and since cholesterol is a lipid, most studies of experimental atherosclerosis have used cholesterol and/or dietary fat. But not all animal species respond to diet in the same way.[5,6] Thus, dietary studies in animals must take into consideration the differing individual metabolic characteristics. Human studies are primarily epidemiologic or retrospective in nature rather than experimental (See Chapter 1). Nutritional characteristics of any given population are based on cultural factors of affluence, religion, geography, and custom. One or more of these factors can come into play in determining coronary disease status.

* Supported, in part, by a Research Career Award (HL-00734) from the National Institutes of Health and by a grant-in-aid from the Commonwealth of Pennsylvania.

Table 2-1. Dietary Cholesterol and Serum Cholesterol[a]

	CHD	Normal
Ten Lowest Serum Cholesterol		
Cholesterol, mg/dl	196 ± 4.5	161 ± 2.4
Cholesterol ingested, g/wk	3.28 ± 0.50	3.84 ± 0.34
Ten Highest Serum Cholesterol		
Cholesterol, mg/dl	416 ± 16.5	313 ± 3.2
Cholesterol ingested, g/wk	4.12 ± 0.55	4.26 ± 0.39
Ten with Highest Ingestion		
Cholesterol, mg/dl	288 ± 21.9	213 ± 11.4
Cholesterol ingested, g/wk	5.67 ± 0.15	6.98 ± 0.31
Ten with Lowest Ingestion		
Cholesterol, mg/dl	271 ± 14.2	222 ± 15.6
Cholesterol ingested, g/wk	1.34 ± 0.10	1.37 ± 0.13

[a]Data from Gertler et al.[7]

In humans, it has been assumed that dietary cholesterol determines cholesterol levels in the blood, and the central theme of much diet therapy is reduction of cholesterol intake. There is no argument regarding the importance of plasma or serum cholesterol level as a risk factor; the controversy centers on the effects of diet—especially dietary lipid—on cholesterol level. Gertler and colleagues, for example[7] in 1950 compared a large group of patients who had coronary disease with a control group and tried to relate their cholesterol intake to their cholesterol level (Table 2-1). The coronary cases exhibited higher cholesterol levels in every subgroup, but there was no direct relationship in this study between cholesterol intake and cholesterol level. In the Framingham Study,[8] it was found that neither cholesterol intake nor other aspects of fat, protein or carbohydrate intake were related to cholesterol levels (Table 2-2). In more recent studies, Nichols and colleagues[8] found no relation between diet and serum cholesterol or triglycerides in over 4000 subjects studied in Tecumseh, Michigan. Slater and colleagues[10] and Porter and colleagues[11] have shown that intake of only one or two eggs daily has little effect on serum cholesterol in free-living men. A recent review[12] of diet and coronary disease in three major prospective heart studies showed significant cor-

Table 2-2. Diet and Serum Cholesterol Level in Men: Framingham Study[a]

	Serum cholesterol, mg/dl		
	<180	180–299	300+
Number	51	329	51
Calories/day	3181	3161	3009
Protein,			
g/day	124	124	125
Animal/vegetable	2.9	3.1	3.3
Fat,			
g/day	130	138	130
Animal/vegetable	2.6	2.5	2.6
Cholesterol, mg	669	714	676
Carbohydrate,			
g/day	354	324	302
Complex/simple	0.88	0.93	0.97

[a]Data from Kannel and Gordon.[8]

Table 2-3. Diet and Coronary Heart Disease in Three Populations[a]

	Framingham[b]		Puerto Rico		Honolulu	
	No CHD	CHD	No CHD	CHD	No CHD	CHD
Number	780	79 (51)	7932	286 (163)	7008	264 (164)
Total calories	2622	2488	2395	2289[c]	2319	2210[c]
Protein, g	101	99	86	85	95	95
Fat, g	114	112	95	94	87	86
P-S ratio	0.39	0.41	0.45	0.49	0.54	0.57
Cholesterol, mg	529	534	417	419	555	549
Carbohydrate, g	252	248	280	262[c]	264	249[c]
Sugar, g	72	78	52	50	46	45
Starch, g	117	118	180	167[c]	165	155[c]
Other, g	61	52[c]	48	45	52	48
Alcohol, g	25	12[c]	12	8	14	8[c]

[a]Data from Gordon et al.[12] Values are age–adjusted means of specified variables.

[b]CHD = coronary heart disease. Number in parentheses = myocardial infarction or coronary death.

[c]p ≤ 0.05.

relations with some carbohydrates and with alcohol intake in one or other of the studies, but not with other dietary factors (Table 2-3). Nutritional factors other than fat also play a role in cholesterolemia (See page 5).

New areas of research and controversy relating diet to plasma lipids and heart disease are emerging.* Research in cardiovascular disease has gone far beyond simple measurement of lipid levels. Gofman and colleagues[13] first pointed out that the particular portion of the lipid-protein continuum in which cholesterol is transported is of greater importance than the total cholesterol level. Barr and colleagues[14] showed that the ratio of lipoprotein fractions could be more indicative of risk. This finding was revived and amplified a few years ago[15] and became the basis of the interest in levels of high-density lipoproteins (HDL). (See Chapters 3, 5) HDL has been subfractionated into HDL_2 and HDL_3 which carry divergent risk status. An even more important development has been the identification of the apolipoproteins and their metabolic roles (Chapter 3). These fractions hold the potential for being more accurate indicators of cardiovascular risk. Results of work on effects of diet on apolipoprotein levels and distribution in lipoproteins is beginning to appear in the literature. (Table 3-2 presents the chemical and physical characteristics of the major lipoprotein classes.)

LIPIDS
(See also Chapters 3, 4, 5, 10)

The hypercholesterolemic effect of intake of saturated fat has been documented amply in man and was characterized by Ahrens,[16] who demonstrated that serum cholesterol levels generally rose as fat saturation increased. Diets containing saturated fat are more atherogenic for rabbits, and many other species of experi-

---

*See Chapter 1 for a discussion of the problems of design and interpretation of epidemiologic studies relating dietary components to plasma lipids and coronary heart disease.

Table 2-4.   Influence of Peanut Oil on Experimental Atherosclerosis in Rabbits[a]

Oil	No.	Serum cholesterol (mg/dl)	Atherosclerosis	
			Arch	Thoracic
Coconut	44	1360	2.15	1.67
Peanut	98	1483	1.89	1.35
PGF[b]	73	1650	1.57	1.11
PGF/R[c]	31	1723	1.40	0.94
PNO/R[d]	31	1833	1.31	1.05
Corn	100	1548	1.52	1.05

[a]Data from Kritchevsky et al.[23,25]

[b]PGF = blend of olive[55] safflower[35] and olive[10] oils whose fatty acid resembles peanut oil less arachidic and behenic acids.

[c]PGF/R = PGF interesterified with arachidic and behenic-rich glycerides to give a fat whose fatty acid spectrum is exactly like that of peanut oil.

[d]PNO/R = randomized (autointeresterified) peanut oil.

mental animals, than diets containing unsaturated fat. This observation in rabbits is true whether the diet contains cholesterol or not.[17–20]

One fat that does not fit into the pattern of saturation effect is peanut oil, a relatively unsaturated vegetable oil. Peanut oil, which has no significant effect on cholesterol levels in man,[16] is inordinately atherogenic for rats,[21,22] rabbits,[23] and rhesus monkeys.[24] Peanut oil may contain up to 7 per cent of long-chain saturated fatty acids (arachidic, behenic, lignoceric), and at one time these were thought responsible for its atherogenicity. Subsequent experiments have shown that the structure of the component triglycerides determine this oil's atherogenic effect. Autointeresterification (randomization) of peanut oil provides a fat with the same fatty acid spectrum and iodine value as those of the starting peanut oil, but with greatly reduced atherogenicity.[25] (Table 2-4). Randomized peanut oil is also less atherogenic than peanut oil in vervet monkeys.[26] Studies of the fine structure of randomized peanut oil and oils from various cultivars of peanut are underway in an effort to find a structural clue to the effects observed.[27,28]

Kummerow[29] has suggested that increasing levels of transunsaturated fatty acids (TFA) in the American diet might explain the increases in coronary disease observed in the United States since 1920. Although TFA occur in nature, their major dietary source is hydrogenated fat, such as in margarines. Studies in rabbits fed cholesterol and elaidic acid or elaidinized olive oil showed that the trans fat increased serum cholesterol levels but did not affect the severity of atherosclerosis.[30,31] Rabbits fed two levels of TFA in semipurified, cholesterol-free diets exhibited higher cholesterol levels but not more severe atherosclerosis than did controls.[32]

The hypothesis was put forth that TFA were less readily metabolized than their cis counterparts and, hence, might affect metabolic processes. There seem to be no differences in the absorption or oxidation of cis or trans unsaturated fatty acids,[33,34] and while cholesteryl esters of TFA are synthesized and hydrolyzed less readily than the cis isomers,[35–37] lipolysis of triglycerides containing cis or trans isomers proceed at the same rate.[38] Once feeding of TFA is stopped, they disappear from the blood and tissues of rats[39] or monkeys.[40]

There are still a few important facets of TFA metabolism that require clarification. Whether all tissues metabolize cis and trans unsaturated fats in the same way is amenable to easy test. Another aspect related to the location of the double bonds is more complicated; that is, What are the metabolic effects in man of the many potential products of hydrogenation? When a fat is hydrogenated, the double bonds tend to migrate, giving rise to both geometric and positional isomers.[41] Thus, a partially hydrogenated fat may contain cis and trans isomers of fatty acids with double bonds anywhere from C4 to C12. Their metabolic effects remain to be elucidated.

CARBOHYDRATE
(See Chapter 6)

Plasma triglyceride levels are elevated in subjects ingesting a high carbohydrate diet.[42–44] While some investigators have found that substitution of dietary starch by sucrose or fructose is hypertriglyceridemic,[45–47] McGandy and colleagues[48] have suggested that sucrose taken in normal quantities has no effect on triglyceride levels, but Yudkin[49,50] insists that sucrose consumption is central to the etiology of coronary disease. Fructose has been shown to be triglyceridemic for rats,[51–53] and baboon,[54,55] and vervet monkeys.[56] When fed to experimental animals as components of a semipurified, cholesterol-free diet, sucrose and fructose are more atherogenic than glucose or lactose[57,58] (Table 2-5). A sucrose-cholesterol diet is more cholesterolemic for chickens[59] or rabbits[60] than is a glucose-cholesterol diet. Wells and Anderson[61] found that lactose was very atherogenic when fed to rabbits as part of a cholesterol-containing diet. Baboons fed a semipurified diet containing lactose exhibit little aortic sudanophilia, but addition of 0.1 per cent cholesterol to the diet renders it atherogenic[62] (Table 2-6). Since the serum cholesterol of the lactose-fed baboons are not significantly different from those of baboons fed other carbohydrates, the lactose-cholesterol effect may be mediated by other metabolic factors, possibly by the synthesis and composition of aortic glycosaminoglycans. (The differences in species response of plasma lipids and lipoproteins to various sugars and the differences observed in normal and hyperlipidemic human subjects are discussed in Chapter 6.)

Table 2-5.   Influence of Carbohydrate on Atherosclerosis in Rabbits[a]

	Cholesterol		Avg. Atherosclerosis
Carbohydrate	Serum (mg/dl)	Liver (g/100 g)	(Arch + Thoracic/2)
Fructose	922	1.99	2.00
Sucrose	520	1.69	1.45
Starch	532	2.01	1.35
Glucose	451	1.62	0.85
Lactose	329	1.81	0.50

[a]Data from Kritchevsky et al.[57,58]

Rabbits fed 40 percent carbohydrate, 25 percent casein, 14 percent coconut oil, 15 percent cellulose, 5 percent salt mix, 1 percent mineral mix for 10 months.

Table 2-6. Influence of Carbohydrate in Baboons Fed Semipurified Diets Containing 0.1 percent Cholesterol[a]

	Carbohydrate					
	Fructose	Sucrose	Starch	Glucose	Lactose	Control
Serum lipids (mg/dl)						
Cholesterol	144 ± 5	143 ± 3	155 ± 5	155 ± 6	170 ± 5	117 ± 3
Triglyceride	122 ± 5	91 ± 4	96 ± 4	105 ± 5	98 ± 3	95 ± 4
HDL/LDL	0.79	0.93	0.93	1.02	1.07	1.56
Liver lipids (mg/g)						
Cholesterol	4.9 ± 0.4	3.7 ± 0.3	4.4 ± 0.6	2.9 ± 0.5	5.1 ± 0.7	2.8 ± 0.3
Triglyceride	25.6 ± 2	41.3 ± 7	27.8 ± 6	13.3 ± 1	28.0 ± 7	15.8 ± 6
Aorta						
Sudanophilia (%)	11 ± 4	10 ± 5	21 ± 9	17 ± 10	66 ± 14	1 ± 0.4
Plaques	3/6	2/6	1/6	0/6	5/6	0/6

[a]Data from Kritchevsky et al.[62] Six baboons/group fed 40 percent carbohydrate, 25 percent casein, 14 percent coconut oil, 15 percent cellulose, 0.1 percent cholesterol for 17 months.

FIBER
(Chapter 6)

Health-promoting properties of fiber have been discussed in the medical literature since the time of Hippocrates, but the public awareness of fiber has been stimulated by discussions in the popular press of the work of Burkitt and colleagues[63] and Trowell.[64] These investigators equated the absence of coronary disease in African black populations with their high fiber diets, a possibility suggested by Walker and Arvidsson[65] in 1954. One suggestion was that the decreased intestinal transit time caused by some types of fiber could result in reduced absorption of nutrients and, thus, lead to hypocholesterolemia. Ponz de Leon and colleagues[66] have recently shown that transit time is inversely correlated with cholesterol absorption in humans; bran, however, which decreases transit time, is virtually without effect on human serum cholesterol levels.[67]

Fiber is a generic term for substances that are not broken down by human intestinal secretions and includes a number of substances of individual chemical structures and unique physiologic effects. With the exception of lignin, most types of fiber are carbohydrate in nature. The major classes of fiber are cellulose, hemicellulose, pectin, and lignin. In man, cellulose has no effect on serum lipids,[68] whereas pectin exhibits definite hypocholesterolemic properties.[68–72] Bran is regarded by many as pure fiber, but it is actually a mixture of several types of fiber and other nutrients.[73] Despite its popularity, bran has no effect on human lipid levels.[67] Addition of fiber to a standard diet for diabetics will reduce cholesterol levels, glycemia, and requirements for insulin or other hypoglycemic agents.[74–77]

Grande[78] has summarized data that show that isocaloric substitution of dietary sucrose by starch (rice, bread, legumes) was uniformly hypocholesterolemic. The substitutions replaced sucrose, but they also added to the fiber content of the diet.

About 20 years ago, it was reported that diets high in saturated fat but devoid of cholesterol could be atherogenic for rabbits.[79,80] A review of the literature[81] revealed that saturated fat was atherogenic when present as part of a semipurified diet, but was without effect when added to a stock diet. The difference was thought to be due to the different fibers present in the two diets. This suggestion was verified by experimental proof.[82,83] Moore[84] fed rabbits semipurified diets containing butter and also showed that severity of atherosclerosis varied significantly with type of dietary fiber. When rats are fed fiber-free diets containing 1 percent cholesterol, their serum cholesterol levels rise by 25 percent but liver cholesterol rises by 500 percent. Addition of 5 to 10 percent pectin or vegetable gum to the diet leads to a dramatic drop in liver cholesterol levels,[85–89] but cellulose,[87,89] agar, or alginic acid[89] will raise cholesterol levels. Pectin is also hypocholesterolemic in rabbits[90–92] and will inhibit cholesterol-induced atherogenesis in chickens.[93]

The mode of action of fiber is still unclear. In rabbits,[94] it decreases sterol absorption and increases excretion. It affects bile acid turnover,[95] which it may do by binding bile acids,[96–99] thus, inhibiting lipid absorption. We need more information concerning the particular aspects of fiber chemistry that account for its specific properties.

PECTIN

The first purely nutritional studies in experimental atherosclerosis were carried out by Ignatowski,[100,101] who was interested in the effects of animal protein. In the 1920s, Newburgh and his colleagues[102–106] found that both casein and meat were atherogenic for rabbits. They showed that the amount of cholesterol present in beef was insufficient to be atherogenic by itself.[107] Nuzum and colleagues[108–110] also found casein or other animal protein to be atherogenic in rabbits. The first comparison of animal and vegetable proteins was carried out by Meeker and Kesten in rabbits,[111,112] who compared casein and soy protein; the latter was significantly more atherogenic. Enselme and colleagues[113] fed rabbits diets containing 8 percent corn oil and 25 percent casein or wheat gluten. They did not find atherosclerotic lesions, but the casein diet was significantly more cholesterolemic. Howard and colleagues[114] fed rabbits casein or soy protein and beef fat and found that casein was about twice as atherogenic. Lactalbumin was more atherogenic in rabbits than wheat gluten or corn protein.[114] Hamilton and Carroll[116] fed rabbits diets containing 30 percent defatted animal or vegetable protein and 1 percent corn oil for a month and found that there was a wide range of cholesterolemic effect in both groups (Table 2-7). Clearly, the effect of protein on atherosclerosis in experimental animals is dependent on more than its origin.

After analyzing epidemiologic data available in 1957, Yudkin[49] and Yerushalmy and Hilleboe[117] concluded that intake of animal protein was better correlated with human coronary disease than the intake of fat. Hodges and colleagues[118] found that a diet containing mixed protein was more lipidemic than one containing vegetable protein. Walker and colleagues[119] found that young women eating 50 g/day of vegetable protein had lower cholesterol levels than women taking a similar amount of animal protein. Sirtori and his colleagues[120,121] reported that subjects with type II hyperlipoproteinemia exhibited lower cholesterol and triglyceride levels ingesting a diet containing soy protein compared to their starting diet containing meat (Table 2-8).

Table 2-7.   Influence of Protein on Serum Cholesterol Level (mg/dl) in rabbits[a]

Protein	Serum Cholesterol
Egg yolk	260
Skim milk	230
Turkey	217
Lactalbumin	210
Casein	200
Whole egg	183
Fish	167
Beef	153
Chicken	147
Pork	107
Egg White	100
Wheat gluten	80
Peanut	80
Oat	77
Cottonseed	73
Sesame seed	70
Alfalfa	67
Soy isolate	67
Sunflower seed	53
Pea	40
Fava bean	30

[a]Data from Carroll and Hamilton.[116] Rabbits fed 30 percent defatted protein and 1 percent corn oil for 28 days.

What is the mechanism of action of vegetable protein? The intestinal flora appear to have no influence on the protein effects.[122] Huff and Carroll[123] found that feeding of partially hydrolyzed casein or soy protein lowered cholesterol levels in rabbits, but feeding of the constituent amino acids did not. In a series of complex feeding experiments, they used various combinations of mixtures of essential or nonessential amino acids plus various other amino acid additions, but no clear-cut suggestions of mechanism emerged.

Another hypothesis concerns the possibility that the ratio of lysine to arginine (2.0 in casein, 0.9 in soy) may play a role in atherogenesis.[124,125] Addition of enough lysine to soy protein to change the lysine/arginine ratio of soy to that of casein enhances atherogenicity in rabbits, and addition of arginine to casein reduces its atherogenicity.[126,127] The changes in atherogenicity are accompanied by changes in lipoprotein spectrum. When three proteins of similar lysine content but different lysine/arginine ratios (fish protein, casein, milk protein) are fed to rab-

Table 2-8.   Influence of Soy Protein Diet on Subjects with Type II Hyperlipoproteinemia[a]

	Type IIA (22)		Type IIB (16)	
	Start	End	Start	End
Total cholesterol, mg/dl	346 ± 22	289 ± 24	326 ± 15	262 ± 10
LDL cholesterol, mg/dl	278 ± 21	224 ± 23	233 ± 14	181 ± 10
VLDL cholesterol, mg/dl	28 ± 2	30 ± 3	56 ± 4	47 ± 5
Triglyceride, mg/dl	134 ± 7	139 ± 9	246 ± 16	221 ± 24
Weight change, kg		−1.2 ± 0.2		−0.6 ± 0.2

[a]Data from Sirtori et al.[121] Subjects fed diet containing 21 percent protein (63 percent soy, 30 percent other vegetable protein, 7 percent animal protein) for 3 weeks.

bits, the extent of atherosclerosis is directly related to the lysine/arginine ratio.[128] Beef protein is much more atherogenic than textured vegetable protein (TVP), but a 1:1 mixture of the two proteins is no more atherogenic in rabbits than TVP alone.[129] The mixture has a lower lysine/arginine ratio than does beef protein. When casein-fed rabbits are placed on a soy protein diet they exhibit a rapid drop in serum cholesterol level. When soy protein is replaced with casein, there is a rapid increase in serum cholesterol level.[130]

Casein-fed rabbits absorb more cholesterol and excrete less than rabbits fed soy protein.[131,132] The disappearance of 14 C-cholesterol from serum of rabbits fed soy protein yields a curve which resembles that seen in rabbits fed commercial ration. The type of fat in the diet has little effect on the cholesterol disappearance curve. Cholesterol turnover in casein-fed rabbits proceeds at a much slower rate. The kinetics of cholesterol turnover in rabbits fed soy protein plus lysine resemble those reported for casein.[133]

The effects of animal and vegetable protein can be vitiated by the type of carbohydrate[116] or fiber[134] present in the diet.

TRACE MINERALS
(Chapter 9)

Water softness has been suggested as an etiologic agent in atherosclerosis,[135–137] and water hardness has been negatively associated with cardiovascular mortality.[138–141] Schroeder[142] found that the chromium level of tissues fell with age and that atherosclerotic aortas contained none of this element. He suggested that chromium deficiency might be a factor in development of atherosclerosis. Klevay[143] has proposed that the dietary ratio of zinc to copper may affect cholesterolemia and atherosclerosis. Mertz[144] recently reviewed the literature on trace minerals and cardiovascular disease and pointed out that deficiency of several trace elements can have a negative effect on metabolic process known to be involved in the atherosclerotic process, but noted that no direct proofs relating trace minerals to the pathogenesis of atherosclerosis were yet available. The elements that Mertz focused on were sodium, calcium, magnesium, zinc, copper, vanadium, chromium, iron, and iodine.

CONCLUSION

The influence of diet on vascular disease is complex. Most dietary intervention in man is aimed at lowering cholesterol levels. A trial in an incarcerated (mental home) population, in which dietary unsaturated fat was increased yielded significant lowering of serum cholesterol levels and decreased mortality.[145] A drug trial in a free-living population yielded significant lowering of mortality, with only minimal decreases in plasma cholesterol levels[146] (See also Chapter 1). Animal experiments can provide data concerning effects of specific nutrients fed under static conditions. Interactions among nutrients can alter the lipidemic or atherogenic propensity of individual substances. In man the situation is even more difficult to assess since dietary effects are modified by interplay with other risk factors as well as by genetic influences.

Armstrong and colleagues[147] surveyed dietary practices in 30 countries and found positive correlations with gross national product, total calories, protein, fat, sugar, eggs, coffee, tea, and cigarettes. They suggested that their findings should be used to investigate avenues for further research. Stavraky[148] has referred to such findings as "hypothesis generating data." The past few decades have seen great advances in our understanding of lipid metabolism and its relation to atherosclerosis. The effects on diet in modifying these interactions are suggestive but not as conclusive as scientists might wish them to be. The truth will yield to perseverance, not polemic!

REFERENCES

1. Truswell AS: Diet and plasma lipids—a reappraisal. Am J Clin Nutr 31:977, 1978.
2. Kagan A, Kannel WB, Dawber TR, Revotskie N: The coronary profile. Ann NY Acad Sci 97:883, 1962.
3. Strasser T: Atherosclerosis and coronary heart disease: The contribution of epidemiology. WHO Chron 26:7, 1972.
4. Hopkins PN, Williams RR: A survey of 246 suggested coronary risk factors. Atherosclerosis 40:1, 1981.
5. Wissler RW, Vesselinovitch D: Differences between human and animal atherosclerosis. In Schettler G, Weizel A (eds): Atherosclerosis III. Berlin, Springer Verlag, 1974, pp 319–325.
6. Kritchevsky D: Animal models for atherosclerosis research. In Kritchevsky D (ed): Hypolipidemic Agents. Berlin, Springer Verlag, 1975, pp 216-228.
7. Gertler MM, Garn SM, White PD: Diet, serum cholesterol and coronary artery disease. Circulation 2:696, 1950.
8. Kannel WB, Gordon T (eds): The Framingham diet study: diet and the regulation of serum cholesterol. United States Department of Health, Education and Welfare, The Framingham Study. Section 24. Washington, 1970.
9. Nichols AB, Ravenscroft C, Lamphiear DE, Ostrander LD Jr: Independence of serum lipid levels and dietary habits, the Tecumseh study. JAMA 236:1948, 1976.
10. Slater G, Mead J, Dhopeshwarkar G, Robinson S, Alfin-Slater RB: Plasma cholesterol and triglycerides in men with added eggs in the diet. Nutr Rep Int 14:249, 1976.
11. Porter MW, Yamanaka W, Carlson SD, Flynn MA: Effect of dietary egg on serum cholesterol and triglyceride of human males. Am J Clin Nutr 30:490, 1977.
12. Gordon T, Kagan A, Garcia-Palmieri M, Kannel WB, Zukel WJ, Tillotson J, Sorlie P, Hjortland M: Diet and its relation to coronary heart disease and death in three populations. Circulation 63:500, 1981.
13. Gofman JW, Lindgren F, Elliott H, Mantz W, Hewitt J, Strisower B, Herring V, Lyon TP: The role of lipids and lipoproteins in atherosclerosis. Science 111:166, 1950.
14. Barr DP, Russ EM, Eder HA: Protein — lipid relationships in human plasma. II. Atherosclerosis and related conditions. Am J Med 11:480, 1951.
15. Miller GJ, Miller NE: Plasma high density lipoprotein concentration and development of ischaemic heart disease. Lancet 1:16, 1975.

16. Ahrens EH Jr: Nutrutional factors and serum lipid levels. Am J Med 23:928, 1957.
17. Kritchevsky D, Moyer AW, Tesar WC, Logan JB, Brown RA, Davies MC, Cox HR: Effect of cholesterol vehicle in experimental atherosclerosis. Am J Physiol 178:30, 1954.
18. Kritchevsky D, Moyer AW, Tesar WC, McCandless RFJ, Logan JB, Brown RA, Englert M: Cholesterol vehicle in experimental atherosclerosis. II. Effect of unsaturation. Am J Physiol 185:279, 1956.
19. Funch JP, Krogh B, Dam H: Effects of butter, some margarines and arachis oil in purified diets on serum lipids and atherosclerosis in rabbits. Br J Nutr 14:355, 1960.
20. Kritchevsky D: Role of cholesterol vehicle in experimental atherosclerosis. Am J Clin Nutr 23:1105, 1970.
21. Gresham GA, Howard AN: The independent production of atherosclerosis and thrombosis in the rat. Br J Exp Pathol 41:395, 1960.
22. Scot RF, Morrison ES, Thomas WA, Jones R, Nam SC: Short term feeding of unsaturated versus saturated fat in the production of atherosclerosis in the rat. Exp Mol Pathol 3:421, 1964.
23. Kritchevsky D, Tepper SA, Vesselinovitch D, Wissler RW: Cholesterol vehicle in experimental atherosclerosis. 11. Peanut oil. Atherosclerosis 14:53, 1971.
24. Vesselinovitch D, Getz GS, Hughes RH, Wissler RW: Atherosclerosis in the rhesus monkey fed three food fats. Atherosclerosis 20:303, 1974.
25. Kritchevsky D, Tepper SA, Vesselinovitch D, Wissler RW: Cholesterol vehicle in experimental atherosclerosis. 13. Randomized peanut oil. Atherosclerosis 17:225, 1973.
26. Kritchevsky D, Davidson LM, Weight M, Kriek NPJ, duPlessis JP: Influence of native and randomized peanut oil on lipid metabolism and aortic sudanophilia in the vervet monkey. Atherosclerosis 42:53, 1982.
27. Myher JJ, Marai L, Kuksis A, Kritchevsky D: Acylglycerol structure of peanut oils of different atherogenic potential. Lipids 12:775, 1977.
28. Manganaro F, Myher JJ, Kuksis A, Kritchevsky D: Acylglycerol structure of genetic varieties of peanut oils of varying atherogenic potential. Lipids 16:508, 1981.
29. Kummerow FA: Current studies on relation of fat to health. J Am Oil Chem Soc 51:255, 1974.
30. Weigensberg BI, McMillan GC, Ritchie AC: Elaidic acid: effect on experimental atherosclerosis. Arch Pathol 72:126, 1961.
31. McMillan GC, Silver MD, Weigensberg BI: Elaidinized olive oil and cholesterol atherosclerosis. Arch Pathol 76:106, 1963.
32. Ruttenberg H, Davidson LM, Little NA, Klurfeld DM, Kritchevsky D: Influence of trans unsaturated fats on experimental atherosclerosis in rabbits. J Nutr (in press).
33. Ono K, Fredrickson DS: The metabolism of ^{14}C-labeled cis and trans isomers of octadecanoic and octadecadienoic acids. J Biol Chem 239:2482, 1964.
34. Anderson RL: Oxidation of the geometric isomers of $\Delta^{9,12}$-octadecadienoic acids by rat liver mitochondria. Biochim Biophys Acta 152:531, 1968.
35. Sgoutas DS: Hydrolysis of synthetic cholesterol esters containing trans fatty acids. Biochim Biophys Acta 164:317, 1968.
36. Sgoutas DS: Effect of geometry and position of ethylenic bond upon acyl coenzyme-cholesterol-cholesterol-O-acyltransferase. Biochemistry 9:1826, 1970.
37. Kritchevsky D, Baldino AR: Pancreatic cholesteryl ester synthetase: Effects of trans unsaturated and long chain saturated fatty acids. Artery 4:480, 1978.
38. Jensen RG, Sampugna J, Pereira RL: Pancreatic lipase: lipolysis of synthetic triglycerides containing a trans fatty acid. Biochim Biophys Acta 84:481, 1964.
39. Moore CE, Alfin-Slater RB, Aftergood L: Incorporation and disappearance of trans fatty acids in rat tissues. Am J Clin Nutr 33:2318, 1980.

40. Kritchevsky D: Trans fatty acid effects in experimental atherosclerosis. Fed Proc 41: 2813, 1982.
41. Dutton HJ: Hydrogenation of fats and its significance. In Emken EA, Dutton HJ (eds): Geometrical and Positional Fatty Acid Isomers. Champaign, Ill, Am Oil Chem Soc pp 1-16, 1979.
42. Albrink MJ, Meigs TW, Man EB: Serum lipids, hypertension and coronary heart disease. Am J Med 31:4, 1961.
43. Knittle JL, Ahrens EH: Carbohydrate metabolism in two forms of hyperglyceridemia. J Clin Invest 43:485, 1964.
44. Bierman EL, Porte D Jr: Carbohydrate intolerance and lipemia. Ann Intern Med 68: 926, 1968.
45. MacDonald I, Braithwaite DM: The influence of dietary carbohydrates on the lipid pattern in serum and in adipose tissue. Clin Sci 27:23, 1964.
46. Kuo PT: Dietary sugar in the production of hypertriglyceridemia in patients with hyperlipemia and atherosclerosis. Trans Assoc Am Physicians 78:97, 1965.
47. Nikkila EA, Pelkonen R: Enhancement of alimentary hypertriglyceridemia by fructose and glycerol in man. Proc Soc Exp Biol Med 123:91, 1966.
48. McGandy RB, Hegsted DM, Stare FJ: Dietary fats, carbohydrates, and atherosclerotic vascular disease. N Engl J Med 277:186, 1967.
49. Yudkin J: Diet and coronary thrombosis: Hypothesis and fact. Lancet 2:155, 1957.
50. Yudkin J: Dietetic aspects of atherosclerosis. Angiology 17:127, 1966.
51. MacDonald I, Roberts JB: The incorporation of various ^{14}C dietary carbohydrates into serum and liver lipids. Metabolism 14:991, 1965.
52. Nikkila EA, Ojala K: Induction of hyperglyceridemia by fructose in the rat. Life Sci 4:937, 1965.
53. Bar-On H , Stein Y: Effect of glucose and fructose administration on lipid metabolism in the rat. J Nutr 94:95, 1968.
54. Coltart TM, Crossley JN: Influence of dietary sucrose on glucose and fructose tolerance and triglyceride synthesis in the baboon. Clin Sci 38:427, 1970.
55. Kritchevsky D, Davidson LM, Shapiro IL, Kim HK, Kitagawa M, Malhotra S, Nair PP, Clarkson TB, Bersohn I, Winter PAD: Lipid metabolism and experimental atherosclerosis in baboons: influence of cholesterol-free, semi-synthetic diets. Am J Clin Nutr 27:29, 1974.
56. Kritchevsky D, Davidson LM, vanderWatt JJ, Winter PAD, Bersohn I: Hypercholesterolemia and atherosclerosis induced in vervet monkeys by cholesterol-free, semi-synthetic diets. S Afr Med J 48:2413, 1974.
57. Kritchevsky D, Sallata P, Tepper SA: Experimental atherosclerosis in rabbits fed cholesterol-free diets. 2. Influence of various carbohydrates. J Atheroscler Res 8:697, 1968.
58. Kritchevsky D, Tepper SA, Kitagawa M: Experimental atherosclerosis in rabbits fed cholesterol-free diets. 3. Comparison of fructose and lactose with other carbohydrates. Nutr Rep Int 7:193, 1973.
59. Kritchevsky D, Grant WC, Fahrenbach MJ, Riccardi BA, McCandless RFJ: Effect of dietary carbohydrate on the metabolism of cholesterol-4-C^{14} in chickens. Arch Biochem Biophys 75:142, 1958.
60. Grant WC, Fahrenbach MJ: Effect of dietary sucrose and glucose on plasma cholesterol in chicks and rabbits. Proc Soc Exp Biol Med 100:250, 1959.
61. Wells WW, Anderson SC: The increased severity of atherosclerosis in rabbits on a lactose-containing diet. J Nutr 68:541, 1959.
62. Kritchevsky D, Davidson LM, Kim HK, Krendel DA, Malhotra S, Mendelsohn D,

vanderWatt JJ, duPlessis JP, Winter PAD: Influence of type of carbohydrate on athero-sclerosis in baboons fed semipurified diets plus 0.1% cholesterol. Am J Clin Nutr 33:1869, 1980.

63. Burkitt DP, Walker ARP, Painter NS: Dietary fiber and disease. JAMA 229:1068, 1974.

64. Trowell H: Ischemic heart disease and dietary fiber. Am J Clin Nutr 25:926, 1972.

65. Walker ARP, Arvidsson UB: Fat intake, serum cholesterol, concentration and athero-sclerosis in the South African Bantu. I. Low fat intake and age trend of serum choles-terol concentration in the South African Bantu. J Clin Invest 33:1358, 1954.

66. Ponz de Leon M, Iori R, Barbolini G, Pompei G, Zaniol P, Carulli N: Influence of small bowel transit time on dietary cholesterol absorption in human beings. N Engl J Med 307:102, 1982.

67. Kay RM, Truswell AS: Dietary fiber: Effects on plasma and biliary lipids in man. In Spiller GA, Kay RM (eds): Medial Aspects of Dietary Fiber. New York, Plenum Press, 1980, pp 153-173.

68. Keys A, Grande F, Anderson JT: Fiber and pectin in the diet and serum cholesterol concentration in man. Proc Soc Exp Biol Med 106:555, 1961.

69. Jenkins DJA, Leeds AR, Newton C, Cummings JH: Effect of pectin, guar gum and wheat fibre on serum cholesterol. Lancet 1:1116, 1975.

70. Durrington PN, Manning AP, Bolton CH, Hartog M: Effect of pectin on serum lipids and lipoproteins, whole gut transit time and stool weight. Lancet 2:394, 1976.

71. Kay RM, Truswell AS: Effect of citrus pectin on blood lipids and fecal steroid excre-tion in man. Am J Clin Nutr 30:171, 1977.

72. Miettinen TA, Tarpila S: Effect of pectin on serum cholesterol, fecal bile acids and biliary lipids in normolipidemic and hyperlipidemic individuals. Clin Chem Acta 79:471, 1977.

73. Mullen JD: Dietary fiber sources for human studies. Am J Clin Nutr 31:5103, 1978.

74. Stone DB, Connor WE: The prolonged effects of a low cholesterol, high carbohydrate diet upon the serum lipids in diabetic patients. Diabetes 12:127, 1963.

75. Kiehm TG, Anderson JW, Ward K: Beneficial effects of a high carbohydrate, high fiber diet on hyperglycemic, diabetic man. Am J Clin Nutr 29:895, 1976.

76. Miranda PA, Horwitz DL: High-fiber diets in the treatment of diabetes mellitus. Ann Intern Med 88:482, 1978.

77. Anderson JW: Dietary fiber and diabetes. In Spiller GA, Kay RM (eds): Medical Aspects of Dietary Fiber. New York, Plenum Press, 1980, pp 193–221.

78. Grande F: Sugars in cardiovascular disease. In Sipple HI, McNutt KW (eds): Sugars in Nutrition. New York, Academic Press, 1974, pp 401–437.

79. Lambert GF, Miller JP, Olsen RT, Frost DV: Hypercholesteremia and atherosclerosis induced in rabbits by purified high fat rations devoid of cholesterol. Proc Soc Exp Biol Med 97:544, 1958.

80. Malmros H, Wigand G: Atherosclerosis and deficiency of essential fatty acids. Lancet 2:749, 1959.

81. Kritchevsky D: Experimental atherosclerosis in rabbits fed cholesterol-free diets. J Athero-scler Res 4:103, 1964.

82. Kritchevsky D, Tepper SA: Factors affecting atherosclerosis in rabbits fed cholesterol-free diets. Life Sci 4:1467, 1965.

83. Kritchevsky D, Tepper SA: Experimental atherosclerosis in rabbits fed cholesterol-free-diets: influence of chow components. J Atheroscler Res 8:357, 1968.

84. Moore JH: The effect of the type of roughage in the diet on plasma cholesterol levels and aortic atherosis in rabbits. Br J Nutr 21:207, 1967.

85. Wells AF, Ershoff BH: Beneficial effects of pectin in prevention of hypercholesterolemia and increase in liver cholesterol in cholesterol-fed rats. J Nutr 74:87, 1961.

86. Ershoff BH, Wells AF: Effects of gum guar, locust bean gum, and carrageenan on liver cholesterol in cholesterol-fed rats. Proc Soc Exp Biol Med 110:580, 1962.

87. Riccardi BA, Fahrenbach MJ: Effect of guar gum and pectin NF on serum and liver lipids of cholesterol-fed rats. Proc Soc Exp Biol Med 124:749, 1967.

88. Kiriyama S, Okozaki Y, Yoshida A: Hypocholesterolemic effect of polysaccharides and polysaccharide-rich foodstuffs in cholesterol-fed rats. J Nutr 97:382, 1969.

89. Tsai AC, Elias J, Kelley JJ, Lin RSC, Robson JRK: Influence of certain dietary fibers on serum and tissue cholesterol levels in rats. J Nutr 106:118, 1976.

90. Ershoff BH: Effects of pectin NF and other complex carbohydrates on hypercholesterolemia and atherosclerosis. Exp Med Surg 21:108, 1963.

91. Berenson LM, Bhandaru RR, Radhakrishnamurthy B, Srinivasan SB, Berenson GS: The effect of dietary pectin on serum lipoprotein cholesterol in rabbits. Life Sci 16:1533, 1975.

92. Hamilton RMG, Carroll KK: Plasma cholesterol levels in rabbits fed low fat, low cholesterol diets. Effects of dietary proteins, carbohydrates and fibre from different sources. Atherosclerosis 24:47, 1976.

93. Fisher H, Soller WG, Griminger P: The retardation by pectin by cholesterol-induced atherosclerosis in the fowl. J Atheroscler Res 6:292, 1966.

94. Kritchevsky D, Tepper SA, Kim HK, Moses DE, Story JA: Experimental atherosclerosis in rabbits fed cholesterol-free diets. 4. Investigation into the source of cholesteremia. Exp Mol Pathol 22;11, 1977.

95. Portman D, Murphy P: Excretion of bile acids and hydroxysterols by rats. Arch Biochem Biophys 76:367, 1958.

96. Eastwood MA, Hamilton D: Studies on the adsorption of bile salts to nonabsorbed components of diet. Biochim Biophys Acta 152:165, 1968.

97. Kritchevsky D, Story JA: Binding of bile salts in vitro by nonnutritive fiber. J Nutr 104:458, 1974.

98. Birkner HJ, Kern F Jr: In vitro adsorption of bile salts to food residues, salicylazosulfapyridine and hemicellulose. Gastroenterology 67:237, 1974.

99. Story JA, Kritchevsky D: Comparison of the binding of various bile acids and bile salts in vitro by several types of fiber. J Nutr 106:1292, 1976.

100. Ignatowski A: Influence de la nourriture animale sur l'organisme des lapins. Arch Med Exp Anat Pathol 20:1, 1908.

101. Igatowski A: Uber die wirkung des tierischen Eiweisses auf die Aorta und die parenchymatosen Organe der kaninchen. Virchows Arch Path Anat Physiol Klin Med 198:248, 1909.

102. Newburgh LH: The production of Bright's disease by feeding high protein diets. Arch Int Med 24:359, 1919.

103. Newburgh LH, Squier TL: High protein diets and arteriosclerosis in rabbits. A preliminary report. Arch Int Med 26:38, 1920.

104. Newburgh LH, Clarkson S: Production of arteriosclerosis in rabbits by diets rich in animal protein. J Am Med Assoc 79:1106, 1922.

105. Newburgh LH, Clarkson S: The production of arteriosclerosis in rabbits by feeding diets rich in meat. Arch Int Med 31:653, 1923.

106. Newburgh LH, Clarkson S: Renal injury produced in rabbits by diets containing meat. Arch Int Med 26:38, 1923.

107. Clarkson S, Newburgh LH: The relation between atherosclerosis and ingested cholesterol in the rabbit. J Exp Med 43:595, 1926.

108. Nuzum FR, Osborne M, Sansum WD: The experimental production of hypertension. Arch Int Med 35:492, 1925.

109. Nuzum FR, Seegal B, Garland R, Osborne M: Arteriosclerosis and increased blood pressure. Arch Int Med 37:733, 1926.
110. Nuzum FR, Elliott AH, Evans RD, Priest BV: The occurrence and nature of spontaneous arteriosclerosis and nephritis in the rabbit. Arch Pathol 10:697, 1930.
111. Meeker DR, Kesten HD: Experimental atherosclerosis and high protein diets. Proc Soc Exp Biol Med 45:543, 1940.
112. Meeker DR, Kesten HD: Effect of high protein diets on experimental atherosclerosis in rabbits. Arch Pathol 31:147, 1941.
113. Enselme J, Cottet J, Fray G: Etude de diverses influences alimentaires sur l'atherosclerose provoquee par une alimentation priovee de cholesterol. Rev de l'Atheroscler 5:52, 1963.
114. Howard AN, Gresham GA, Jones D, Jennings IW: The prevention of rabbit atherosclerosis by soya bean meal. J Atheroscler Res 5:330, 1965.
115. Kritchevsky D, Tepper SA, Czarnecki SK, Story JA, Marsh JB: Experimental atherosclerosis in rabbits fed cholesterol-free diets. II. Corn protein, wheat gluten and lactalbumin. Nutr Rep Int 26:931, 1982.
116. Carroll KK, Hamilton RMG: Effects of dietary protein and carbohydrate on plasma cholesterol levels in relation to atherosclerosis. J Food Sci 40:18, 1975.
117. Yerushalmy J, Hilleboe HE: Fat in the diet and mortality from heart disease: a methodologic note. NY State J Med 57:2343, 1957.
118. Hodges RE, Krehl WA, Stone DB, Lopez A: Dietary carbohydrates and low cholesterol diets: effects on serum lipids of man. Am J Clin Nutr 20:198, 1967.
119. Walker GR, Morse EH, Oversley VA: The effect of animal protein and vegetable protein diets having the same fat content on the serum lipid levels of young women. J Nutr 72:317, 1960.
120. Sirtori CR, Agradi E, Conti F, Mantero O, Gatti E: Soybean protein in the treatment of type II hyperlipoproteinaemia. Lancet 1:275, 1977.
121. Sirtori CR, Gatti E, Mantero O, Conti F, Agradi E, Tremoli E, Sirtori M, Fraterrigo L, Tavazzi L, Kritchevsky D: Clinical experience with the soybean protein diet in the treatment of hypercholesterolemia. Am J Clin Nutr 32:1645, 1979.
122. Kritchevsky D, Kolman RR, Guttmacher RM, Forbes M: Influrence of dietary carbohydrate and protein on serum and liver cholesterol in germ-free chickens. Arch Biochem Biophys 85:444, 1959.
123. Huff MW, Carroll KK: Effects of dietary proteins and amino acid mixtures on plasma cholesterol levels in rabbits. J Nutr 110:1676, 1980.
124. Kritchevsky D, Tepper SA, Story JA: Influence of soy protein and casein on atherosclerosis in rabbits. Fed Proc 37:747, 1978.
125. Kritchevsky D: Vegetable protein and atherosclerosis. J Am Oil Chem Soc 56:135, 1979.
126. Czarnecki SK, Kritchevsky D: The effect of dietary proteins on lipoprotein metabolism and atherosclerosis in rabbits. J Am Oil Chem Soc 56:388A, 1979.
127. Kritchevsky D: Dietary protein in atherosclerosis. In Noseda G, Lewis B, Paoletti R (eds): Diet Drugs and Atherosclerosis. New York, Raven Press, 1980, pp 9–14.
128. Kritchevsky D, Tepper SA, Czarnecki SK, Klurfeld DM: Atherogenicity of animal and vegetable protein: influence of the lysine to arginine ratio. Atherosclerosis 41:429, 1982.
129. Kritchevsky D, Tepper SA, Czarnecki SK, Klurfeld DM, Story JA: Experimental atherosclerosis in rabbits fed cholesterol-free diets. 9. Beef protein and textured vegetable protein. Atherosclerosis 39:169, 1981.
130. Terpstra AHM, Woodward CJH, West CE, Van Boven HG: A longitudinal cross-over study of serum cholesterol and lipoproteins in rabbits fed on semi-purified diets containing either casein or soya-bean protein. Br J Nutr 47:213, 1982.
131. Fumagalli R, Paoletti R, Howard AN: Hypocholesterolaemic effect of soy. Life Sci 22:

947, 1978.

132. Huff MW, Carroll KK: Effects of dietary protein on turnover, oxidation and absorption of cholesterol and on steroid excretion in rabbits. J Lipid Res 21:546, 1980.

133. Kritchevsky D: Unpublished obervation.

134. Kritchevsky D, Tepper SA, Williams DE, Story JA: Experimental atherosclerosis in rabbits fed cholesterol-free diets. 7. Interaction of animal or vegetable protein with fiber. Atherosclerosis 26:397, 1977.

135. Schroeder HA: Relation between mortality from cardiovascular disease and treated water supplies: variations in states and 163 largest municipalities of the United States. J Am Med Assoc 172:1902, 1960.

136. Morris JN, Crawford MD, Heady JA: Hardness of local water supplies and mortality from cardiovascular disease in county boroughs of England and Wales. Lancet 1:860. 1961.

137. Crawford MD: Hardness of drinking water and cardiovascular disease. Proc Nutr Soc 31:347, 1972.

138. Anderson TW, ¹∍ Riche WH, MacKay JS: Sudden death and ischemic heart disease. N Engl J Med 280:805, 1969.

139. Peterson DR, Thompson DJ, Nam JM: Water hardness, arteriosclerotic heart disease and sudden death. Am J Epidemiol 92:90, 1970.

140. Masironi R: Cardiovascular mortality in relation to radioactivity and hardness of local water supplies in the USA. Bull WHO 43:687, 1970.

141. Masironi R, Miesch AT, Crawford MD, Hamilton EI: Geochemical environments, trace elements and cardiovascular diseases. Bull WHO 47:139, 1972.

142. Schroeder HA, Nason AP, Tipton IH: Chromium deficiency as a factor in atherosclerosis. J Chronic Dis 23:123, 1970.

143. Klevay LM: Coronary heart disease: The zinc/copper hypothesis. Am J Clin Nutr 28:764, 1975.

144. Mertz W: Trace minerals and atherosclerosis. Fed Proc 41:2807, 1982.

145. Turpeinen O: Effect of cholesterol–lowering diet on mortality from cardiovascular heart disease and other causes. Circulation 59:1, 1979.

146. Committee of Principal Investigators. A cooperative trial in the primary prevention of ischaemic heart disease using clofibrate. Br Heart J 40:1069, 1978.

147. Armstrong BK, Mann JI, Adelstein AM, Esken F: Commodity consumption and ischemic heart disease mortality with special reference to dietary practices. J Chronic Dis 28:455, 1975.

148. Stavraky KM: The role of ecological analysis in the etiology of disease: a discussion with reference to large bowel cancer. J Chronic Dis 29:435, 1976.

3 | Diet and Plasma Lipids and Lipoproteins

Elaine B. Feldman

The lipid hypothesis promotes the concept that elevations in blood lipids induce atherosclerosis or that they are directly responsible for the process of atherogenesis. Dietary excesses lead to hyperlipidemia, which in turn promotes atherogenesis. Acceptance of this theory implies that atherosclerosis might be prevented by appropriate dietary modification. The hypothesis has been supported by the observation that patients with familial hypercholesterolemia have a 50 percent risk of myocardial infarction occurring in their mid-40s.[1]

The average American diet contains 450 mg cholesterol daily, and 40 percent of the calories are derived from fat. Populations characterized by high average serum cholesterol levels and high atherosclerotic disease rates have saturated fat intakes amounting to 15 percent of total calories. Populations with low coronary heart disease prevalence and low serum cholesterol ingest diets in which saturated fat contributes 10 percent or less of calories.[2] In the usual diet, polyunsaturated fatty acids contribute about 9 percent of calories.

Dietary factors associated with atherosclerosis that influence plasma lipids and lipoproteins will be reviewed in this chapter (see Chapter 7 for a discussion of excess calories and obesity). Primary attention will be paid to fats (saturated, polyunsaturated) (see Chapter 4), cholesterol (see Chapter 5), fiber and refined carbohydrates (see Chapter 6), protein and alcohol (see Chapter 8). This chapter will also review briefly the roles of vitamins and minerals in atherogenesis via their influence on plasma lipids and lipoproteins (see also Chapter 9). A recent survey of 246 suggested coronary risk factors yelded 21 dietary excesses and positive associations and 23 dietary deficiencies and inverse associations or possible protective factors.[3] The specifics of dietary intervention to normalize serum lipids are provided in Chapter 10.

CHOLESTEROL

Hypercholesterolemia may be defined using the 95 percent confidence limits of circulating cholesterol levels (Table 3-1). In the United States, these statistical norms provide high levels that may be unhealthy. Serum cholesterol levels increase with advancing age and differ between men and women (see also Chapter 10, Table 10-1). The risk of atherosclerosis increases linearly as cholesterol levels increase above 180 mg or 200 mg/dl. It may be desirable to control serum cholesterol at these levels throughout adult life. There is some evidence, however, that risk of cancer is increased at lower cholesterol levels,[4] implying that there is an optimal cholesterol level.

The level of plasma cholesterol is determined in part by the dietary intakes of cholesterol, saturated and polyunsaturated fats, and calories (Chapter 5). Dietary cholesterol intake influences plasma cholesterol most profoundly as intake is increased from 0 to about 300 mg.[5] The increase in plasma cholesterol is about 9 mg per 100 mg in the diet up to 300 mg/1,000 kcal. Thereafter, the increase in plasma cholesterol is about 2 mg per 100 mg/1,000 kcal.[2] Dietary saturated fatty acids tend to elevate plasma cholesterol levels, whether they are of vegetable or animal origin (coconut oil, palm oil, cocoa butter versus beef tallow and lard).[6] The highly saturated fats are usually solid at room temperature, with the more unsaturated fats tending to be liquid (oils). Fish oils, of animal origin, are highly polyunsaturated, with longer chain fatty acids, many of which have four and five double bonds (see Chapters 4 and 10). Vegetarian populations with low intakes of cholesterol and saturated fats tend to have lower plasma cholesterol levels and less coronary heart disease.[7] One predictive equation of blood cholesterol levels indicates that dietary saturated fat is twice as powerful in increasing plasma cholesterol as is polyunsaturated fat in decreasing plasma cholesterol. This effect of fat on blood cholesterol occurs in addition to the significant effect of dietary cholesterol (Chapters 5 and 10).[2]

LIPOPROTEINS

Cholesterol and triglycerides are transported in plasma as lipoproteins (Table 3-2). Lipoproteins are classified according to their physical-chemical properties.

Table 3-1. Plasma Cholesterol Levels, mg/dl

Age (years)	Men		Women		Safe
	Mean	Abnormal	Mean	Abnormal	
20	170	220	170	220	175
30	195	255	180	230	185
40	205	270	195	250	220
50	215	275	220	285	220
60	215	275	230	300	220
70	205	270	230	295	220
80	205	260	225	290	220

Values are adapted from the mean values of the Lipid Research Clinics Program Prevalence Study. Abnormal values are the 95th percentile. "Safe" values are estimated not to increase the risk of atherosclerosis. Values have been rounded out to the nearest 5 mg.

Lipoproteins transport dietary and endogenous lipids, and are related in various ways to atherogenesis. Diets high in saturated fat and cholesterol produce alterations in plasma lipoproteins, and these alterations cause certain lipoproteins to deliver cholesterol to the arterial wall. Other compensatory changes in lipoproteins then occur. Atherosclerosis occurs when the influx of cholesterol into the artery exceeds the efflux of cholesterol from tissues (Chapter 5).[8]

CHYLOMICRONS AND CHYLOMICRONEMIA

Chylomicrons are intestinal particles that are formed when fat is ingested, and are present normally only after a fatty meal. Serum lipids should therefore be screened in samples drawn in the morning, 12 to 14 hours after the evening meal. Chylomicrons add turbidity to plasma. Turbidity of plasma is observed when triglycerides exceed 200 mg/dl, and is obvious at triglyceride levels of 500 mg/dl. In the plasma sample placed in the refrigerator overnight, chylomicrons will rise to the top to form a creamy layer. Agarose gel electrophoresis may detect chylomicronemia more efficiently than the standing plasma test.[9]

The chylomicron (Table 3-2) is a large particle that floats, and consists predominantly of triglyceride with small amounts of phospholipids, esterified and free cholesterol, and specific proteins (apolipoproteins). Chylomicrons formed in the small intestine after a fatty meal are absorbed into the lymphatics. The particles then enter the circulation where they are removed by the action of lipoprotein lipase, an enzyme located in the capillary endothelium of extrahepatic tissues.

Inborn errors of metabolism, either lipoprotein lipase deficiency or absence of the enzyme activator C-II apolipoprotein, result in chylomicronemia, a form of hypertriglyceridemia (Table 3-3).[10] This hyperlipoproteinemia is treated by reducing dietary fat intake to less than 20 g/day.[11] It is not clear whether patients with chylomicronemia are at increased risk for atherosclerosis. These patients develop recurrent abdominal pain, at times caused by acute pancreatitis.[12] Elevated triglyceride levels may be manifested overtly by eruptive xanthomas of the skin of extremities, neck, back, or buttocks. When circulating triglyceride levels exceed 3,000 mg/dl, lipemia retinalis may be observed on funduscopic examination. Chylomicronemia may be secondary to diabetic ketoacidosis, alcoholic pancreatitis (Chapter 8) and dysglobulinemia in autoimmune diseases such as disseminated lupus erythematosus or multiple myeloma. The lipolytic action of lipoprotein lipase activity produces the chylomicron remnant, which is taken up by the liver. The remnant particle may be atherogenic.[13]

VLDL

The very low-density lipoprotein (VLDL) is produced in the liver and intestine (small chylomicron or smaller intestinal particle). VLDL (Table 3-2) is the main transporter of endogenous triglyceride, which is synthesized when there is excessive intake of carbohydrate calories. VLDL particles are smaller than chylomicrons. They lend turbidity to plasma, but instead of floating to the top of the test

Table 3-2. Plasma Lipoproteins

| | | | | | | Chemical Composition | | | | |
| | | | | | | Surface | | | Core | |
Class	Particle Diameter (nm) (nm)	Flotation Density	Electrophoretic Mobility	Apoproteins	Proteins	Phospho-lipids	Cholesterol % %	Cholesterol Esters	Triglyc-erides
Chylomicrons	80–500	0.93	α2	B, E, A-I, A-IV, C	2	7	2	3	86
VLDL	30–80	0.95–1.006	pre-β	B, E, C	8	18	7	12	55
IDL	25–35	1.006–1.019	slow pre-β	B, E	19	19	9	29	23
LDL	22	1.019–1.063	β	B	22	22	8	42	6
HDL$_2$	10	1.063–1.125	α1	A-I, A-II, C, E	40	33	5	17	5
HDL$_3$	7.5	1.125–1.210	α1	A-I, A-II, C	55	25	4	13	3

Adapted from Havel RJ, Goldstein JL, Brown MD: Lipoproteins and lipid transport. In Bondy PK, Rosenberg LE (eds): Metabolic Control and Disease, 8th ed. Philadelphia, WB Saunders, 1980, p 398.

Table 3-3. Types of Primary Hyperlipoproteinemias

Lipid Abnormality in Plasma	Lipoprotein Abnormality	Common Term	Classification	Hereditary Forms	Mechanisms
Hypercholesterolemia	$\uparrow$LDL	Familial hyper-cholesterolemia	2a	FH	defective LDL receptor
C 350–600 mg/dl				autosomal dominant heterozygous homozygous	
C > 600 mg/dl					
C < 600 mg/dl	$\uparrow$LDL			familial multiple lipoprotein type hyper-lipidemia (polygenic hypercholesterolemia)	?overproduction apo-B
Hypertriglyceridemia	Chylomicronemia	exogenous hyperlipemia	1	familial — LPL deficiency C-II deficiency	
TG 250–500 mg/dl	$\uparrow$VLDL	endogenous hyperlipemia	4	familial hypertriglyc-eridemia (mild) monogenic hyper-triglyceridemia	
TG 500–1,500 mg/dl					clearance defect + overproduction VLDL-TG
TG 2,000–10,000 mg/dl	Chylo + VLDL	mixed hypertriglyc-eridemia	5	familial hypertriglyc-eridemia (severe) ? E^4 phenotype ? E^4 phenotype	defective clearance TG + overproduction VLDL-TG
Combined hyperlipidemia (C & TG) C & TG ~	$\uparrow$IDL (β-VLDL)	dysbetalipoproteinemia broad-beta disease	3	familial dysbetalipo-proteinemia	abnormal E isoform(s) with defective clearance
C < 350, TG > 250	$\uparrow$LDL + $\uparrow$VLDL		2b, 4	familial multiple lipoprotein type hyper-lipidemia	? overproduction TG + apo-B
TG > 500	$\uparrow\uparrow$VLDL (extreme)	endogenous hyperlipidemia (severe)	4	familial multiple lipoprotein type hyper-lipidemia	? overproduction TG + apo-B

tube as a layer on standing in the cold, VLDL particles become distributed throughout, leading to diffuse turbidity. Compared with chylomicrons, VLDL contain more protein and less triglyceride. VLDL is also removed from plasma via the activity of lipoprotein lipase. Excess production of VLDL triglyceride is usually secondary to high caloric intake, especially of carbohydrate and alcohol, and is associated with obesity. These dietary influences are described in detail in Chapters 6, 7, and 8. VLDL triglycerides are often increased in renal failure, hypothyroidism, diabetes, and dysglobulinemias.[14] Hyperlipidemia with increased levels of VLDL is termed endogenous hyperlipemia (Table 3-3). There are familial forms of mild hypertriglyceridemia (triglyceride levels between 250 and 500 mg/dl).

TRIGLYCERIDES

In the absence of chylomicrons, VLDL levels in plasma are synonymous with fasting triglyceride levels, for practical purposes. Circulating triglyceride levels increase with age (Table 3-4), and are lower in men than in women. Triglyceride values increase with weight gain[15]; they are higher in postmenopausal women, and they increase with administration of estrogens. Elevation of plasma triglycerides is common in patients with coronary heart disease, but the role of plasma triglyceride as an independent risk factor is in dispute.[14]

Levels of serum VLDL respond in proportion to intake of dietary carbohydrate, particularly refined carbohydrate. The specific effects of fructose, sucrose, starch, and fiber on lipoproteins, the mechanisms of effects, and the metabolic control of plasma triglycerides and VLDL—all are described in Chapter 6. Alcohol is particularly contraindicated in patients with elevated VLDL; triglyceride levels may not be normalized unless alcohol is eliminated from the diet (Chapter 8).

LDL

Removal of triglyceride from VLDL by lipoprotein lipase generates low-density lipoprotein (LDL). LDL is the main transporter of cholesterol in plasma (Table 3-2). LDL is about 50 percent cholesterol. LDL is taken up by peripheral

Table 3-4.   Plasma Triglyceride Levels, mg/dl

Age (years)	Men		Women	
	Mean	Abnormal	Mean	Abnormal
20	100	200	75	135
30	130	320	80	145
40	150	320	100	185
50	155	310	110	220
60	140	270	120	230
70	135	260	130	230
80	130	255	130	130

See footnote to Table 3-1.

tissues and liver by the specific cell-surface lipoprotein receptor (Chapter 5). The absence or malfunction of this receptor is the genetic defect in familial hypercholesterolemia (Table 3-3).[16,17] Familial hypercholesterolemia is associated with external signs of eyelid xanthelasmas, tendon xanthomas, and premature corneal arcus.[1] The plasma cholesterol level should be measured in subjects with these physical signs, and also in their family members. In this and other forms of primary hyperlipidemia, about half are familial (Table 3-3) and the remainder are diet induced.

LDL may be the "villain" in atherosclerosis; it is the most atherogenic of all the lipoproteins. Increased plasma levels of LDL are correlated strongly with manifestations of atherosclerosis. It is not clear how LDL is atherogenic. It may be that chemically modified high levels of LDL have longer half-lives. They may also stimulate cell growth and proliferation and thereby initiate atherogenesis.[8] LDL cholesterol levels in plasma vary with age and sex, and parallel total cholesterol (Table 3-1). LDL cholesterol can be estimated by subtracting from the value for total cholesterol the triglyceride value divided by 5 and the value for HDL cholesterol. This calculation is not useful when triglyceride levels exceed 400 mg/dl or in dysbetalipoproteinemia.[18] About half of the patients with familial hypercholesterolemia or their family members sustain a myocardial infarction by the mid-40s; by age 60 years, 85 percent have had a myocardial infarction.

DIET TO REDUCE LDL

The dietary factors that decrease circulating cholesterol (reduce intake of saturated fat and cholesterol, increase intake of polyunsaturated fats, substitute soy protein for meat protein,[19] substitute complex for simple carbohydrate[20]) also decrease LDL (Chapter 10). Both VLDL and LDL will be lowered with reduction of calories in the obese and resultant weight loss. Cholesterol absorption (50 percent of that ingested) contrasts with over 95 percent absorption of dietary long chain fatty acid esters. Unabsorbed dietary cholesterol, along with fats secreted into the intestine and bile, is excreted in the feces along with bile acids not reabsorbed in the enterohepatic circulation. Factors that enhance cholesterol turnover and its concentration in bile, such as polyunsaturated fat and some lipid-lowering drugs, may induce gallstone formation. It may be that colon cancer is promoted by increasing the enterohepatic circulation of cholesterol and bile acids (Chapter 5).

COMBINED HYPERLIPIDEMIA

Familial combined hyperlipidemia (monogenic) and *multiple lipoprotein-type hyperlipidemia* are terms describing families with hypercholesterolemia (non-FH), hypertriglyceridemia, or both (Table 3-3).[14] In these families, about one-third have an increase of plasma LDL (type IIa), one-third have an increase of LDL and VLDL (type IIb), and one-third have an increase in VLDL (type IV). It is not certain if the primary defect is overproduction of apo-B, with an increase in lipoprotein particles secreted by the liver. If triglyceride is overproduced, or if the patient is obese or glucose intolerant, VLDL triglyceride secretion is increase along with apo-B, and the result is mild hypertriglyceridemia.[14]

IDL

Intermediate-density lipoprotein (IDL), an intermediary in the catabolism of VLDL to LDL, is not normally present in the circulation. IDL may be increased in an inborn error of metabolism, dysbetaglobulinemia, or type III hyperlipoproteinemia (Table 3-3).[21] IDL in type III hyperlipoproteinemia is characterized by enrichment of apoprotein E and abnormal E isoforms, with defective clearance, or absence of apo E.[22] Patients with dysbetaglobulinemia have characteristic palmar xanthomas and tuberous xanthomas. These patients may also have premature and severe peripheral vascular disease. They may respond to dietary restriction of cholesterol, saturated fats, and calories.[11] This disorder may be suspected when the elevated levels of cholesterol and triglycerides in plasma are approximately equal. By ultracentrifugation, the triglyceride-containing lipoproteins (IDL) have a relatively higher proportion of cholesterol to triglycerides than do VLDL (Table 3-2). This finding, along with the demonstration of a floating β-lipoprotein band on electrophoresis, should lead to the demonstration of the apoprotein E abnormality by electrophoresis using isoelectric focusing.[22–24]

Atherogenic diets may give rise to the so-called β-VLDL,[8] which is related to IDL (Chapter 5). β-VLDL is cholesterol rich, contains apo-B and apo-E, and interacts with a specific high-affinity receptor on the suface of macrophages. This interaction results in an increase in cholesterol esters in macrophages, the precursor of lipid-laden foam cells in the arterial wall. Diet-induced β-VLDL, which may represent either chylomicron remnants or hepatic lipoprotein, may be the atherogenic particle postulated by Zilversmit.[13]

MIXED HYPERLIPOPROTEINEMIA

Increased levels of VLDL and chylomicrons produce mixed hyperlipoproteinemia (Table 3-3), commonly associated with insulin-dependent diabetes mellitus and characterized by premature vascular disease. These subjects may develop recurrent abdominal pain, similar to patients with chylomicronemia.[25] The abdominal pain is often due to acute pancreatitis, which may not be accompanied by the usual increase in serum amylase. The incidence of abdominal pain is directly related to the level of triglycerides, and occurs most often when triglyceride levels exceed 2,000 mg/dl. Eruptive xanthomas and lipemia retinalis may be observed in these patients. Many patients are obese, and lipemia subsides with weight reduction. The dietary management includes limitation of dietary fat and carbohydrate, particularly refined carbohydrate (Chapter 10). Cholesterol levels normally are not as high as in familial hypercholesterolemia or dysbetaglobulinemia unless the triglyceride levels are greatly increased. The defect in these patients is a combination of defective clearance of triglyceride and overproduction of VLDL triglyceride (Table 3-3). Recently, investigators demonstrated an increase in the E_4 phenotype, which suggests that apo-E_4 may play a role in the etiology of type V hyperlipoproteinemia.[26]

HDL

High-density lipoprotein (HDL) is a small particle generated in the intestine or the liver. HDL is about half protein and half lipid, of which the predominant lipid component is phospholipid (Table 3-3). HDL transports about half as much of the total plasma cholesterol as does LDL. HDL consists of several subfractions. Among these the protein content can vary from 40 to 60 percent. Cholesterol esters range from 10 to 20 percent; triglycerides make up less than 4 percent. The proportion of free cholesterol and phospholipids are increased as the density is less. There are also differences in the ratio of A-I and A-II apoproteins, with the A-I–A-II ratio being higher in HDL_2.[18] The amount of apo-C in HDL depends on the flux of triglyceride-rich lipoproteins. The cholesterol-triglyceride ratio increases in HDL as the dietary cholesterol is increased. This ratio in HDL is decreased in hypertriglyceridemia, uremia, and ischemic heart disease.

Other subfractions of HDL in addition to HDL_2 (the major antiatherogenic subfraction of HDL), include HDL_3, HDL_{2a}, HDL_{2b} and HDL_c. The feeding of cholesterol results in the production of HDL_c. This particle is enriched in cholesterol ester and is larger, measuring 16 to 24 nm in diameter; it floats at a lower density (even at 1.006), and is progressively enriched in apo-E. It is assumed that HDL acquires cholesterol from peripheral tissues to form HDL_c. Cholesterol esters are acquired via lecithin cholestlerol acyltransferase (LCAT) and the cholesterol ester-enriched particle controls the acquisition of apo-E from other lipoproteins (Chapter 5).

HDL arises from the interaction of nascent particles secreted by the liver and intestine with lipids and proteins released during catabolism of triglyceride-rich lipoproteins.[18] A portion of lipid is acquired from transfer and uptake of free cholesterol from cell membranes. Lipoprotein lipase transfers surface lipids from HDL_3 to HDL_2. Therefore, HDL levels correlate with levels of LPL and the fractional catabolic rate of plasma triglycerides. HDL lipids are the substrate for

Table 3-5.   Mean Plasma HDL Cholesterol Levels, mg/dl

Age (years)	Men			Women		
	HDL_2	HDL_3	HDL	HDL_2	HDL_3	HDL
20	15	28	44	20	31	53
30			45			56
40	12	30	45	17	34	57
50	15	30	44	20	35	61
60			44			61
70			52			61

See footnote to Table 3-1.

Table 3-6.   Factors Affecting Plasma HDL

Increases	Decreases
Female	Male
Weight loss	Obesity
Running	Physical inactivity
Genetic	Genetic
Alcohol	Cigarette Smoking
Black (U.S.)	Antihypertensive drugs
Triglycerides	Hypertriglyceridemia
LDL cholesterol	Uremia
Age (survival)	Androgens
Estrogens	Progestins (OC)
Insulin	Diabetes mellitus

hepatic lipase activity. Hepatic lipase has been reported to be decreased when HDL_2 is increased. Factors regulating the primary synthesis of HDL particles and the major HDL apoproteins, and thereby regulating levels of HDL, are poorly understood.

HDL has been called the ''good'' lipoprotein, since HDL cholesterol levels (especially HDL_2) are inversely related to the risk of atherosclerosis.[27] HDL carries out reverse cholesterol transport, taking cholesterol away from cells and delivering it to the liver for catabolism to bile acids and resultant loss from the body (Chapter 5). HDL was discovered in the early 1950s. Interest was renewed when laboratories became able to measure HDL cholesterol without use of the ultracentrifuge.[28] Various metals and polyanions combine to precipitate apo-B–containing lipoproteins (VLDL and LDL). This procedure leaves HDL in the supernatant, where its cholesterol can be measured easily. An alternative method is to carry out ultracentrifugation to float VLDL, and then to precipitate LDL and measure HDL cholesterol in the supernatant.

HDL cholesterol levels are higher in women (Tables 3-5 and 3-6). Women also have higher levels of apo–A-I. HDL cholesterol levels are increased by estrogens and may be decreased by progestogens. Thus, the effect of oral contraceptives may depend on the level of estrogen, the level of progestogen, and some influence of the ratio of the two hormones. In uremia there is a decrease in HDL cholesterol associated with low levels of LPL. HDL cholesterol levels may be raised in these patients by oral carnitine.[18] The role of androgens and HDL concentration is conflicting. HDL cholesterol is increased with increase in FSH and LH gonadotropins.

DIET AND HDL

There are a variety of dietary effects on HDL with changes also observed in other lipoproteins.[8] An increase in simple sugars or a high carbohydrate diet for short periods results in a decrease in HDL cholesterol and apo–A-I, presumably by accelerating removal of HDL cholesterol.[18] These diets also increase VLDL triglycerides. An increase in polyunsaturated fat or decrease in saturated fat results in a decrease in HDL cholesterol and apo–A-I. These results vary depending on the P-S ratio. These diets also decrease LDL cholesterol, and may thereby result in a more favorable (less atherogenic) ratio of LDL cholesterol to HDL cholesterol. Diets high in fat and cholesterol increase LDL. These LDL particles are larger in diameter and of increased molecular weight. They are enriched in cholesterol esters, and stimulate cholesterol esterification and accumulation in smooth muscle cells.[8] Increases in saturated fats and cholesterol in the diet result paradoxically in an increase in HDL cholesterol, especially HDL_2.[29] Lipoprotein changes with a high-fat, high-cholesterol diet include a decrease in the typical HDL and an increase in HDL_c (HDL with apo-E), which delivers cholesterol to cells. There is also an increase in LDL and the appearance of β-VLDL (the lipoprotein of < 1.006, like chylomicrons of VLDL, but with β rather than pre-β mobility on electrophoresis).[8] (See Chapter 5.)

Other dietary influences on HDL include increased intake of vitamin E, resulting in increased levels of HDL cholesterol; increased dietary intake of zinc, resulting in decreased HDL cholesterol level; an intake of brewer's yeast containing chromium, resulting in increased levels of HDL cholesterol.[18] HDL levels may also be increased by modest amounts of alcohol (two to three drinks per day), leanness or weight loss, and a vigorous, maintained exercise program (Table 3-6).[20] Other specific dietary manipulations that may increase (or decrease) HDL cholesterol remain to be demonstrated unequivocally. Genetic factors may be involved in the absence of or excessive amounts of any of the lipoproteins.[10]

Lp(a)

Lp(a) is a B apoprotein containing lipoprotein with additional unique antigen determinants.[8] It is floated at a density of 1.063 to 1.125, similar to HDL_2. Dietary, genetic, and other factors influencing the level of Lp(a) and its relation to atherosclerosis remain to be elucidated.

APOPROTEINS

The lipoprotein apoproteins play an important role in lipid transport.[8,30] Apoproteins regulate the metabolism of specific classes of lipoproteins and determine their roles in lipid metabolism. There are at least eight different apoproteins (Table 3-2). Apoprotein B is present in chylomicrons, VLDL, and LDL. The C apoproteins (I, II, III) are in chylomicrons, VLDL, and HDL. A and D apoproteins are in HDL. Apoprotein E is in VLDL, HDL, and other lipoproteins. The concentrations of the different apoproteins in plasma can be measured by specific assays. The apoprotein B in LDL arises from the VLDL form, with a precursor product relationship. The molecular weight of apo-B is an indication of its origin from liver or intestine. Most lymph chylomicron apo-B is composed of lower molecular weight apo-B, ''B-48.'' C apoproteins in VLDL and HDL are related to one another; the C apoproteins are either secreted alone or with HDL, and are readily exchanged between HDL and triglyceride-rich VLDL and chylomicrons. The A apoproteins are found almost exclusively in HDL. Apo-E is exchanged between VLDL and HDL.

The apoprotein structure in solution explains its ability to bind lipids. The apoproteins have specific functions in addition to carrying lipid in the circulation. Apo-A-I is the specific cofactor for LCAT, which produces esterified cholesterol by transfer of fatty acid from lecithin to cholesterol. Apo–C-II is a specific coenzyme for LPL. The A and B apoproteins are made by both intestine and liver; C apoproteins are made only by the liver. Some inborn errors of metabolism are associated with abnormalities in the apoproteins (Table 3-3). Absence of apo–C-II is associated with excess apo-E and absence of one or more E isoforms.[21] Thus many of the lipid transport disorders may be translated to apoprotein disorders. Future treatments may be based on influencing the levels and types of apoprotein rather than lipids.[30]

THE PATIENT WITH HYPERLIPIDEMIA

When patients with hyperlipidemia are recognized, it is important to initiate the appropriate diet to lower their lipids and thereby decrease the risk of atherosclerosis (Chapter 10). Since many individuals are asymptomatic, it is useful to measure circulating lipids as part of the general medical evaluation of all adults. Lipid levels should probably be measured every 2 years as part of routine health evaluation in adults over the age of 40 years. When increased levels of circulating cholesterol or triglycerides are reported, the values should be confirmed in another sample. The patient's dietary habits should be ascertained, preferably with the assistance of a nutritionist trained in this area. If the patient is overweight, reduction to ideal body weight should improve the abnormal lipid pattern. More restrictive diets may be needed for more serious abnormalities (Chapter 10). Dietary manipulations of calories, cholesterol, animal products, alterations in type of fat, type of protein, fiber content,[31] minerals, and vitamins all influence serum lipids. Whatever the dietary intervention, the effect must be monitored. The patient-to-patient response to a given diet is highly variable. The genetic and metabolic mechanism underlying this variability are unknown.

If diet is not adequate to control hyperlipidemia, it may be necessary to add a lipid-lowering drug.[11] In most instances, for drug therapy to be effective it is necessary that the patient continue on the lipid-lowering diet. This diet should be nutritionally adequate. If calories are reduced below 1,300 kcal/day a multivitamin supplement should be added. For menstruating women it may also be necessary to add supplemental iron.

OTHER NUTRIENTS

Other nutrients that may influence plasma lipids include calcium (2 g/day), vanadium, silicate, copper, and vitamin C, all of which have been shown to lower plasma cholesterol (Chapter 9).[32] Excessive vitamin D may increase plasma cholesterol. Diet can also influence platelet aggregation and thrombosis (Chapter 4). Deficiency of vitamin E and essential fatty acids (linoleic, ? linolenic) may be atherogenic, perhaps via effects on serum lipids or lipoproteins, but the evidence for such a process in humans is tenuous.

SUMMARY

Levels of plasma lipids and lipoprotein composition and concentration are regulated by genetic and environmental influences, especially diet. Calories, alcohol, macronutrients and micronutrients exert their individual and collective interactive effects on many parameters influencing plasma lipids and lipoproteins. While the etiologic agent of atherosclerosis remains unidentified, "lipid" risk factors play a prominent role for populations and should be considered for individuals. Hyperlipidemia should be identified, quantified, investigated, characterized, and controlled by appropriate dietary measures. Response must be monitored. Identification and understanding of inborn errors of lipoproteins involves sophisticated demonstration of missing or abnormal cell-surface receptors, apoprotein deletions, or charge differences. Despite controversy over whether a "prudent" diet should be ingested by all adult Americans, appropriate diet modification is effective and safe in patients with hyperlipidemia and should be prescribed.

REFERENCES

1. Feldman EB: Familial hypercholesterolemia—Predecessor of coronary heart disease. Res Staff Phys 6:70, 1978.
2. Blackburn H: Diet and mass hyperlipidemia: a public health view. In Levy R, Rifkind B, Dennis B, Ernst N (eds): Nutrition, Lipid and Coronary Disease. New York, Raven Press, 1979.
3. Hopkins PN, Williams RR: A survey of 246 suggested coronary risk factors. Atherosclerosis 40:1, 1981.
4. Cholesterol and noncardiovascular mortality. JAMA 244:25, 1980.
5. Mattson FH, Erickson BA, Kligman AM: Effect of dietary cholesterol on serum cholesterol in man. Am J Clin Nutr 25:589, 1972.
6. Feldman EB: Saturated fats. In Feldman EB (ed): Nutrition and Cardiovascular Disease. New York, Appleton-Century Crofts, 1976.
7. Keys A, Grande F, Anderson JT: Fiber and pectin in diet and serum cholesterol concentration in man. Proc Soc Exp Biol Med 106:555, 1961.
8. Mahley RW: Atherogenic hyperlipoproteinemia. Med Clin North Am 66:375, 1982.
9. McNeely S, Seatter K, Yuhaniak J, Kashyap ML: The 16-hour-standing test and lipoprotein electrophoresis compared for detection of chylomicrons in plasma. Clin Chem 27:731, 1981.
10. Havel RJ, Goldstein JL, Brown MS: Lipoproteins and lipid transport. In Bondy PK, Rosenberg, LE (eds): Metabolic Control and Disease, 8th ed. Philadelphia, WB Saunders, 1981.
11. Havel RJ, Kane JP: Therapy of hyperlipidemic states. Ann Rev Med 33:417, 1982.
12. Brunzell JD, Bierman EL: Chylomicronemia syndrome. Med Clin North Am 66:455, 1982.

13. Zilversmit DB: Role of triglyceride-rich lipoproteins in atherogenesis. Ann NY Acad Sci 275:138, 1976.

14. Grundy SM: Hypertriglyceridemia: Mechanisms, clinical significance and treatment. Med Clin North Am 66:519, 1982.

15. Feldman EB, Benkel P, Nayak RB: Physiologic factors influencing circulating triglyceride concentration in women: Age, weight gain and ovarian function. J Lab Clin Med 62:437, 1963.

16. Goldstein JL, Brown MS: Familial hypercholesterolemia: Identification of defect in the regulation of 3-hydroxy-3-methylglutaryl coenzyme A reductase activity associated with overproduction of cholesterol. Proc Nat Acad Sci 70:2804, 1973.

17. Goldstein JL, Brown MS: LDL receptor defect in familial hypercholesterolemia. Med Clin North Am 66:335, 1982.

18. Krauss RM: Regulation of high density lipoprotein levels. Med Clin North Am 66:403, 1982.

19. Sirtori CR, Agradi E, Conti F, et al: Soybean-protein diet in the treatment of Type II hyperlipoproteinemia. Lancet 1:275, 1977.

20. Grundy SM, Bilheimer D, Blackburn H, et al: Rationale of the diet-heart statement of the American Heart Association. Circulation 65:839A, 1982.

21. Havel RJ: Familial dysbetalipoproteinemia. Med Clin North Am 66:441, 1982.

22. Ghiselli G, Schaefer EJ, Gascon P, Brewer HB: Type III hyperlipoproteinemia associated with apo-lipoprotein E deficiency. Science 214:1239, 1981.

23. Weidman SW, Suarez B, Falko JM, et al: Type III hyperlipoproteinemia: development of a VLDL Apo E gel isoelectric focusing technique and application in family studies. J Lab Clin Med 93:549, 1979.

24. Zannis VI, Breslow JL: Human very low density lipoprotein apolipoprotein E isoprotein polymorphism is explained by genetic variation and post translational modification. Biochemistry 20:1033, 1981.

25. Feldman EB: Patient management problem 3. In Bollet AJ (ed): Principles of Internal Medicine, Patient Management Problems: Pre-Test Self-Assessment and Review. New York, McGraw-Hill, 1981.

26. Ghiselli G, Schaefer EJ, Zech LA, et al: Increased prevalence of apolipoprotein E_4 in Type V hyperlipoproteinemia. J Clin Invest 70:474, 1982.

27. Gordon T, Castelli WP, Hjorland MC, et al: HDL cholesterol and coronary heart disease risk: The Framingham Study. Am J Med 62:707, 1977.

28. Lipid and lipoprotein analyses. In: Manual of Laboratory Operations, Lipid Research Clinics Program. United States Department of Health, Education and Welfare Publication (NIH) 75-628, 1974.

29. Schonfeld G, Patsch W, Rudel LL, et al: Effects of dietary choleseterol and fatty acids on plasma lipoproteins. J Clin Invest 69:1072, 1982.

30. Levy RI: Cholesterol, lipoproteins, apoproteins, and heart disease: Present status and future prospects. Clin Chem 27:653, 1981.

31. Chen WL, Anderson JW: Effect of plant fiber in decreasing plasma total cholesterol and increasing high density lipoprotein cholesterol and increasing high density lipoprotein cholesterol. Proc Soc Exp Biol Med 162:310, 1979.

32. Ginter E, Cerna O, Budlovsky J, et al: Effects of ascorbic acid on plasma cholesterol in humans in a long-term experiment. Int J Vit Nutr Res 41:123, 1977.

4 | Dietary Fats, Platelets, Prostaglandins, and Plasma Lipids

William S. Harris
Scott H. Goodnight, Jr.
William E. Connor

Arteriosclerotic vascular disease is the primary cause of morbidity and mortality in the United States today. Dietary intervention is believed to be helpful in the prevention and treatment of the disease, and the replacement of saturated fats by polyunsaturated oils is one of the most common recommendations[1,2] (see Chapters 1, 3, 5, and 9). This dietary modification may favorably influence two of the primary metabolic mediators of the disease, the thrombotic tendency and the level of the plasma lipids and lipoproteins.[3–5]

This chapter will explore in depth the actions of the principal polyunsaturated fatty acids on thrombosis and the plasma lipids, and, in particular, will differentiate the effects of the two different families of essential fatty acids: those derived from vegetable oils (chiefly the omega (ω)-6 fatty acids) and those derived mainly from fish oils (the ω-3 fatty acids) (Table 4-1). In past studies of the effects of feeding

Supported by research grants (HL25687, AM29930, HL22906, and HL00953) from the National Heart, Lung, and Blood Institute; the Clinical Research Center Grant (RR334) from the Division of Research Resources of the National Institutes of Health; and a grant from the Medical Research Foundation of Oregon (26.57).

Table 4-1.   Major Families of Polyunsaturated Fatty Acids

Family	Parent	Major metabolites	Characteristic structure	Principal sources
ω-9	C18:1 ω-9 oleic acid	C20:3 ω-9[a] eicosatrienoic acid	$H_3C\text{-}C\text{-}C\text{-}C\text{-}C\text{-}C\text{-}C\text{-}C\text{-}C^9 =$ C-RCOOH	Synthesis from acetate; animal and vegetable fats
ω-6	C18:2 ω-6 linoleic acid	C20:4 ω-6 arachidonic acid	$H_3C\text{-}C\text{-}C\text{-}C\text{-}C\text{-}C^6 =$ C-R'COOH	Many vegetable oils
ω-3	C18:3 ω-3 linolenic acid	C20:5 ω-3 eicosapentaenoic acid	$H_3C\text{-}C\text{-}C^3 = C\text{-}R''COOH$	Some vegetable oils, (18:3)
		C22:6 ω3 docosahexaenoic acid		Marine oils (20:5,22:6)

(Reprint by permission of the American Heart Association Inc. from Goodnight SH, Harris WS, Connor WE, Illington DR: Polyunsaturated fatty acids, hyperlipidemia and thrombosis. Arteriosclerosis 2:78–113, 1982.)

A fourth family of polyunsaturated fatty acids (ω-7) can be synthesized from palmitoleate (C16:1 ω-7), but only trace amounts of ω-7 polyunsaturated fatty acids are present in the tissues. The omega (ω) number indicates the location of the first double bond counting from the methyl end of the fatty acid (ω is the last character of the Greek alphabet). An alternative nomenclature frequently used is the "n" system, where "n" replaces the ω (e.g., 18:2 ω-6 = 18:2 n-6).

[a]Accumulates only in essential fatty acid deficiency.

polyunsaturated fats, the possible metabolic differences between these two structurally different families of polyunsaturated fatty acids have not been evaluated.

Suggestions that dietary fat might affect thrombosis date back to studies conducted over 20 years ago, in which saturated fat was considered "thrombogenic," and polyunsaturated fat, "nonthrombogenic."[7–9] Recently, with the discovery of platelet and vessel-wall prostaglandins, a more precise mechanism of how dietary fatty acids might affect thrombosis has been elucidated. Twenty-carbon fatty acids of both the ω-6 and ω-3 families serve as substrates for the synthesis of different prostaglandins with diverse activities. The thromboxanes induce platelet aggregation and vasoconstriction; the prostacyclins inhibit platelet aggregation and produce vasodilation.[10] Currently there is great interest in the possibility that dietary ω-3 polyunsaturated fatty acids may alter platelet function in antithrombogenic direction.

Since 1952, the plasma cholesterol lowering effects of polyunsaturated fat in the human diet have been demonstrated by many investigators[11,12] (see Chapters 3 and 5). On a gram-for-gram basis, saturated fat is twice as effective in raising plasma cholesterol levels as is polyunsaturated fat in lowering cholesterol.[13,14] The precise mechanisms by which dietary fats affect the plasma lipid levels, and therefore the arteriosclerotic risk, are still unknown and are the subject of intensive study.

DIETARY FAT, PLATELETS, AND A PREDISPOSITION TO THROMBOSIS

A large number of studies have been carried out in which certain dietary fats were fed to experimental animals and the predisposition of the animals to thromboses produced by biologic or mechanical stimuli were determined. For example, when a diet rich in butter fat was fed to rats, they developed larger hepatic thrombi, following the infusion of an endotoxin, than did controls.[15,16] Platelets from rats fed saturated-fat diets showed increased sensitivity to thrombin-induced platelet aggregation, and were able to release platelet Factor III more readily than controls.[16–18]

Further studies have examined whether different dietary fatty acids may influence the number of platelet-derived pulmonary thrombi produced by an infusion of adenosine diphosphate (ADP) into the inferior vena cava of rats.[19] After the saturated fat diet, the ADP infusion led to the immediate formation of thrombi in 90 percent of the animals, whereas the incorporation of polyunsaturated fatty acids into the diet (replacing 20 percent of the saturated fat) significantly reduced, but failed to eliminate, pulmonary thrombi.

Additionally, following surgical insertion of a small polyethylene cannula into the abdominal aorta of male rats, the number of hours required for occlusion of the cannula by a platelet thrombus was recorded.[20,21] There was a direct relationship between the dietary linoleic acid content and prolongation of the aortic occlusion time. Conversely, the ingestion of saturated fatty acids of increasing chain length was associated with a progressive shortening of the occlusion time. The platelet count was higher and the platelets more sensitive to aggregation by ADP in the animals fed the saturated-fat diet.

These and other experiments indicate that the chronic feeding of diets rich in saturated fat to experimental animals increased their tendency toward thrombosis. Although the dietary manipulations resulted in increased platelet reactivity by various in vitro measurements, it remains to be proven that the increased propensity to thrombosis was actually caused by dietary-induced alterations in platelet reactivity.

PROSTAGLANDINS DERIVED FROM POLYUNSATURATED FATTY ACIDS IN PLATELETS AND BLOOD VESSELS

Our understanding of polyunsaturated fatty acids and their roles in platelet and vascular function has been aided greatly by the recent identification and characterization of platelet and endothelial cell prostaglandins[10,22,23] (Fig. 4-1). Since these potent substances (that is, thromboxane A_2 and prostaglandin I_2)* are ultimately derived from dietary fatty acids, it is possible that manipulation of dietary fat content might alter prostaglandin synthesis and subsequent platelet-vessel interactions.

Arachidonic acid ($C20:4\omega6$) may be transported in the circulation either as the free fatty acid bound to albumin or esterified in lipoprotein phospholipids and cholesterol esters.[24] Direct uptake of free arachidonic acid by platelets or the vessel wall leads to its incorporation into membrane phospholipids;[25,26] the latter

---

* The prostaglandins have been named in the order of their discovery beginning with A and proceeding to I (for example, PGI_2). The numerical subscript refers to the number of double bonds in the prostaglandin side chain.

also exchange with plasma phospholipids. Following activiation of one or more phospholipases, arachidonic acid becomes available to the enzyme cyclooxygenase and is rapidly converted to the labile cyclic endoperoxides, PGG_2 and PGH_2.[27] Enzymes such as thromboxane synthetase in the platelet or prostacyclin synthetase in the endothelial cell convert the endoperoxides to biologically active thromboxane A_2 or PGI_2 (prostacyclin).[28–30] The potent vasoconstricting and platelet-aggregating effects of thromboxane A_2 and the vasodilating and platelet inhibitory effects of prostacyclin are now well known and have been studied extensively.[29]

Other polyunsaturated fatty acids besides arachidonic acid may serve as substrates for prostaglandin synthesis[23] (Fig. 4-2). For example, dihomo-gamma-linolenic acid (C20:3ω6) acts as a substrate for prostaglandins of the "1" series, such as the classical prostaglandin PGE_1 (thromboxane A_1 or PGI_1, if formed at all, appear to be inactive).[23] Eicosapentaenoic acid (C20:5ω3) is the substrate for prostaglandins of the "3" series, and, under certain conditions, leads to the production of thromboxane A_3 and PGI_3.[23]

The biochemical relationships and metabolic pools of the polyunsaturated fatty acids in the human require further study. For example, the essential fatty acid linoleic acid is converted to C20:3ω6 and ultimately to archidonic acid in the liver.[23] Although the feeding of diets rich in linoleic acid regularly leads to its accumulation in platelet membrane phospholipids, archidonate levels are unchanged or may even be decreased in platelets.[30] Similarly, feeding of linolenic acid (C18:3ω

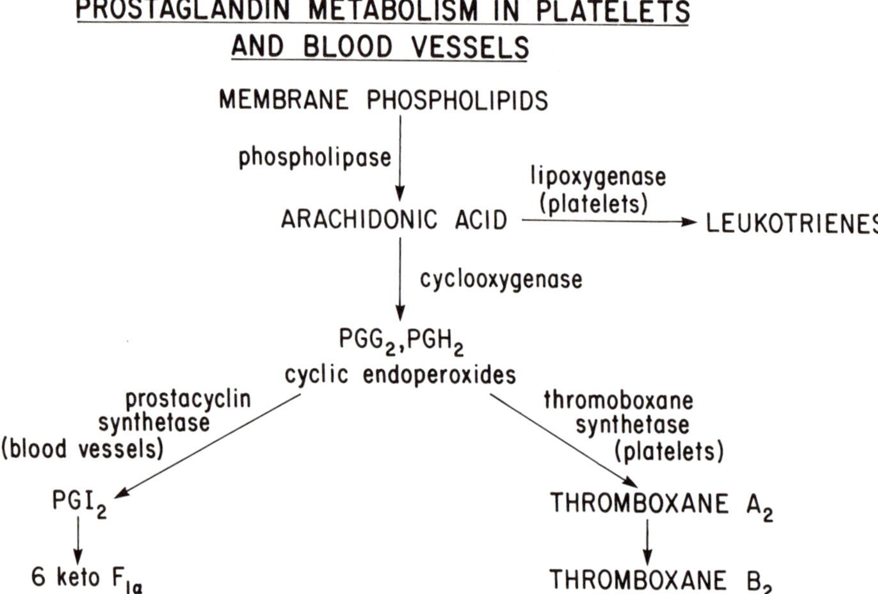

Fig. 4-1.   The conversion of arachidonic acid to PGI_2, thromboxane A_2, and leukotrienes. (Reprinted by permission of the American Heart Association Inc. from Goodnight SH, Harris WS, Connor WE, Illingworth DR: Polyunsaturated fatty acids, hyperlipidemia and thrombosis. Arteriosclerosis 2:78–113, 1982.)

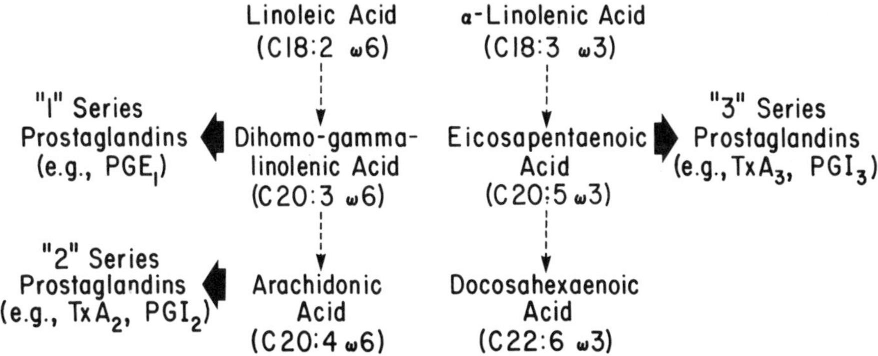

Fig. 4-2. Conversion of ω-6 and ω-3 fatty acids to various prostaglandins. The dotted lines indicate that the elongation and desaturation steps depicted occur in some but not all tissues. (Reprinted by permission of the American Heart Association Inc. from Goodnight SH, Harris WS, Connor WE, Illingworth DR: Polyunsaturated fatty acids, hyperlipidemia and thrombosis. Arteriosclerosis 2:78–113, 1982.)

3) does not appear to lead to significant increases of eicosapentaenoic acid in adult human plasma.[31] The feeding of marine foods rich in eicosapentaenoic acid, however, leads to rapid incorporation of this fatty acid into both platelet and endothelial cell membranes.[32–38]

Recent studies have shown that arachidonic acid can also be converted by the lipoxygenase pathway to a new class of compounds, the leukotrienes. Since leukotrienes have been shown to have bronchoconstrictive properties (that is, slow reacting substance of anaphylaxis, [SRS-A], chemotactic activity, and possible influences on thromboxane and prostacyclin synthesis), they will provide a fertile area for future biochemical and clinical research.[39,40]

The rapidly increasing knowledge of prostaglandin and leukotriene metabolism will allow reinterpretation of older studies of the effect of dietary fatty acids on platelet function. More importantly, it will enable future investigators to construct more rational attempts to manipulate cellular prostaglandin synthesis by dietary or other therapeutic means.

THE EFFECTS OF ω-6 FATTY ACIDS ON PLATELET AND VASCULAR COMPOSITION AND FUNCTION

Linoleic Acid

The early studies of fatty acids and thrombosis generally supported the hypothesis that replacement of saturated by polyunsaturated fatty acids in the diet might be protective against thromboembolic events and that this protective effect might be mediated through an inhibition of platelet function. Consequently, during the last decade a number of investigators have examined the effects of diets containing large amounts of polyunsaturated fatty acids (especially linoleic acid) on platelet lipid composition and hemostatic function. Evaluation of these studies has been somewhat difficult because of marked variations in experimental design, dietary control, lipid analyses, and tests of platelet function. However, some important generalizations can be made in spite of these drawbacks.

Platelet and Vessel Lipid Composition. Although linoleic acid is converted rapidly to arachidonic acid in the liver and in cells such as fibroblasts, similar elongation and desaturation does not occur in platelet membranes. Indeed, studies in which linoleic acid was fed to rabbits in the form of corn oil led to a reproducible increase in the precentage concentration of linoleic acid in platelet membrane phospholipids, compared with the fatty acid composition with a butter-fat diet.[30,41] Platelet arachidonic acid, however, was *decreased* in the corn-oil–fed animals compared with the butter-fat group. Similar findings were observed in rats fed diets containing combinations of corn oil and hydrogenated coconut oil.[42] The arachidonic acid content of aortic phospholipids was also increased in butter-fed rabbits.[41]

A recent study in human volunteers showed that feeding supplemental linoleic acid in the form of corn oil (25 ml/day) for 6 weeks led to an increase in the linoleate content of the phosphatidylcholine component of platelet phospholipids but not of the phosphatidylethanolamine or phosphatidylinositol fractions.[38] Total platelet arachidonate levels were unchanged.

Some additional experimental data clarifying this question has become available recently using cultured endothelial cells or platelets incubated with various fatty acids for 1 to 72 hours.[44,45] When the incubation medium was enriched with linoleic acid, the phospholipids in endothelial cells and platelets increased their linoleic acid content from 5 to 25 percent, but arachidonic acid levels fell by 25 to 40 percent. This reduction may be due in part to a $\Delta 6$ desaturase deficiency in endothelial cells, which prevents conversion of C18:2 to C20:4 by interfering with the desaturation of C18:2 to C18:3. In addition, high concentrations of linoleic acid may simply reduce arachidonic acid levels by competing for esterification sites in phospholipids.

Therefore, in at least some experimental situations, feeding a diet very rich in linoleic acid may lead to a selective decrease in arachidonic acid, whereas diets containing saturated fatty acids may lead to the opposite effect. Whether these changes in arachidonic acid content will regularly translate into equivalent changes in thromboxane or prostacyclin release remains to be determined.[45]

Platelet and Vessel-wall Function. Changes in platelet function have been studied after the chronic feeding of diets rich in polyunsaturated vegetable oils. When bleeding times in human subjects ingesting a diet rich in ω-6 polyunsaturated fatty acids were compared with these measurements during a control dietary period, no significant differences were found either in our studies (unpublished observations) or in those of others.[38,46,47] Despite this lack of prolongation in the bleeding times, some tests of platelet aggregation have been affected by dietary linoleic acid.

In rabbits fed corn oil, the sensitivity for arachidonic acid and collagen-induced platelet aggregation was lowered when compared with aggregation in butter-fed animals.[48] In humans, Renaud reported that platelet aggregation in response to thrombin and ADP (but not collagen or epinephrine) was increased in a group of French farmers with a high saturated fat intake, compared with a second group eating a diet containing less saturated fat.[50] Similarly, platelet aggregation induced by low concentrations of collagen was decreased in a group of Norwegian subjects given a corn oil supplement.[38] In contrast to these studies, a group of normal American men given dietary supplements of margarine and vegetable oils failed to show differences in platelet aggregation but did show a significant reduction in platelet retention on glass bead columns.[51]

Two rather large studies have used the filtragometer to measure the time taken for platelets to occlude a microfilter inserted in a closed in vitro system containing flowing blood. In one study, patients in a Finnish chronic care hospital were given a diet high in linoleic acid. The occlusion time in the filtragometer was lengthened in these patients during this dietary period.[47,52] In another study, circulating platelet aggregates decreased in the plasma after switching from saturated fat to a margarine-based diet.[51]

In summary, supplementing or replacing saturated fat with oils rich in linoleic acid apparently result in mild and variable effects on platelet function. Although the bleeding time is not significantly prolonged, platlet retention on glass beads is reduced and the time to platelet aggregation in the filtragometer is prolonged. Platelets also appear less reactive, as evidenced by a reduction in circulating platelet aggregates.

Mechanisms.   The mechanisms underlying the changes in platelet function and proposed antithrombitic effects of dietary ω-6 polyunsaturated fatty acids are not understood completely. Recent studies examining prostaglandin synthesis and other biochemical pathways of platelets and vessel walls provide some insight and future directions for study.

In one experiment rabbits were fed a diet containing 8 percent of their calories as corn oil for 3 weeks, and the conversion of exogenous radiolabeled arachidonic acid to labeled thromboxane B_2 in platelet rich plasma was examined. Platelet thromboxane production was significantly lowered in the corn-oil–fed animals.[48] The decrease in thromboxane production was associated with less platelet aggregation following stimulation by arachidonic acid or low doses of collagen.

In a second study from the same laboratory, rabbits were fed diets enriched in or depleted of linoleic acid for 3-month periods.[41] The linoleate-rich diet led to an increase in linoleic acid and a decrease in arachidonic acid in platelet phospholipids. This change was paralleled by a reduced production of thromboxane B_2 from exogenous radiolabeled arachidonic acid, but collagen-induced thromboxane production from endogenous arachidonic acid was not changed. Recently, a preliminary report indicated that arachidonic acid content of rat platelets was correlated directly with changes in thromoboxane B_2 production after stimulation of the platelets by collagen.[49]

After human volunteers were fed relatively low amounts (for example, 25 ml/day) of a corn oil supplement, collagen-induced thromboxane B_2 production decreased significantly (60 to 20 ng/ml) even though the arachidonic acid content of platelet phospholipids was unchanged.[38] Therefore, after corn-oil feeding, platelet thromboxane production apparently is decreased. This occurs when arachidonic acid is added to the prostaglandin pathway from exogenous sources, or when arachidonate is released from endogenous pools of phospholipid after stimulation with low concentrations of collagen. It is currently unclear whether the decreased prostagladin synthesis is a result of decreased precursor fatty acids, alterations in the activity of platelet enzyme systems such as pholspholipase, cyclooxygenase, or thromboxane sythetase, or is related to other remote factors such as a possible effect on thromboxane production by dietary cholesterol.[53]

Dietary fatty acids could influence platelet reactivity in ways other than acting directly on thromboxane synthesis. One study examined the half-life of thromboxane A_2 in a buffer test system containing albumin.[54] The addition of a mixture of free fatty acids extracted from human plasma to the test system led to accelerated destruction of thromboxane A_2, presumably by interfereing with the thromboxane-stabilizing effects of albumin. Another report suggested that the feeding of linoleic acid resulted in increased levels of platelet cyclic AMP which in turn could lead to decreased platelet reactivity.[42] Finally, a recent study from Japan found that polyunsaturated fatty acids (especially linoleic and arachidonic acids) markedly inhibited platelet phosphodiesterase in vitro which could prolong the effectiveness of cyclic AMP.[55]

Platelet reactivity could also be altered by variations in vascular prostaglandin synthesis (that is, prostacyclin). Only a few studies are currently available to examine this important question, and unfortunately variations in methodology and experimental design have made a general interpretation of the results difficult. In 1979, the investigative group from Unilever in Holland examined the PGI_2-like acitivity generated from perfused segments of rat aorta taken form animals that had been fed a diet high in sunflower seed oil.[56] Aortas from several animals fed this vegetable oil produced somewhat less PGI_2-like activity than did those from animals ingesting 35 percent of their calories as hydrogenated coconut oil, but the differences were not statistically significant. A study from Italy using pieces of aorta taken from butter– or corn-oil–fed rabbits also documented decreased production of PGI_2-like activity in the animals fed the polyunsaturated fat diet.[41] The increased production of PGI_2 in the saturated fat group correlated well with the increase in the arachidonic acid in the phosphatidylinositol fraction of the aortic phospholipids. In contrast to these studies, a second study by the Dutch workers showed a slightly increased aortic production of PGI_2 in linoleic-acid–fed rats; this change correlated with the increased C18:2ω6 in the diet.[57]

A series of experiments have been carried out using human umbilical endothelial cells cultured in vitro.[44,58] Enrichment of these cells with linoleic acid led to a significant decrease in spontaneous or stimulated PGI_2 production. This effect may be due to a competitive inhibition of endothelial cell cyclooxygenase by linoleic acid or to a linoleic-acid–induced reduction in phospholipid arachidonic acid content.[43]

To summarize the potential mechanisms of action, feeding diets high in linoleic acid to animals or humans apparently leads to increased concentrations of linoleic acid in the platelet membrane and decreased concentrations of arachidonic acid.

Thromboxane production is decreased from platelets after they are stimulated with low doses of collagen. PGI_2 production from blood vessels may also decrease because of the reduced arachidonic acid content of the vascular phospholipids or the inhibition of endothelial cell cyclooxygenase.

Dihomo-Gamma-Linolenic Acid (C20:3ω6)

The effects of dihomo-gamma-linolenic acid (DHLA) on platelets and blood vessels have been of interest because this 20 carbon fatty acid is the precursor to the "1" series of prostaglandins, such as PGE_1. The latter has an inhibitory effect on platelet function. Since naturally occurring fats and oils contain only minute amounts of DHLA,[23] purified DHLA (usually as the ethyl or methyl ester) must be given to experimental subjects to increase its concentration in plasma or tissues. If radiolabeled DHLA is given to an experimental animal, it is largely converted to arachidonic acid (its natural endproduct) by the liver and other tissues, although it is possible to "load" plasma, platelets, and, most likely, endothelial cells by DHLA feeding.[59] Endothelial cells do contain the Δ5-desaturase necessary to convert C20:3ω6 to C20:4ω6.[60] The increased concentration of DHLA in platelets and endothelial cells (from feeding purified DHLA) is associated, however, with a decrease in the content of linoleic acid and a significant reduction in arachidonic acid.[61,62]

Feeding purified DHLA to humans or animals has led to conflicting results with respect to its effects on platelet function. One study showed decreased platelet aggregation in response to collagen or ADP, but a second study showed little effect.[62,63] One human subject fed DHLA had no prolongation of the bleeding time.[64] The direct addition of DHLA to platelet-rich plasma does not lead to platelet aggregation, and, in fact, may be inhibitory.[63]

The mechanism for the putative decrease in platelet reactivity to aggregating agents could reflect decreased thromboxane A_2 production from arachidonic acid by the platelets. Needleman has shown that incorporation of DHLA into platelets does not lead to the formation of PGE_1; rather, DHLA is converted by thromboxane synthetase to hydroxyheptadecadienoic acid, which is a functionally inactive compound.[65] Thromboxane B_1, PGE_1, and PGD_1 are not formed in appreciable amounts.

The effects of free or albumin-bound DHLA added to endothelial cell cultures was studied recently by Nordy and colleagues,[58] who showed that endothelial cell enrichment with C20:3 led to a marked reduction of synthesized PGI_2-like material. In contrast, the addition of arachidonic acid led to the endothelial cell production of a factor (presumably prostacyclin) that strikingly inhibited ADP-induced platelet aggregation.

In summary, feeding purified methyl or ethyl DHLA to humans or animals leads to the incorporation of this fatty acid into platelets and vascular cells, where it is associated with decreased amounts of arachidonic acid in membrane phospholipids. Consequently, "2"-series prostaglandin synthesis (such as thromboxane A_2) may be diminished due to a decrease in arachidonate availability or possible competitive inhibition of thromboxane synthetase. Whether the prostaglandin inhibitory effects of DHLA are relatively more pronounced in platelets or in vascular endothelium is not known.

THE EFFECTS OF ω-3 FATTY ACIDS ON PLATELET AND VASCULAR COMPOSITION AND FUNCTION

Linolenic Acid (C18:3ω3)

In most tissues (except, for example, platelets and red blood cells) or in vitro systems, linolenic acid (C18:3ω3) may be desaturated and elongated to eicosapentaenoic acid.[23] The feeding of oils rich in linolenic acid (such as linseed oil, which contains 53 percent C18:3ω3) to animals or humans might theoretically lead to the accumulation of eicosapentaenoic acid in tissues such as platelets or endothelial cells. One study showed that feeding rats up to 4 percent of the calories as purified methyl linolenate led to a decrease in arachidonic acid (23 percent to 11 percent) and an increase in eicosapentaenoic acid from 0.1 to 3–4 percent in liver and serum lipids.[66] The production of thromboxane B_2 from platelets, as measured by radioimmunoassay in serum, substantially declined (130 ng/ml to 27 ng/ml) as the linolenate content of the diet was increased. In contrast, Dyerberg fed a normal volunteer 45 ml/day of linseed oil and failed to detect any increase in eicosapentaenoic acid in serum lipids.[31] Platelet or vascular concentrations of C20:5ω3 were not measured.

A few studies have examined the effects of feeding C18:3ω3 on platelet or endothelial cell function. Borchgrevink and colleagues found no changes in platelet adhesiveness or bleeding times in humans after dietary supplements of linseed oil.[67] Recently ten Hoor and coworkers fed a diet containing 25 percent C18:3ω3 to rats and noted that collagen-induced platelet malondialdehyde production and aortic vascular production of PGI_2-like material with this diet were lower than in a group of rats fed a diet high in linoleic acid.[57]

Eicosapentaenoic Acid (C20:5ω3)

Recent reports from Denmark have linked the low incidence of cardiovascular diseases among Greenland Eskimos to their high intake of fish and marine oils.[68–71] The presence of elevated levels of ω-3 fatty acids in their diets and plasma lipids has led to the hypothesis that ω-3 fatty acids may be protective against arteriosclerotic disease.[71,72]

A bruising or bleeding tendency had been described among the Greenland Eskimos and was also noted in the 1930s by a French explorer who visited the northern Canadian Eskimos who were eating a similar diet.[69,74] Pursuing these leads, the Danish investigators studied the bleeding times of their Eskimo subjects and found them to be prolonged in comparison to a control population living in Denmark.[73] These and other observations have stimulated a growing interest in the effects of ω-3 fatty acids derived from marine oils on the composition and function of platelets and on cellular prostaglandin metabolism.

Platelet Lipid Composition. The changes in platelet phospholipid composition brought about by feeding dietary supplements of fish oils to animals or humans are now well documented. The concentrations of both linoleic acid and arachidonic acid were decreased in platelet phospholipids of the Eskimo. Observations were similar in volunteers fed mackerel oil, cod liver oil, or salmon oil and in animals given menhaden or cod liver oils.[32,33,38] This reduction in linoleic acid could be a reflection of the low linoleate intake (most fish oils contain only 1 to 2 percent linoleic acid) or may relate to the displacement of linoleate by other fatty acids.[5] The mechanism responsible for the reduction in the arachidonic acid content of platelets is not known, but it is possible that the decreased dietary linoleic acid may lead to reduced arachidonic acid levels in plasma and, hence, in platelet membrane phospholipids. Alternatively, arachidonic acid simply may be displaced by other fatty acids.

As might be expected, the consumption of ω-3–rich fish oils led to a marked incorporation of eicosapentaenoic acid and even longer chain polyunsaturated ω-3 fatty acids in the platelet membrane phospholipids.[32,37,38] The reduction in arachidonic acid and increase in eicosapentaenoic acid led to a marked increase in the C20:5/C20:4 ratio (for example, 0.0043 to 0.3) which may interfere with cellular prostaglandin metabolism.[37,38]

Platelet and Vascular Function. Both platelet function and platelet–vessel-wall interactions have been altered by diets enriched in ω-3 fatty acids. With one exception, bleeding times invariably were prolonged by 30 to 40 percent in humans ingesting fish oils for several weeks or longer, although a bleeding tendency was not observed clinically.[32,33,37,38] Brox and colleagues[38] failed to show a lengthening of the bleeding time, but this may have been due to the lesser quantity (25 ml/day) of fish oil that was administered.

Platelet aggregation in response to ADP was impaired in the Eskimos and in the residents of a fishing village in Japan, as well as in human subjects fed salmon and cod liver oils.[32,37,38,75] In other studies, aggregation induced by low doses of collegen was also diminished.[32,37,38] Platelet retention on glass beads (which may reflect platelet aggregation as well as platelet adhesion) was significantly decreased in subjects receiving a diet containing supplemental salmon oil.[37] In addition, the occlusion time of vascular prostheses inserted into the aorta of rats was prolonged when the animals were fed cod liver oil.[19]

Decreased platelet counts were observed in subjects ingesting large amounts of ω-3 fatty acids. These include the early observations in the Eskimo, as well as a recent study of the effects of salmon oil feeding in volunteers.[37,73] In general, the reduced platelet count, while of statistical significance, remained within the normal range and was not low enough to affect the bleeding times (for example, less that $100,000/mm^3$). In several individuals, however, the platelet count fell more markedly. After the salmon oil feeding was discounted, the platelet count rose rapidly to normal levels. In one subject, a repeat study feeding salmon oil led to a second reduction in platelet count, although platelet survival using ^{51}Chromium was similar before and during fish oil feeding.[76] At present it is not clear whether the thrombocytopenia is related to the ω-3 fatty acids in the fish oil, other natural components, or contaminants.

In summary, feeding ω-3 fatty-acid–rich fish oils to humans leads to a reproducible prolongation of the Ivy bleeding time, inhibition of platelet aggregation by ADP and collagen, and a decrease in platelet retention on glass beads. In some settings there may also be reduction in platelet count. The mechanisms for these functional alterations may reside in changes in platelet and endothelial cell prostaglandin synthesis induced by alterations in dietary fatty acid composition.

Mechanism of ω-3 Fatty Acid Effects.   In two studies in which fish oils were fed to humans, thromboxane B_2 production (the stable metabolite of thromboxane A_2) was decreased following stimulation of platelets by collagen or ADP.[32,38] In a study in rats, no appreciable production of thromboxane A_3 from platelets was observed after feeding cod liver oil.[36] Thus, it seems more likely that reduced thromboxane A_2 levels, rather than increased production of the inactive thromboxane A_3, are responsible for the observed antithrombotic effects.

The production of PGI_2-like activity from vessel walls after fish-oil feeding has also been examined.[36] Incubated segments of rat aorta from animals ingesting cod liver oil produced less platelet inhibitory activity (presumed to be PGI_2) compared with results of feeding sunflower seed oil. In addition, the production of prostaglandin 6-keto-$F_{1\alpha}$ (the stable, inactive breakfdown product of PGI_2) was decreased in the fish-oil–treated animals, as was Δ17-6-keto-$F_{1\alpha}$ (the breakdown product of PGI_3). It seems clear that feeding of fish oils containing ω-3 fatty acids leads to a reduction in prostacyclin-like activity from the walls of blood vessels.

Biochemical explanations for these findings have been sought by a number of in vitro experiments using purified fatty acids and specific assays for prostaglandin metabolites. For example, Dyerberg and colleagues have shown that eicosapentaenoic acid will not induce platelet aggregation when added to platelet-rich plasma and will inhibit the second wave of platelet aggregation that follows the addition of ADP.[70]

One explanation for the reduced formation of thromboxane B_2 from platelets enriched in eicosapentaenoic acid may involve competitive inhibition of cyclooxygenase by eisapentaenoic acid, which leads to reduced thromboxane A_2 synthesis from arachidonic acid[77,78] (Fig. 4-3). In addition, eicosapentaenoic acid is a relatively poor substrate for cyclooxygenase, and consequently only very small amounts of thromboxane A_3 (a weak platelet-aggregating substance) are produced.[77,79] It is also possible that prostaglandins of the D series (such as PGD_3) may be formed from eicosapentaenoic acid, and that these may also inhibit platelet aggregation.[80]

Several other hypotheses for the decreased platelet responsiveness that follows ω-3 fatty acid ingestion are possible. These include the blockade of thromboxane receptors on platelets[81] by eicosapentaenoic acid, replacement of arachidonic acid by eicosapentaenoic acid in platelet phospholipids with a concomitant reduction in the amount of arachidonate available for prostaglandin synthesis, or an inhibitory effect of eicosapentaenoic acid on phospholipase A_2 leading to a reduced release of arachidonic acid from platelet phospholipids.

The effects of eicosapentaenoic acid on prostaglandin production by endothelial cells has received less attention. Preliminary evidence indicates that both PGI_2 and PGI_3 are decreased, although some platelet inhibitory activity may still be present.[82] If it should be shown conclusively that vascular PGI_2 as well as platelet thromboxane production is diminished, then further studies on the magni-

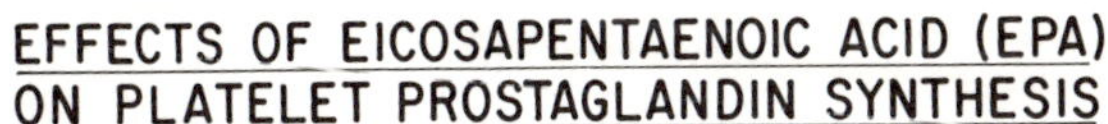

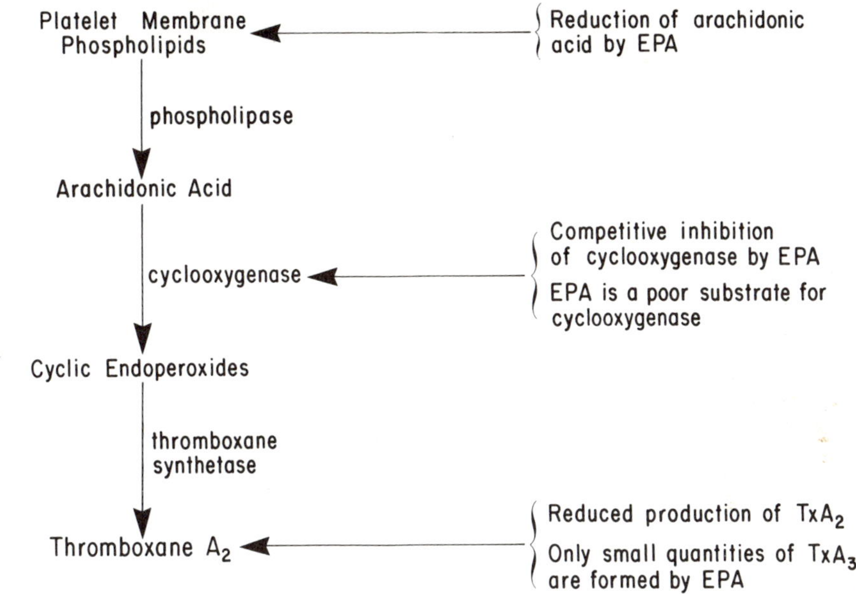

Fig.4-3.   Possible sites of action of eicosapentaenoic acid (EPA) on the conversion of arachidonic acid to thromboxane A_2. (Reprinted by permission of the American Heart Association Inc. from Goodnight SH, Harris WS, Connor WE, Illingworth DR: Polyunsaturated fatty acids, hyperlipidemia and thrombosis. Arteriosclerosis 2:78–113, 1982.)

tude of these decreases will be required. Since the bleeding time is prolonged in humans fed fish oil, it may be that there is a relatively greater decrease in thromboxane generation than in prostacyclin production.

In summary, the ingestion of dietary fish oils containing the ω-3 fatty acid eicosapentaenoic acid may have profound effects on platelet or vessel composition and function. Concentrations of arachidonic acid in cellular phospholipids are decreased, bleeding times are prolonged, and various in vitro tests of platelet function are inhibited. One explanation for the platelet inhibition may be the significant reduction in platelet thromboxane synthesis that has been demonstrated repeatedly. More data are needed on the vascular production of prostacyclin, and particularly on the balance between thromboxane and PGI_2 effects under various experimental or clinical conditions in vivo.

THE EFFECTS OF DIETARY FATS ON PLASMA LIPID LEVELS

Dietary fats also influence another factor in the development of heart disease, namely, the plasma lipid levels. This section briefly reviews the effects of the two major classes of polyunsaturated fatty acids on plasma lipid and lipoprotein levels (see also Chapters 3 and 5).

ω-6 Fatty Acids and Plasma Lipids

The hypocholesterolemic effect of the polyunsaturated fatty acids present in vegetable oils has been appreciated for 30 years.[83–90] In 1952 Kinsell and colleagues[11] suggested that it was not simply the amount of fat in the diet but the *type* of fat (animal or vegetable) that affected the plasma cholesterol levels. Later, this point was demonstrated clearly by Ahrens and colleagues,[12] who subsequently showed that feeding two *vegetable* fats (coconut oil and corn oil) led to vastly different plasma cholesterol levels.[91] The iodine number (total unsaturation) of the oil, rather than its source, was strongly correlated with the degree of cholesterol lowering. About the same time, it was shown that the addition of polyunsaturated fat to a fat-free diet resulted in a reduction in plasma cholesterol levels of the same magnitude as the rise in cholesterol when saturated fats were substituted.[11] The possibility that hypercholesterolemia resulted from essential fatty acid deficiency was discounted when it was shown that a fish oil, high in ω-3 polyunsaturates but low in linoleic acid, effectively reduced plasma cholesterol levels.[103] On the basis of this and similar studies, Keys and colleagues[14] and Hegsted and colleagues[13] developed predictive equations of the magnitude of change in plasma cholesterol after substitutions in the cholesterol or fatty acid composition of the diet. Both equations predict that, gram-for-gram, saturated fatty acids raise cholesterol levels about twice as much as polyunsaturated fatty acids lower them. These equations, derived from studies in which linoleic acid was the polyunsaturated fat acid fed, may not apply to fish oil feeding studies.

Previous studies demonstrated that polyunsaturated fatty acids derived from vegetable oils (principally linoleic acid) reduce plasma cholesterol levels in healthy volunteers.[13,14,86,92–109] Typically, vegetable oils comprised 40 percent of the total calories, and the cholesterol intake was about 400 mg/day. The average decline in plasma cholesterol levels in these studies was about 13 percent (range 0 to 28 percent).

The extent of cholesterol lowering was related to at least two factors: (1) the magnitude of the difference between the P-S ratios (polyunsaturated to saturated fatty acids as a percent of total calories) of the diets; and (2) the presence of cholesterol in the diet. For example, in eight studies the P-S ratio of the polyunsaturated diet averaged about seven-fold higher than that of the saturated diet (1.5 versus 0.2); these studies reported an average decrease in plasma cholesterol levels of only 8 percent. In six other studies, the P-S ratio of the polyunsaturated diet averaged 27-fold higher than that of the saturated diet (4.6 versus 0.17); this difference was associated with an average cholesterol decrease of 20 percent (see ref. 5).

In hyperlipidemic patients, the effects of polyunsaturated vegetable oils were similar to, or in some case greater than, those reported in normal subjects.[84,93,103–112] The average percent decrease was somewhat higher than that of normal subjects (22 percent; range 13 to 33). Even in these hypercholesterolemic patients, however, those fed diets with the smallest difference in P-S ratios (2.0 versus 0.2) experienced the smallest decrease in plasma cholesterol levels (13 percent).[105]

All phenotypic forms of hyperlipidemia showed some hypolipidemic response

to dietary polyunsaturated fats. In the 17 type IIa patients reported, the average decline in plasma cholesterol levels was 19 percent; in 15 type IIb patients, 21 percent; in 29 type IVs, 15 percent; and in seven type Vs, 16 percent. Thus, no particular phenotype was unusually responsive or resistant to changes in the amount of polyunsaturated fat in the diet (see ref. 5).

In summary, there is universal agreement that a high intake of polyunsaturated vegetable oils reduces plasma cholesterol and LDL levels. There is probably little effect of ω-6 polyunsaturated fatty acids on plasma triglyceride and VLDL levels, although the data in this area is not clearcut.[5] HDL cholesterol levels sometimes fall, but usually remain unaffected by linoleic acid.[5] Future studies must be careful to allow adequate time for plasma lipids to stabilize on different dietary regimens; they must control caloric intake to prevent the confounding influences of body weight changes on lipid metabolism; and they should examine how plasma lipids are affected by reasonable changes in the amount of polyunsaturated fat in the diet.

The mechanisms by which polyunsaturated ω-6 fatty acids exert their hypolipidemic effects have been examined extensively, but to date no unifying mechanism operative in all situations has been found. Proposed mechanisms include (1) decreased cholesterol absorption, (2) increased fecal excretion of neutral and acidic steroids, (3) decreased cholesterol synthesis, (4) transfer of cholesterol from plasma to tissues, (5) changes in the cholesterol-to-protein ratio in LDL, and (6) changes in the rates of synthesis or catabolism of individual lipoproteins. In addition, the changes in the fatty acid composition of membrane lipids (fluidity) may affect lipoprotein metabolism in two ways:

1. The changes in the lipoprotein particle may make it a better substrate for catabolic enzymes, or for binding to cellular receptors.

2. Changes in cellular membranes may affect the local milieu of receptors and membrane-bound enzymes, thereby increasing their reactivity toward their lipoprotein substrates. (See ref. 5 for discussion of mechanisms.)

ω-3 Fatty Acids and Plasma Lipid Levels

Between 1956 and 1963, seven studies of fish-oil feeding were carried out in humans.[103,115–120] Although they varied in the kind of subjects studied, the degree of dietary control, the sources of fish-oil fatty acids, and duration, there was good agreement that fish oils were at least as hypocholesterolemic as polyunsaturated vegetable oils. The principal intent of these studies was to demonstrate that polyunsaturated fats from *any* source (fish or vegetable) were hypocholesterolemic. There was no indication from these studies that fish oils had any unique properties not shared by other polyunsaturated oils from vegetable sources.

Two interesting features of these studies may not have been appreciated at the time. First, since fish oils contain large amounts of cholesterol (300 to 500 mg/100 g) and vegetable oils contain none, the majority of these investigators fed higher levels of cholesterol during the fish oil phase than during the vegetable oil phase. Thus, the finding of similar hypocholesterolemic effects of these two types of fat implied that the fish oils might have been even more hypocholesterolemic if they had not contained cholesterol. Second, the daily intake of ω-6 fatty acids was invariably greater than the intake of ω-3 fatty acids, and yet similar or greater reductions in plasma cholesterol levels occurred with ω-3 fatty acids. Thus, gram-for-gram, the ω-3 fatty acids were considerably more hypocholesterolemic than linoleic acid. Others showed that tetraenes, pentaenes, and hexaenes produced 2 to 3 times greater cholesterol lowering than did the dienes or trienes.[117]

More recently, dramatic reductions in the concentrations of plasma triglycerides and VLDL were observed in both normolipidemic[35,121,122,125] and hyperlipidemic subjects[34,124] fed diets supplemented with fish oils. In one study, normal subjects were fed diets enriched with salmon oil, polyunsaturated vegetable oils, and a relatively saturated control diet each for periods of 4 weeks.[125] Plasma cholesterol levels were reduced similarly with both the salmon-oil and vegetable-oil diets (190 to 170 mg/dl). In contrast, however, plasma triglyceride levels fell 33 percent (77 to 48 mg/dl) with the salmon-oil diet but were unchanged after the vegetable-oil diet.

This direct comparison provides the first demonstration that ω-3 fatty acids possess unique hypotriglyceridemic properties not found in the polyunsaturated ω-6 fatty acids of vegetable oils. In these studies it was further demonstrated that dietary ω-3 fatty acids significantly decreased plasma VLDL (50 percent) and LDL (16 percent) levels but did not change the concentrations of HDL. The fact that HDL levels were not depressed has been confirmed by others,[122] and in some studies HDL cholesterol levels have actually increased with the diets rich in ω-3 fatty acid.[121,123]

The effects of fish oils in hypercholesterolemic and hypertriglyceridemic patients have been reported in only two studies. Ahrens and colleagues[103] examined two subjects (probably type IIb) given isocalroic amounts of either corn oil or menhaden oil at 40 percent of calories. Plasma cholesterol and triglyceride levels were both reduced more by the fish oil than by the vegetable oil. Phillipson and colleagues[34,124] reported the effects of feeding diets rich in salmon oil, polyunsaturated vegetable oils, and saturated fats to hyperlipidemic subjects. In patients with type IIb hyperlipidemia, plasma cholesterol levels (mg/dl) decreased from 294 to 239 (ω-6 diet) and to 200 (ω-3 diet). Thus, the fish oil diet was significantly more hypolipidemic than the polyunsaturated vegetable oil diet.

The effects of dietary fish oil on the plasma lipids of patients with severe hypertriglyceridemia (type V phenotype) were first reported in 1981.[124] These patients, in whom hypertriglyceridemia normally is exacerbated by even moderate intakes of dietary fat, were able to consume up to 30 percent of calories as fish oil, with a concomitant lowering of their plasma lipid levels. The ω-3 fatty acid–rich diet resulted in 46 percent decline in plasma cholesterol levels and a 77 percent drop in triglyceride levels, compared with a control diet containing only 5 percent fat. Comparative diets containing 30 percent of calories as ω-6 fatty acids caused rapid increase in the concentrations of plasma cholesterol and triglycerides; it became necessary to stop these diets after 14 days because of the increasing risk of abdominal pains, hepatomegaly, and acute pancreatitis. ω-3 Fatty acids had effects on plasma lipid levels that were distinctly different from the effects of ω-6 fatty acids, and may be of substantial therapeutic benefit in hypertriglyceridemic patients.

A few attempts have been made to determine the minimum intake of ω-3 fatty acids necessary to produce significant changes in plasma lipid levels.[121–123] Although dose-responses have not been acertained fully, it was shown that approximately 4g/day of ω-3 fatty acids from 20 ml of cod liver oil produced greater cholesterol lowering than did 16 g of linoleic acid.[119,121] In another study, however, the addition of up to 8 grams of ω-3 fatty acids (from cod liver oil) did not change the plasma cholesterol levels but resulted in a significant reduction in plasma triglycerides.[122] A further study showed that 4 g of ω-3 fatty acids per day reduced the levels of plasma triglycerides but not of cholesterol.[123] A major problem with many of these studies was that the fish oils were simply given as supplements and were not incorporated into a metabolic diet as a replacement for a portion of the customary dietary fat. In addition, the cholesterol intake was usually higher during the fish oil phase. For these reasons it seems likely that more significant hypocholesterolemic effects might have occurred if the dietary periods had been more rigorously matched in terms of both fat and cholesterol content.

In summary, although relatively few studies have examined the effects of ω-3 polyunsaturated fatty acids plasma lipids and lipoproteins, the findings of lipid lowering are consistent not only in metabolic studies but also with free-living human beings consuming high levels of ω-3 fatty acids. Fish oils have always been at least as effective as vegetable oils (if not more so) in lowering plasma cholesterol levels. These reductions occurred when ω-3 fatty acids constituted from 1 to 8 percent of total calories. In light of the fact that linoleic acid intakes of 15 to 20 percent of calories were needed to achieve similar depressions in plasma cholesterol levels, the dietary ω-3 fatty acids were roughly 2 to 5 times more potent than the ω-6 acids.

The most striking effects of fish oil feeding have been the rapid and dramatic decrease in the levels of plasma triglyceride and VLDL. Since vegetable oils produce little or no depression in plasma triglyceride concentrations, it is evident that ω-3 fatty acids have unique effects not shared with the ω-6 fatty acids. Studies in hyperlipidemic subjects have demonstrated that small quantitites of ω-3 fatty acids are much more hypolipidemic than larger amounts of linoleic acid. Thus, dietary ω-3 fatty acids may prove to be very effective in the treatment of hyperlipidemia.

The mechanism of the ω-3 induced hypocholesterolemia has not been studied as extensively as that resulting from ω-6 fatty acid ingestion. Nevertheless, there are data to suggest the following mechanisms: (1) increased fecal steroid excretion; (2) changes in the fatty acid composition (fluidity) of lipoproteins; (3) changes in the rates of synthesis and/or catabolism of VLDL and LDL. Reductions in the concentrations of plasma triglycerides and VLDL may result from lower rates of synthesis of the triglyceride or apoprotein B moieties of VLDL, or may result from an increased rate of clearance of VLDL from the plasma. (See reference 5 for discussion of mechanisms.)

SUMMARY

Polyunsaturated fat has an antithrombotic action in the body when it is substituted for saturated fat in the diet. The antithrombotic effects may result from either the simple reduction of more thrombogenic saturated fat by substitution with polyunsaturated fat in the diet, or, alternatively, from an independent modification of platelet or vessel-wall membrane function via perturbations of prostaglandin metabolism. While experimental feeding of both ω-6 and ω-3 fatty acids leads to clear inhibition of platelet aggregation in vitro, only fish-oil feeding reliably leads to a significant prolongation of the Ivy bleeding time in humans. These effects may reflect the changes in the fatty acids composition that occur with polyunsaturated-fat feeding (vegetable or fish oils). High levels of either linoleic acid or fish oil ω-3 fatty acids appear to reduce the levels of arachidonic acid in membranes. This would tend to reduce both thromboxane A_2 and prostacyclin production to unknown extents. A further inhibition of prostaglandin synthesis, however, may be expected from fish oils containing eicosapentaenoic acid. This fatty acid will compete with arachidonic acid for cyclooxygenase and block the production of (presumably) both thromboxane A_2 and prostacyclin. Since only fish oils prolong bleeding times, the balance between these two compounds appear to be more favorable with fish oils than with vegetable oils. There remains a great need for studies to characterize the in vivo production of platelet thromboxane and vessel wall prostacyclin during fish-oil and vegetable-oil feeding.

The substitution of polyunsaturated fat in the diet for saturated fat also has a hypolipidemic effect that has been demonstrated in a variety of experiments in both animals and humans. Both the ω-6 and ω-3 families of fatty acids are hypocholesterolemic and both reduce the plasma concentrations of LDL. Only the ω-3 fatty acids from fish oils, however, have a pronounced hypotriglyceridemic effect in both normal and hypertriglyceridemic subjects. ω-6 Fatty acids may have a mild hypotriglyceridemic action in some subjects with no demonstrable effect on plasma triglyceride concentrations in others. In patients with severe hypertriglyceridemia (type V hyperlipidemia), dietary ω-3 fatty acids are remarkably hypolipidemic and much more effective than ω-6 fatty acids.

The recommended dietary changes that fit the experimental evidence presented in this review are the following: Reduce saturated fat in the diet, because of its thrombogenic and hyperlipidemic effects, from the current American intake of well over 20 percent of the total calories to less than 8 percent of the total calories. If dietary linoleic acid is at the level of 6 to 8 percent of the total calories (the present United States intake), there is little indication that increasing linoleate further would result in significant health benefits. On the other hand, there are indications that benefit would be obtained and no harm produced by the ingestion of moderate amounts (4 to 8 g/day) of ω-3 fatty acids derived from fish. The effects of dietary polyunsaturated fatty acids of both the ω-6 and the ω-3 families continue to be the object of intensive research. The antithrombotic and hypolipidemic properties of fish oils must be characterized further and translated into specific nutritional interventions that may be helpful in the prevention and treatment of atherosclerotic diseases.

ACKNOWLEDGMENT

Material for this chapter was derived in part from a review (ref. 5), and is used by permission of the American Heart Association Inc.

REFERENCES

1. Report of the American Heart Association Nutrition Committee: Rationale of the diet-Heart Statement of the AHA. Arteriosclerosis 4:177–191, 1982.

2. Connor WE: The relationship of hyperlipoproteinemia to artherosclerosis: the decisive role of dietary cholesterol and fat. In Scanu AM (ed): The Biochemistry of Atherosclerosis. New York, Marcel Dekker, 1979, pp 371–418.

3. Davignon J: The lipid hypothesis: pathophysiological basis. Arch Surg 113:26–34, 1978.

4. Ross R: Atherosclerosis—A problem of the biology of the arterial wall cells and their interactions with blood components. Arteriosclerosis 1:293–311, 1981.

5. Goodnight SH, Harris WS, Connor WE, Illingworth DR: Polyunsaturated fatty acids, hyperlipidemia and thrombosis. Arteriosclerosis 2:78–113, 1982.

6. French JE: Atherogenesis and thrombosis. Semin Hematol 8:84–94, 1971.

7. Connor WE, Poole JCF: The effect of fatty acids on the formation of thrombi. Quart J Exptl Physiol 46:1–7, 1961.

8. Connor WE: The acceleration of thrombus formation by certain fatty acids. J Clin Invest 41:1199–1205, 1962.

9. Connor WE, Hoak JC, Warner ED: Massive thrombosis produced by fatty acids infusion. J Clin Invest 42:860–866, 1963.

10. Malmsten C: Prostaglandins, thromboxanes, and platelets. Brit J Haematol 41:453–458, 1979.

11. Kinsell LW, Partridge J, Boling L, Margen S, Michaels GP: Dietary modification of serum cholesterol and phospholipid levels. J Clin Endocrinol 12:909–913, 1952.

12. Ahrens EH, Blankenhorn DH, Tsaltas TT: Effect on human serum lipids of substituting plant for animal fat in the diet. Proc Soc Exp Biol Med 86:872–878, 1954.

13. Hegsted DM, McGandy RB, Myers ML, Stare FJ: Quantitative effects of dietary fat on serum cholesterol in man. Am J Clin Nutr 17:281–295, 1965.

14. Keys A, Anderson JT, Grande F: Prediction of serum cholesterol responses of man to change in fats in the diet. Lancet ii:959–966, 1957.

15. Gutheron P, Renaud S: Hyperlipemia-induced hypercoagulable state in rat. Role of an increased activity of platelet phosphatidyl serine in response to certain dietary fatty acids. Thromb Res 1:353–370, 1972.

16. McGregor L, Morazain R, Renaud S: A comparison of the effects of dietary short and long chain saturated fatty acids on platelet functions, platelet phospholipids, and blood coagulation in rats. Lab Invest 43:438–442, 1980.

17. Renaud S, Kuba K, Goulet C, Lemire Y, Allard C: Relationship between fatty acid composition of platelets and platelet aggregation in rat and man. Circulation Res 26:553–563, 1970.

18. Nordy A, Hamlin JT, Chandler AB, Newland H: The influence of dietary fats on plasma and platelet lipids and ADP–induced platelet thrombosis in the rat. Scand J Haemat 5:458–473, 1968.

19. Hornstra G: Dietary fats and arterial thrombosis. Haemostasis 2:21–52, 1973/74.

20. Hornstra G: Dietary fats and arterial thrombosis: Effects and mechanism of action. Prog Biochem Pharmacol 14:326–338, 1977.

21. Hornstra G, Lussenburg RN: Relationship between the type of dietary fatty acid and arterial thrombosis tendency in rats. Atherosclerosis 22:499–516, 1975.

22. Moncada S, Vane JR: Arachidonic acid metabolites and the interactions between platelets and blood vessel walls. N Engl J Med 300:1142–1147, 1979.

23. Willis AL: Nutritional and pharmacological factors in eicosanoid biology. Nutr Rev 39:289–301, 1981.

24. Bills TK, Smith JB, Silver MJ: Metabolism of (^{14}C) arachidonic acid by human platelets. Biochim Biophys Acta 303–314, 1976.
25. Bills TK, Smith JB, Silver MJ: Selective release of archidonic acid from the phospholipids of human platelets in response to thrombin. J Clin Invest 60:1–6, 1977.
26. Hamberg M, Samuelsson B: prostaglandin endoperoxides. Novel transformations of arachidonic acid in human platelets. Proc Nat Acad Sci 71:3400–3404, 1974.
27. Hamberg M, Svensson J, Samuelsson B: Thromboxanes: A new group of biologically active compounds derived from prostaglandin endoperoxides. Proc Nat Acad Sci 72: 2994–2998, 1975.
28. Moncada S, Gryglewski R, Bunting S, Vane JR: An enzyme isolated from arteries transforms prostaglandin endoperoxides to an unstable substance that inhibits platelet aggregation. Nature 263:663–665, 1976.
29. Moncada S, Vane JR: The role of prostacyclin in vascular tissue. Fed Proc 38:66–71, 1979.
30. Galli C, Agradi E, Petroni A, Socini A: Modulation of prostaglandin production in tissues by dietary essential fatty acids. Acta Med Scand (suppl) 642:171–179, 1980.
31. Dyerberg J, Bang HO, Aagaard O: α-Linolenic acid and eicosapentaenoic acid. Lancet 1:199, 1980.
32. Siess W, Scherer B, Bohlig B, Roth P, Kurzmann I, Weber PC: Platelet-membrane fatty acids, platelet aggregation, and thromboxane formation during a mackerel diet. Lancet 1:441–444. 1980.
33. Sanders TAB, Naismith DJ, Haines AP, Vickers M: Cod-liver oil, platelet fatty acids, and bleeding time. Lancet 1:1189, 1980.
34. Phillipson BE, Connor WE, Illingworth DR: Effectiveness of low fat, high carbohydrate diets in type V hyperlipidemia. Clin Res 29:418A, 1981.
35. Harris WS. Connor WE: The effects of salmon oil upon plasma lipids, lipoproteins and triglyceride clearance. Trans Assoc Am Phys 43:148–155, 1980.
36. Hornstra G, Christ-Hazelhof E, Haddeman E, ten Hoor F, Nugteren DH: Fish oil feeding lowers thromboxane- and prostacyclin production by rat platelets and aorta and does not result in the formation of prostaglandin I_3. Prostaglandins, 21:727–738, 1981.
37. Goodnight SH, Harris WS, Conner WE: The effects of dietary ω3 fatty acids on platelet composition and function in man: A prospective, controlled study. Blood 58:880–885, 1981.
38. Brox JH, Killle JE, Gunnes S, Nordy A: The effect of cod liver oil and corn oil on platelets and vessel wall in man. Thrombos Haemostas 46:604–611, 1981.
39. Samuelsson B, Hammarstrom S: Nomenclature for Leukotrienes. Prostaglandins 19: 645–648, 1980.
40. Samuelsson B: Prog Lipid Res Leukotrienes: A novel group of compounds including SRS-A. 20:23–30, 1981.
41. Galli C, Agradi E, Petroni A, Tremoli E: Differential effects of dietary fatty acids on the accumulation of arachidonic acid and its metabolic conversion through the cyclooxygenase and lipoxygenase in platelets and vascular tissue. Lipids 16:165–172, 1981.
42. McGregor L, Renaud S: Effect of dietary linoleic acid deficiency on platelet aggregation and phospholipid fatty acid of rats. Thromb Res 12:921–927, 1978.
43. Fine KM, Dupont J, Mathias MM: Rat platelet prostaglandin, cyclic AMP, and lipid response to variations in dietary fat. J Nutr 111:699–707, 1981.
44. Spector AA, Hoak JC, Fry GL, et al: Effect of fatty acid modification on prostacyclin production by cultured human endothelial cells. J Clin Invest 65:1003–1012, 1980.
45. Needleman SW, Spector AA, Hoak JC: Enrichment of human platelet phospholipid with linoleic acid diminishes arachidonic acid content and thromboxane release. Blood 58:(suppl 1): 201A, 1981.

46. O'Brien JR, Etherington MD, Jamieson S, Vergroesen AJ, Ten Hoor F: Effects of a diet of polyunsaturated fats on some platelet–function tests. Lancet 2:995–996, 1976.

47. Hornstra G, Chait A, Karvonen MJ, Lewis B, Turpeinen O, Vergroesen AJ: Influence of dietary fat on platelet function in men. Lancet 1:1155–1157, 1973.

48. Agradi E, Tremoli E, Colombo C, Galli C: Influence of short term dietary supplementation of different lipids on aggregation and arachidonic acid metabolism in rabbit platelets. Prostaglandins 16:973–984, 1978.

49. Hornstra G, Haddeman E, Don JA: Relationship between arachidonic acid content of blood platelets and their TxA$_2$-production upon stimulation (abst). Thrombosis and Haemostasis 46:208, 1981.

50. Renaud S, Dumont E, Godsey F, Suplisson A, Thevenon C: Platelet functions in relation to dietary fats in farmers from two regions of France. Thrombos Haemostas 40: 518–531, 1978.

51. Fleischman I, Justice D, Bierenbaum ML, Stier A, Sullivan A: Beneficial effect of increased dietary linoleate upon in vivo platelet function in man. J Nutr 105:1286–1290, 1975.

52. Jakubowski JA, Ardlie NG: Modification of human platelet function by a diet enriched in saturated or polyunsaturated fat. Atherosclerosis 31:335–344, 1978.

53. Stuart MJ, Gerrard JM, White JG: Effect of cholesterol on production of thromboxane B$_2$ by platelet in vitro. N Engl J Med 302:6–10, 1980.

54. Lagarde M, Velardo B, Blanc M, Dechavanne M: Fatty acids bound to serumalbumin decrease the half-life of thromboxane A$_2$. Prostaglandins 20:275–283, 1980.

55. Hirose S, Asano T, Hidaka H: Effect of unsaturated fatty acids on separated form of human platelet cyclic nucleotide phosphodiesterase. Thromb Res 12:701–706, 1978.

56. de Deckere EAM, Nugteren DH, ten Hoor F: Influence of type of dietary fat on the prostaglandin release from isolated rabbit and rat hearts and from rat aortas. Prostaglandins 17:947–955, 1979.

57. ten Hoor F, de Deckere EAM, Haddeman E, Hornstra G, Quadt JFA: Dietary manipulation of prostaglandin and thromboxane synthesis in heart, aorta and blood platelets of the rat. Adv Prostaglandin Thromboxane Res 8:1771–1781, 1980.

58. Nordy A, Svensson B, Hoak JC: The effects of albumin bound fatty acids on the platelet inhibitory function of human endothelial cells Eur J Clin Invest 9:5–10, 1979.

59. Effects of feeding dihomo-γ-linolenic acid (20:3ω6) in man. Nutr Rev 37:286–288, 1979.

60. Spector AA, Kaduce TL, Hoak JC, Fry GL: Utilization of arachidonic and linoleic acids by cultured human endothelial cells. J Clin Invest 68:1003–1011, 1981.

61. Stone KJ, Willis AL, Hart M, Kirtland SJ, Kernoff PBA, McNicol GP: The metabolism of dihomo-γ-linolenic acid in man. Lipids 14:174–180, 1980.

62. Oelz O, Seyberth HW, Knapp HR, Sweetman BJ, Oates JA: Effects of feeding ethyl-dihomo-γ-linolenate on prostaglandin biosynthesis and platelet aggregation in the rabbit. Biochim Biophys Acta 431:268–277, 1976.

63. Willis AL, Comai K, Kuhn DC, Paulsrud J: Dihomo-γ-linolenate suppresses platelet aggregation when administered in vitro or in vivo. Prostaglandins 8:509–519, 1974.

64. Kernoff PBA, Willis AL, Stone KJ, Davies JA, McNicol GP: Antithrombotic potential of dihomo-γ-linolenic acid in man. Brit Med J 2:1441–1444, 1977.

65. Needleman P, Whitaker MO, Wyche A, Watters K, Sprecher H, Raz A: Manipulation of platelet aggregation by prostaglandins and their fatty acid precursors: Pharmacological basis for a therapeutic approach. Prostaglandins 19:165–181, 1980.

66. Hwang DH, Carroll AE: Decreased formation of prostaglandins derived from arachidonic acid by dietary linolenate in rats. J Clin Nutr 33:590–597, 1980.

67. Borchgrevink F, Berg KJ, Skjaeggestad Ø, Skaga E, Stormorken H: Effect of linseed oil on platelet adhesiveness and bleeding-time in patients with coronary heart-disease. Lancet 2:980–981, 1965.
68. Arthrand JB: Cause of death in 339 Alaskan Natives as determined by autopsy. Arch Path 90:433–438, 1970.
69. Bang HO, Dyerberg J: Lipid metabolism and ischemic heart disease in Greenland eskimos. Adv Nutr Res 3:1–22, 1980.
70. Dyerberg J, Bang HO, Stofferson E, Moncada S, Vane JR: Eicosapentaenoic acid and prevention of thrombosis and atherosclerosis. Lancet ii:117–119, 1978.
71. Dyerberg J, Bang HO, Hjørne N: Fatty acid composition of the plasma lipids in Greenland Eskimos. Am J Clin Nutr 28:958–966, 1975.
72. Bang HO, Dyerberg J, Hjørne N: The composition of food consumed by Greenlandic Eskimos. Acta Med Scand 200:69–73, 1976.
73. Dyerberg J, Bang HO: Hemostatic function and platelet polyunsaturated fatty acids in Eskimos. Lancet ii:433–435, 1979.
74. de Poncins G Kabloona: Time-Life Books, Inc. Alexandria, VA, 1941, p 225.
75. Hirai A, Hamazaki T, Terano T, et al: Eicosapentaenoic acid and platelet function in Japanese. Lancet 2:1132–1133, 1980.
76. Goodnight SH, Howard J: unpublished data.
77. Needleman P, Raz A, Minkes MS, Ferrendelli JA, Sprecher H: Triene prostaglandins: Prostacyclin and thromboxane biosynthesis and unique biological properties. Proc Natl Acad Sci 76:944–948, 1979.
78. Culp BR, Titus BG, Lands WEM: Inhibition of prostaglandin biosynthesis by eicosapentaenoic acid. Prostaglandins and Medicine 3:269–278, 1979.
79. Smith DR, Weatherly BC, Salmon JA, Ubatuba FB, Gryglewski RJ, Moncada S: Preparation and Biochemical Properties of PGH_3. Prostaglandins 18:423–438, 1979.
80. Whitaker MO, Wyche A, Fitzpatrick F, Sprecher H, Needleman P: Triene prostaglandins: Prostaglandin D_3 and icosapentaenoic acid as potential antithrombotic substances. Proc Natl Acad Sci 76:5919–5923, 1979.
81. Gryglewski RJ, Salmon JA, Ubatuba FB, Weatherly BC, Moncada S, Vane JR: Effects of all cis-5,8,11,14,17 eicosapentaenoic acid and PGH_3 on platelet aggregation. Prostaglandins 18:453–478, 1979.
82. Dyerberg J, Jorgensen KA: The effect of arachidonic- and eicosapentaenoic acid on the synthesis of prostacyclin-like material in human umbilical vasculature. Artery 8:12–17, 1980.
83. Jackson RL, Taunton OD, Morrisett JD, Gotto AM: The role of dietary polyunsaturated fat in lowering blood cholesterol in man. Circ Res 42:447–453, 1978.
84. Grundy SM, Ahrens EH: The effects of unsaturated dietary fats on absorption, excretion, synthesis, and distribution of cholesterol in man. J Clin Invest 49:1135–1152, 1970.
85. Schlierf G: Polyunsaturated fatty acids and atherosclerosis. In Kuneau WH, Holman RT(eds): Polyunsaturated Fatty Acids. Champaign, Ill, American Oil Chemists Society, 1977, pp 183–191.
86. Connor WE, Witiak DT, Stone DB, Armstrong ML: Cholesterol balance and fecal neutral steroid and bile acid excretion in normal men fed dietary fats of different fatty acid composition. J Clin Invest 48:1363–1375, 1969.
87. Illingworth DR: Present status of polyunsaturated fats in the prevention of cardiovascular disease. In Santos W, Lopus N, et al (eds): Nutrition and Food Science, vol 3. New York, Plenum Press, 1980.

88. Paul R, Ramesha CS, Ganguly J: On the mechanism of hypocholesterolemic effects of polyunsaturated lipids. Adv Lip Res 17:155–171, 1979.

89. Keys A, Grande F, Anderson JT: Bias and misrepresentation revisited: Perspective "On saturated fat." Am J Clin Nutr 27:188–212, 1974.

90. Glueck CJ: Dietary fat and atherosclerosis. Am J Clin Nutr 32:2703–2711, 1979.

91. Ahrens EH, Hirsch J, Insull W, et al: The influence of dietary fats on serum lipid levels in man. Lancet i:943–953, 1957.

92. Shepherd J, Packard CJ, Grundy SM, Yeshurun D, Gotto AM, Taunton OD: Effects of saturated and polyunsaturated fat diets on the chemical composition and metabolism of low density lipoproteins in man. J Lip Res 21:91–99, 1980.

93. Chait A, Onitiri A, Nicoll A, Rabaya E, Davis J, Lewis B: Reduction of serum triglyceride levels by polyunsaturated fat. Studies on the mode of action and on very low density lipoprotein composition. Atherosclerosis 20:347–364, 1974.

94. Illingworth DR, Sundberg EE, Becker N, Connor WE, Alaupovic P: Influence of saturated, monounsaturated and ω-6 polyunsaturated fatty acids on low density lipoprotein metabolism in man. Arteriosclerosis 1:380A, 1981.

95. Beveridge JMR, Connell WF, Mayer GA: Dietary factors affecting the level of plasma cholesterol in humans: the role of fat. Can J Biochem Physiol 34:441–455, 1956.

96. Nestle PJ, Havenstein N, Scott TW, Cook LJ: Polyunsaturated ruminant fats and cholesterol metabolism in man. Aust NZJ Med 4:497–501, 1974.

97. Turner JD, Le NA, Brown WV: Effect of changing dietary fat saturation on low-density lipoprotein metabolism in man. Am J Physiol 241:E57–E63, 1981.

98. Connor WE, Lin DS, Harris WS: A comparison of dietary polyunsaturated ω-6 and ω-3 fatty acids in humans: Effects upon plasma lipids, lipoproteins and sterol balance. Arteriosclerosis 1:363a, 1981.

99. Moore RB, Anderson JT, Taylor HL, Keys A, Frantz ID: Effect of dietary fat on the fecal excretion of cholesterol and its degradation on products in man. J Clin Invest 47:1517–1531, 1968.

100. Nestel PJ, Havenstein N, Homma Y, Scott TW, Cook LJ: Increased sterol excretion with polyunsaturated fat, high-cholesterol diets. Metabolism 24:189–198, 1975.

101. Stein EA, Mendelsohn D, Fleming M, et al: Lowering of plasma cholesterol levels in free-living adolescent males; use of natural and synthetic polyunsaturated foods to provide balanced fat diets. Am J Clin Nutr 28:1204–1216, 1975.

102. Shepherd J, Packard CJ, Taunton D, Gotto AM: Effects of dietary-fat saturation on the composition of very-low-density lipoproteins and on the metabolism of their major apoprotein, apolipoprotein B. Biochem Soc Trans 6:779–781, 1978.

103. Ahrens EH, Insull W, Hirsch J, et al: The effect on human serum lipids of a dietary fat, highly unsaturated, but poor in essential fatty acids. Lancet i:115–119, 1959.

104. Grundy SM: Effects of polyunsaturated fats on lipid metabolism in patients with hypertriglyceridemia. J Clin Invest 55:269–282, 1975.

105. Vessby B, Gustafson IB, Boberg F, Karlstrom B, Lithell H, Werner I: Substituting polyunsaturated for saturated fat as a single change in a Swedish diet: effects on serum lipoprotein metabolism and glucose tolerance in patients with hyperlipidemia. Eur J Clin Invest 10:193–202, 1980.

106. Vega GL, Groszek E, Wolf R, Grundy SM: Influence of polyunsaturated fats on composition of plasma lipoproteins and apoproteins. J Lipid Res 23:811–822, 1982.

107. Spritz N, Ahrens EH, Grundy S: Sterol balance in man as plasma cholesterol concentrations are altered by exchanges of dietary fats. J Clin Invest 44:1482–1493, 1965.

108. Spritz N, Mishkel MA: Effects of dietary fats on plasma lipids and lipoproteins: an hy-

pothesis for the lipid lowering effect of unsaturated fatty acids. J Clin Invest 48:78–86, 1969.

109. Connor WE, Stone DB, Hodges RD: The interrelated effects of dietary cholesterol and fat upon human serum lipid levels. J Clin Invest 43:1691–1696, 1964.

110. Lewis B: Plasma-lipoprotein interrelationships. Biochem Soc Trans 5:589–601, 1977.

111. Nestel PJ, Haverstein N, Whyte HM, Scott TW, Cook LJ: Lowering of plasma cholesterol and enhanced sterol excretion with the consumption of polyunsaturated ruminant fats. N Engl J Med 288:379–382, 1973.

112. Shepherd J, Packard CJ, Patsch JR, Gotto AM, Taunton OD: Effects of dietary polyunsaturated and saturated fat on the properties of high density lipoproteins and the metabolism of apolipoprotein A-I. J Clin Invest 61:1582–1592, 1978.

113. Shore VG, Krauss RM, Butterfield G, Deshaies Y, Lindgren FT: Effects of dietary polyunsaturated:saturated fat ratio of human serum lipoproteins. Arteriosclerosis 1:386a, 1981.

114. Illingworth DR, Sundberg EE: The influence of dietary fats on lipid synthesis by human mononuclear cells. Biochem Soc Trans 9:49, 1981.

115. Bronte-Stewart B, Antonis A, Easles L, Brock JF: Effects of feeding different fats on serum cholesterol levels. Lancet i:521–526, 1956.

116. Keys A, Anderson JT, Grande F: "Essential" fatty acids, degree of unsaturation and effects of corn (maize) oil on the serum cholesterol level in man. Lancet i:66–68, 1957.

117. Worne HE, Smith LW: Effects of certain pure long chain polyunsaturated fatty acids esters on blood lipids of man. Am J Med Sci 237:710–721, 1959.

118. Kinsell LW, Michaels GD, Walker G, Visintine RE: The effect of a fish-oil fractin on plasma lipids. Diabetes 10:316–318, 1961.

119. Kingsbury KJ, Morgan DM, Aylott C, Emmerson R: Effects of ethyl arachidonate, cod liver oil and corn oil on plasma cholesterol levels. Lancet i:739–741, 1961.

120. Imaichi K, Michaels GD, Gunning B, Grasso S, Fukayama G, Kinsell LW: Studies with the use of fish oil fractions in human subjects. Am J Clin Nutr 13:158–168, 1963.

121. von Lossonczy TO, Ruiter A, Bronsegeest-Schoute HC, van Gent CM, Hermus RJJ: The effect of a fish diet on serum lipids in healthy human subjects. Am J Clin Nutr 31:1340–1346, 1978.

122. Bronsgeest-Schoute HC, van Gent CM, Luten JB, Ruiter A: The effects of various intakes of ω-3 fatty acids on the blood lipid composition in healthy human subjects. Am J Clin Nutr 34:1752–1757, 1981.

123. Sanders TB, Vickers M, Haines AP: Effect on blood lipids and haemostasis of a supplement of cod liver oil, rich in eicosapentaenoic and docosahexaenoic acids, in healthy young men. Clin Sci 61:317–324, 1981.

124. Phillipson BE, Harris WS, Connor WE: Reduction of plasma lipids and lipoproteins in hyperlipidemic patients by dietary ω-3 fatty acids. Clin Res 29:628A, 1981.

125. Harris WS, Connor WE, McMurry MP: The comparative reductions of the plasma lipids and lipoproteins by dietary polyunsaturated fats: salmon oil vs. vegetable oils. Metabolism 32:179–184, 1983.

5 | Cholesterol and Other Sterols: Absorption, Metabolism, Roles in Atherogenesis

Linda L. Gallo

Sterols are biologically important components of cells. Cholesterol is the major sterol in humans and other animals. It is also the major sterol in most marine life, although specific marine organisms contain significant amounts of brassicasterol, 22-dehydrocholesterol, and 24-methylene cholesterol. The major plant sterols are β-sitosterol, stigmasterol, fucosterol, and campesterol (Fig. 5-1).[1] With cholesterol taken as the reference compound, the other marine and plant sterols are distinguished only by side-chain modifications.

Among these sterols, cholesterol has been studied the most widely. These studies have revealed both favorable functions and unfavorable outcomes. Cholesterol, which is required for cell membrane biogenesis, steroid hormone production and bile acid synthesis, can be synthesized by the body; therefore, there is no dietary requirement for cholesterol. Unfavorably, cholesterol, in excess in the diet and in the circulation, increases the risk of atherosclerosis (see Chapters 1 and 2). Atherosclerosis results when influx of cholesterol into the arterial wall exceeds efflux. This aspect of the disease is part of a larger picture in which cholesterol influx into the body exceeds efflux. Interest in the plant and marine sterols is related to their ability to interfere with cholesterol influx and, as a consequence, to aid in either the prevention or treatment of atherosclerosis.

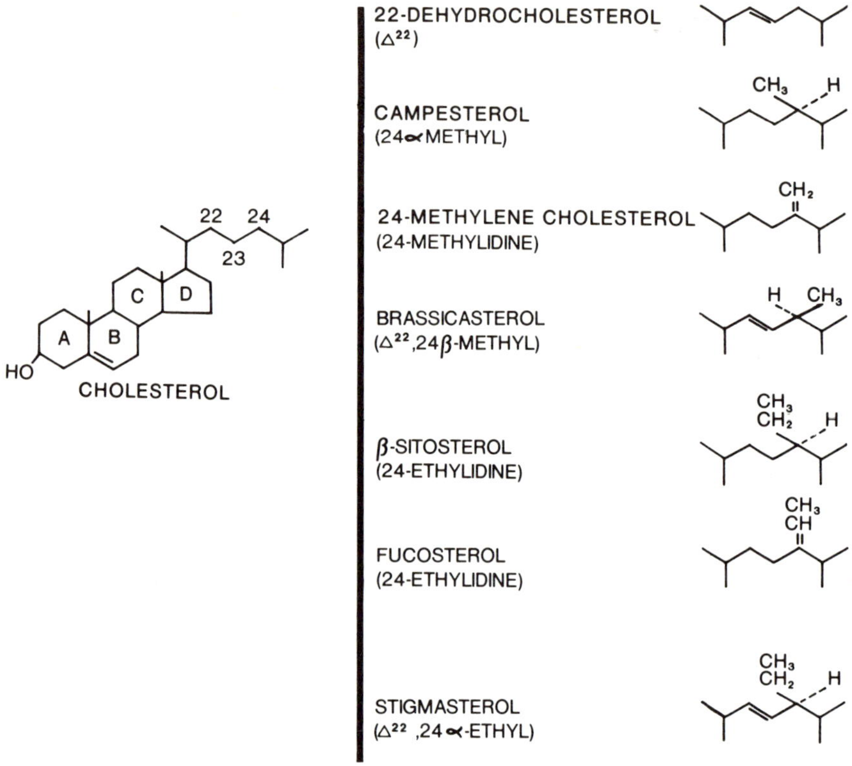

Fig. 5-1.   Side-chain modifications of major plant and marine sterols. (Reproduced with permission from Vahouny GV, and Kritchevsky D: Plant and marine sterols and cholesterol metabolism. In Spiller G (ed): Nutritional Pharmacology. New York, Alan R Liss, 1981)

This chapter will address the normal processes that add and remove body cholesterol, the balance of these processes, how excess cholesterol alters balance and leads to atherosclerosis, a cholesterol-lowering diet, dietary sources of cholesterol, and the effect of plant and marine sterols on cholesterol absorption and metabolism.

PROCESSES THAT ADD AND REMOVE CHOLESTEROL

Two systems add body cholesterol: cholesterol absorption from the intestinal lumen, and cholesterol biosynthesis by the tissues. Luminal cholesterol is derived from the diet, the bile, and the cells lining the digestive tract that may secrete cholesterol or are sloughed during cell turnover with their cholesterol content. About equal amounts of cholesterol are derived from the diet and the bile, 500 to 1,000 mg/day from each source in the human. Biosynthesized cholesterol is contributed by all tissues, although the liver and the intestine are the major sources, which together contribute 500 to 1,000 mg/day.

One major system, fecal excretion, removes cholesterol from the body. Cholesterol removed by this means includes chemically unaltered cholesterol and products of cholesterol metabolism. The chemically unaltered cholesterol is contributed from a portion of the nonabsorbed luminal sources, namely, diet, bile, and cells. Chemically altered cholesterol results from other portions of the luminal sources and bile. Intestinal bacteria convert cholesterol to coprostanol, which is a nonabsorbable saturated analog of cholesterol, and cholesterol is converted to bile acids in the liver. Cholesterol metabolites enter the intestine in the biliary secretion, and they represent a daily sterol removal of 250 to 600 mg. A minor system, desquamation of skin cells, removes 80 to 100 mg of cholesterol daily.

Cholesterol Addition

Absorption.   Cholesterol absorption is an inefficient process. In one study of human subjects consuming diets containing from 401 to 1,214 mg cholesterol as an integral part, absorption averaged 37 ± 5 percent. The highest dietary cholesterol contribution (1,214 mg/day) together with the biliary cholesterol produced a luminal cholesterol input of about 2,300 mg/day. At this daily input, absorption was still linear. This suggests that cholesterol absorption is proportional to dietary intake at the levels normally present (0.3 to 1.0 g) in the human diet.[2]

The site of cholesterol absorption is the proximal third of the small intestine.[3] Within this region, there may be differential uptake of the two major luminal sources of cholesterol. This is suggested from absorption studies in experimental animals in which dietary or biliary cholesterol is isotopically labeled.[4] The basis for such a difference is temporal, that is, biliary cholesterol is secreted in a properly solubilized state for uptake, whereas dietary cholesterol prior to uptake must undergo proper solubilization in the lumen (see micelle formation, below). For this reason biliary cholesterol, requiring no additional processing, may be absorbed without delay higher in the proximal third of the small intestine. There is no evidence that the mechanism of absorption differs in any other respect for the varied luminal sources of cholesterol.

The absorption process, defined as the transfer of cholesterol from the lumen of the small intestine to the lymph, may be considered in four phases: luminal, cell surface, intracellular, and transport (Fig. 5-2).

Phase one (luminal).   Two criteria must be satisfied in the intestinal lumen for successful absorption of cholesterol. One, cholesterol must be present as unesterified or free cholesterol.[5] Two, cholesterol, a highly nonpolar, water insoluble lipid, must be solubilized in molecular aggregates called micelles.[6]

The cholesterol that enters the intestinal lumen from the bile, from the cells lining the digestive tract, and 85 to 90 percent of the cholesterol from the diet is unesterified. The 10 to 15 percent from the diet, which enters the lumen as cholesterol ester, undergoes hydrolysis; hydrolysis is catalyzed by the enzyme cholesterol esterase, present in pancreatic juice, to yield free cholesterol and fatty acid. This enzyme has been purified and fully characterized in the rat, and is secreted as an inactive subunit that undergoes aggregation and activation in the presence of the specific bile salt,

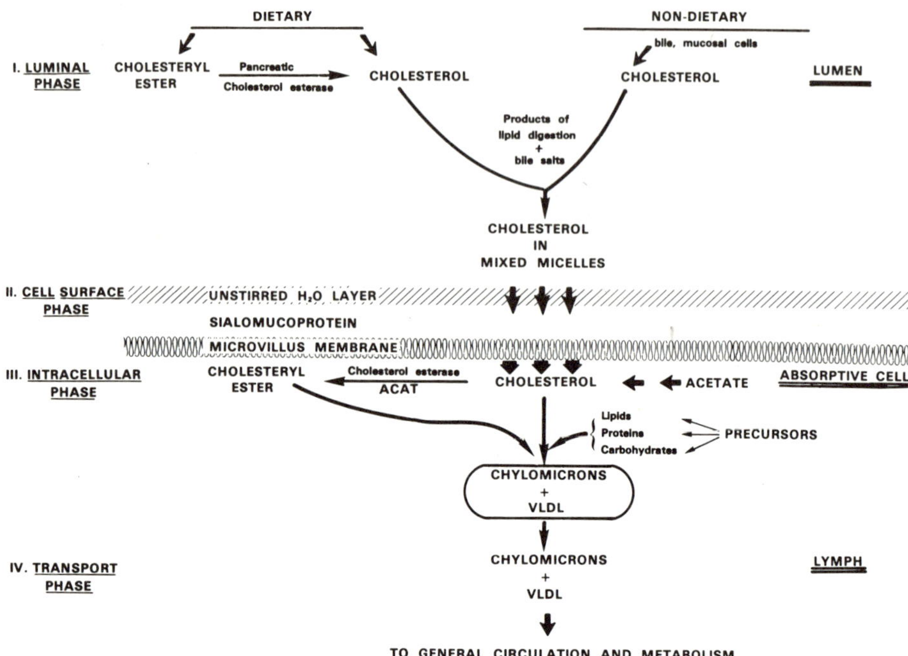

Fig. 5-2.   Schematic representation of cholesterol absorption.

taurocholate.[7] Physiologically, the interaction of the pancreatic enzyme and taurocholic acid occurs in the proximal small intestine.

The solubilization in micelles of luminal free cholesterol is an integrated process that requires bile salts and is optimal in the presence of dietary fat. Bile salts are unique detergents present in the lumen of the small intestine in all vertebrates. The two primary bile salts in humans and most experimental animals are the taurine and/or glycine conjugates of cholic and chenodeoxycholic acids (Fig. 5-3). Their special detergent action resides in the possession of both nonpolar (hydrophobic) and polar (hydrophilic) regions that correspond to similar regions in the fat they solubilize. Their initial detergent function is to emulsify dietary fat (triglycerides, phospholipids), which provides substrates in smaller particulate size which the lipolytic enzymes of pancreatic juice act on. The products of dietary fat lipolysis are monoglycerides, fatty acids, and lysophosphatides (Fig. 5-3). These lipolytic products largely explain the role of dietary fat as an aid to cholesterol absorption by amplifying a second detergent function of bile salts, that is, solubilization of cholesterol in bile salt micelles. The mechanism by which other lipids increase solubilization of cholesterol in the micelle has not been elucidated; however, they play a major role in effecting this process. For example, one molecule of cholesterol is solubilized per 12 molecules of taurocholate in a monoglyceride-containing micelle; that ratio is 1 to 25 in the absence of monoglyceride. In general, monoglycerides and phosphatides expand the nonpolar core of the micelle where cholesterol is located. Variable combinations of cholesterol, fatty acids, phosphatides, and monoglycerides with bile salts are termed mixed micelles. Their structure is depicted in Figure 5-3. The physiologic occurrence of micelles was demonstrated by isolating a micellar phase containing the lipid components, from human jejunum during fat digestion.[8] This phase increases the aqueous concentration of lipolytic products from 100 to 1,000 fold, and provides for cholesterol delivery to the absorptive cell surface.[6]

Phase two (cell surface). A major but ill-defined requirement for cholesterol uptake through the luminal facing membranes (microvilli or brush border) of the intestinal absorptive cells involves the movement of cholesterol across three muco-

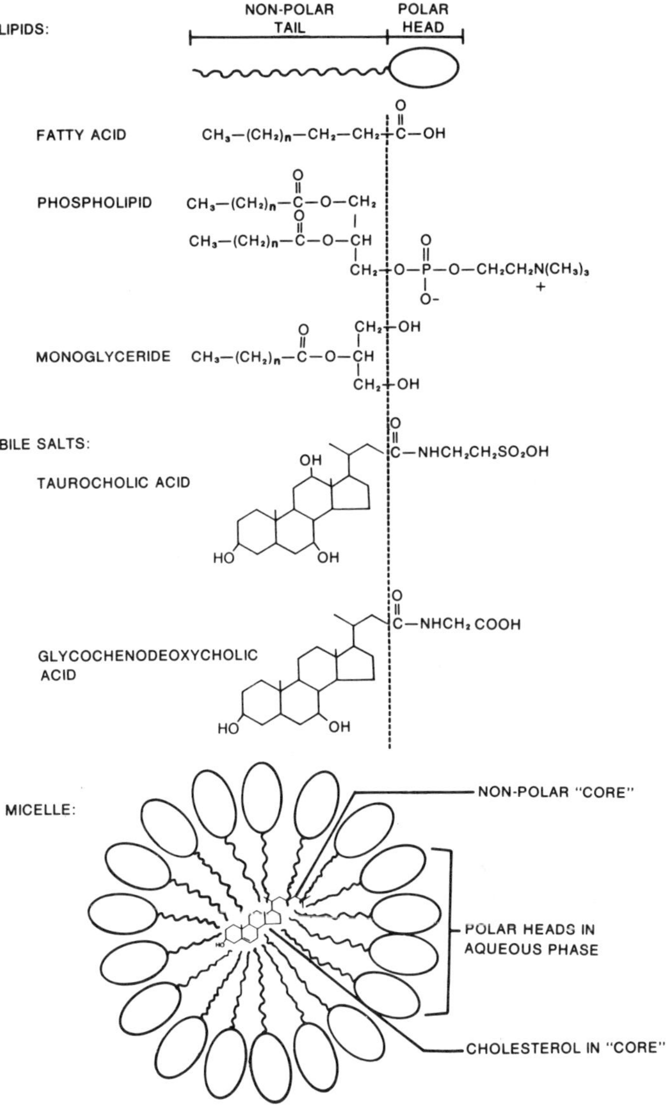

Fig. 5-3. Components and structural organization of mixed micelles.

sal cell barriers: the unstirred water layer, the sialomucoprotein layer, and the membrane itself. The unstirred water layer represents the first barrier to cholesterol uptake. This aqueous phase offers resistance to the movement of nonpolar cholesterol from the bulk luminal phase on its approach to the cell surface, with the extent of the resistance related to the thickness of the layer. The bile salt micelle overcomes the resistance to cholesterol diffusion through the unstirred water layer.[9] Cholesterol binds to the mucoproteins of the sialomucoprotein layer; such binding can be reversed by micellar concentrations of bile salts.[10] The significance of this layer in the overall resistance to cholesterol uptake is undetermined. The final barrier to cholesterol uptake is the cell surface membrane. The membrane lipids, mainly amphiphilic, form an organized bilayer structure, which includes protein. In rabbit jejunum, this membrane is relatively polar. The total resistance to cholesterol uptake is, therefore, the sum of the three barriers. The driving force that opposes this resistance is a function of the concentration of cholesterol in the lumen relative to that in the cell cytoplasm, which interfaces with the cell surface membrane.

The physiochemical state of the cholesterol reaching the membrane and during the time of uptake has been studied. Evidence dictates against the uptake of the intact cholesterol-containing micelle.[11] Alternatively, cholesterol in a monomolecular state may either be taken up from the micelle during its "collision" with the membrane or when the aqueous phase comes into contact with the membrane.[9] The latter possibility is favored. There is evidence neither of a requirement for specific binding sites on the membrane for cholesterol uptake nor for energy.

Phase three (intracellular).   Two criteria must be satisfied in the intestinal cells for successful exit of cholesterol into lymph. First, the free cholesterol that enters from the lumen must be largely (70 to 90 percent) esterified with fatty acids.[5] Second, the cholesterol ester must be assembled with other lipids and specific proteins to form lipoprotein packages (see Chapter 3).

Efficient cholesterol esterification is important and probably essential to cholesterol transport into the lymph. Two enzymatic activities in the intestinal mucosa are candidates for this role: cholesterol esterase (CE'ase) and acyl coenzyme A: cholesterol acyl transferase (ACAT). The reactions catalyzed by each are shown in Fig. 5-4.

CE'ase is secreted in the pancreatic juice,[5] is protected against proteolysis while in the lumen by taurocholic acid,[5] and is taken up by the absorptive cells[12,13] that line the midvillus and villus-tip region of the proximal small intestine.[13] In a broken cell preparation, CE'ase is found in the soluble fraction, and displays maximal esterifying activity at pH 6.2. The activity in vivo and in vitro is dependent on cholic acid or its conjugates (glycine, taurine).[5] The pancreas is the source of the intestinal CE'ase as demonstrated by the finding that esterifying activity and immunocytochemical staining for the enzyme are lost from the mucosa of experimental animals that have undergone pancreatectomy or surgical diversion of pancreatic juice.[5,12,13] The physiologic importance of pancreatic juice as a regulator of cholestrol absorption is apparent from studies in both humans and experimental animals. In pancreatectomized humans, plasma cholesterol levels decrease to about half of presurgery values. On administration of pancreatin, a freeze-dried prepara-

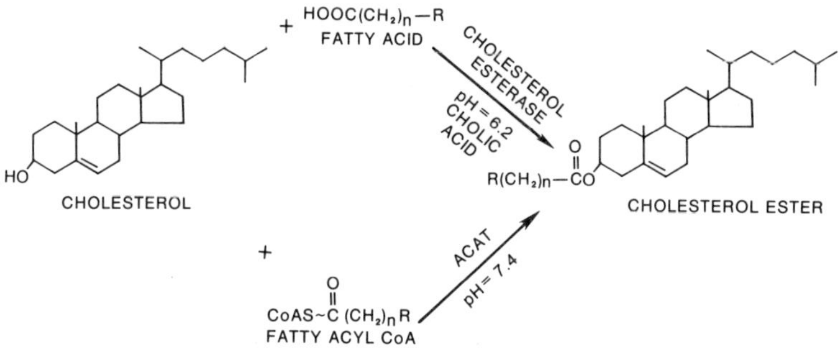

Fig. 5-4. Cholesterol esterification reactions in the intestinal mucosa.

tion of pancreas, plasma cholesterol levels are restored to normal.[14] Pancreatic cholesterol esterase has been demonstrated in the rat[15] as the important component in juice for mucosal esterification and absorption of cholesterol. In this study, the activity of cholesterol esterification enzymes within the intestinal mucosa and cholesterol absorption were compared in lymph-fistula rats in which pancreatic juice had been surgically diverted and replaced by duodenal infusion of either complete pancreatic juice, pancreatic juice devoid of cholesterol esterase (immunoprecipitated), or physiologic saline. Cholesterol absorption and mucosal cholesterol esterase activity were not detectable in the juice-diverted rats nor in the rats that were infused with either cholesterol-esterase–deficient juice or saline. Both processes were restored to control levels in rats infused with complete pancreatic juice. The activity of mucosal ACAT was not altered from normal in any of the experimental conditions.

Intestinal ACAT activity is a product of the mucosal cells. This enzyme is most active in the middle third of small intestine and in cells isolated from the crypt zones.[16] In a broken cell preparation, ACAT is localized in the microsomal fraction and displays maximal activity in vitro over the broad pH range of 6.4 to 7.4.[17] The in vitro activity is inhibited by bile salts. Thus, ACAT is concentrated in cells that are not involved in the absorption of luminal cholesterol; is inhibited by bile salts, which are obligatory for cholesterol absorption and cholesterol-esterase activity; and is unaffected by the removal of pancreatic juice, which is inhibitory to cholesterol absorption. For these reasons, a significant role for ACAT in the absorption of luminal sources of cholesterol is questionable, while such a role is well-founded for cholesterol esterase.

The newly formed cholesterol esters are assembled with other lipids and proteins to form lipoproteins (Chapter 3, Table 3-2). Primarily, two lipoproteins contain these cholesterol esters, chylomicrons and very low density lipoprotein(s) (VLDL). Qualitatively, the two are similar: Both contain a core of nonpolar lipids (cholesterol esters, triglycerides) and a surface coat of both polar lipids (cholesterol, phospholipids) and specific apoproteins (primarily B_{small} [B_{48}]), A-I, A-IV).[18] Quantitatively, the lipoproteins differ in the amount of lipid carried per particle and in their lipid protein ratio, accounting for the lower density of chylomicrons relative to VLDL.

Lipoprotein synthesis and secretion require a sequential participation of several subcellular organelles. The organelles are organized functionally to synthesize the lipid and protein components and add carbohydrate in proper sequence and topographically to provide an avenue by which lipoproteins reach secretory sites on the cell surface membrane. In the synthetic process, fatty acids are re-esterified with monoglycerides to form triglycerides, with lysophosphatides to form phospholipids, and with cholesterol to form cholesterol esters. These reactions are associated with the smooth endoplasmic reticulum.[19] The resynthesized lipids are joined by apoproteins synthesized in the rough endoplasmic reticulum. Of the three major intestinal apoproteins, B_{small} must be added, since it is required in some manner for lipoprotein secretion. The lipid-apoprotein complex undergoes final processing in the Golgi apparatus, which may include glycosylation. In the secretory process, the smooth and rough endoplasmic reticulum and the Golgi apparatus, in this order, are regarded as a more or less continuous tubular channel that not only contains the synthetic machinery described above, but also traverses the length of the cell.[20] Near the plasma membrane, the Golgi membranes are pinched off to form secretory vesicles containing either nascent chylomicrons or VLDL. These secretory vesicles fuse with the basolateral plasma membrane and release the lipoproteins.

The contribution of chylomicrons and VLDL to cholesterol transport from the intestine varies with dietary state (see Chapter 3). During fasting, cholesterol is equally divided between the two lipoproteins. During fat absorption, when chylomicron secretion increases, cholesterol shifts toward greater chylomicron transport. Not only dietary fat load but also the unsaturation of the fatty acids in the dietary fat enhances this shift. In addition to these dietary variables, there is evidence that sex differences influence the partition of cholesterol between the two transport forms.

Phase four (transport).   Cholesterol-containing lipoproteins are secreted by intestinal cells into the spaces between the cells. Then they penetrate, first, the basement membrane and, second, the lymphatic lacteals found in the center of the lamina propria of each intestinal villus. From the intestinal lymphatics, they are transported through the thoracic duct to the blood where metabolism begins.

Biosynthesis.   Cholesterol biosynthesis is a process common to all body tissues. The liver and the intestine are the most active and are calculated to contribute 82 percent and 11.4 percent of the whole body sterol synthesis, respectively.[21] The major steps in the common biosynthetic pathway are represented in Figure 5-5. Acetate is the starting substrate.

There are several controls over biosynthesis. The pathway is feedback-regulated by its end product, cholesterol. This control is exerted on the rate-limiting enzyme, HMG-CoA reductase, which converts β-hydroxy-β-methylglutaryl CoA (HMG-CoA) to mevalonate. Additional controls over this step in the pathway vary with the specific tissues. For example, in the liver the absorption of dietary cholesterol is inhibitory, whereas in the intestine the extent of inhibition varies with animal species with minimal or no effect in humans.[22] In addition, cholesterol from the plasma in lipoprotein form (LDL) inhibits biosynthesis in the rat intestine[23] and perhaps in the human intestine. Similarly, cholesterol biosynthesis is inhibited in

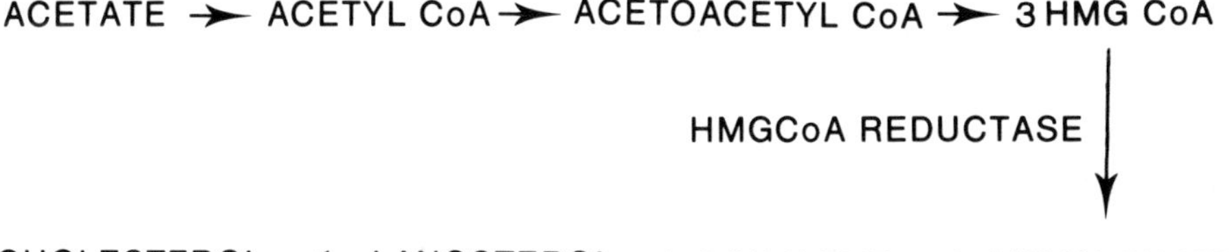

Fig. 5-5.   Outline of cholesterol biosynthesis. Only the major intermediates are shown.

other extrahepatic tissues by lipoprotein cholesterol delivered from the plasma. Fasting reduces hepatic synthesis of cholesterol but produces a much lesser effect in extrahepatic tissues. Conversely, either reduced caloric intake or high fat diets, which decrease fatty acid synthesis and increase catabolism, increase cholesterol synthesis in the liver and extrahepatic tissues.

In addition to dietary factors, bile acids inhibit cholesterol synthesis in the liver and to an uncertain extent in the intestine. Bile acids are synthesized exclusively in the liver to form a bile acid pool which is secreted in the biliary secretion, efficiently reabsorbed in the intestine, and recirculated to the liver (the enterohepatic circulation). Thus, the liver and intestine are regularly exposed to bile acid flux. In the liver, the inhibitory action of the bile acids on cholesterogenesis has been conceptualized as a double feedback process in which the returning bile acids inhibit the conversion of cholesterol to bile acids, and the spared cholesterol inhibits its own synthesis in the feedback manner described previously. In the intestine, which does not synthesize bile acids, an inhibitory effect cannot be explained in a similar way. In fact, while biliary diversion is reported to increase intestinal cholesterogenesis and bile restoration is reported to suppress the increase,[21] suppression of cholesterol synthesis occurs only under conditions in which HMG-CoA reductase activity exceeds basal levels, and then only to and not below basal levels.[24]

Cholesterol biosynthesis in the liver predominates in parenchymal cells from which cholesterol may be excreted either in the bile or secreted as lipoproteins into the blood. Cholesterol biosynthesis in the intestine occurs in the ileum in both crypt and villus cells.[25] It is assumed that the biosynthesized cholesterol not used for membrane biogenesis is processed in the same qualitative manner, with respect to an esterification requirement and lipoprotein transport (as described earlier for luminal cholesterol), while in the mucosal cells and after secretion. The evidence suggests, however, that luminal cholesterol and biosynthesized cholesterol exist in seperate intestinal pools,[26] and that their quantitative distribution between the chylomicron and the intestinal VLDL differs.[27]

Cholesterol Removal

Conversion to Bile Acids.   The conversion of cholesterol to bile acids (acidic sterols) contributes about 40 percent to the total sterol output and represents a daily removal of 250 to 600 mg of sterol in the human. This loss of bile acids is matched by an equal synthesis of them. The liver is the site of synthesis, and the major steps in the pathway are shown schematically in Fig. 5-6. Cholesterol which originates from absorption or biosynthesis is the starting substrate. The initial conversion of cholesterol to 7α-hydroxycholesterol is catalyzed by the rate-limiting enzyme 7α-hydroxylase. At this point, the pathway branches, with one limb giving rise to cholic acid (a trihydroxy bile acid) and the other to chenodeoxycholic acid (a dihydroxy bile acid), the primary bile acids. They feedback to inhibit their own synthesis, are produced in about equal amounts, and are conjugated with taurine or glycine prior to secretion. The glycine conjugates predominate in the human. The newly synthesized bile acids join the bile acid pool (2 to 4 g) and are concentrated in the gallbladder. After a meal, the bile acid pool is expelled into the intestinal lumen, is mostly reabsorbed in the intestine, and is returned via the portal circulation to the liver; the process is repeated one to two times (enterohepatic circulation). If three meals are eaten per day, this enterohepatic circulation represents six to ten cycles or 12 to 40 g of bile acid entering the intestine. Clearly, intestinal reabsorption of bile acids is efficient since 5 percent or less of the bile acids are excreted. The prevailing view is that reabsorption of bile acids occurs predominately by an active transport mechanism confined to the ileum. This position needs reconsideration in light of information that demonstrates in vitro and in vivo that total reabsorption is about equally divided between the proximal and distal small intestine of the rat, and is predominantly a passive process.[28] Only small amounts of bile acids may reach the terminal ileum, where they may be actively reabsorbed or may undergo bacterial alterations. Alterations include deconjugation of glycine or taurine or removal of the hydroxyl group from cholic and chenodeoxycholic acids (see Fig. 5-6), which gives rise to deoxycholic and litho-

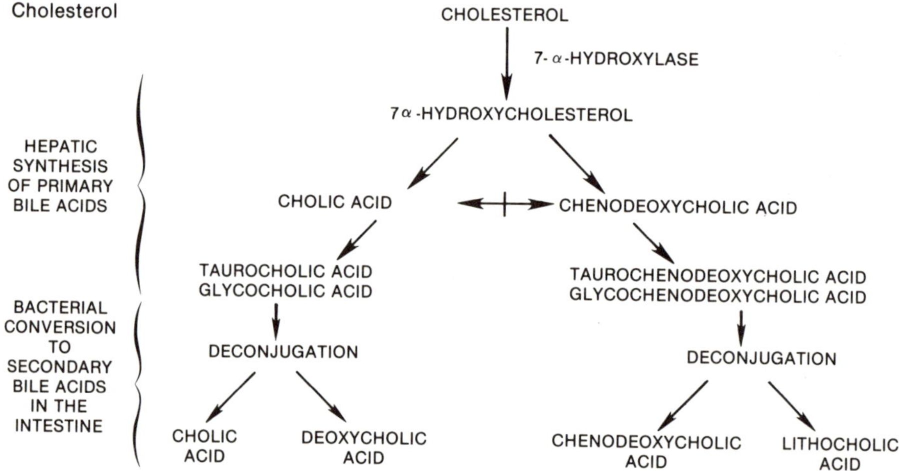

Fig. 5-6.   Outline of the biosynthesis of primary and secondary bile acids. (Reproduced with permission from Vahouny GV, Treadwell CR: Cholesterol: Some aspects of its metabolism and balance in man. In Feldman EB (ed): Nutrition and Cardiovascular Disease, New York, Appleton-Century-Crofts, 1976.)

cholic acids, respectively. These products, termed secondary bile acids, are reabsorbed, and thus they also become a part of the bile acid pool. In this regard, deoxycholic acid predominates. Thus, cholic, chenodeoxycholic, and deoxycholic acids are the major human bile acids, and are secreted in bile in an approximate ratio of 1.1: 1.0: 0.6. Hepatic removal of bile acids is also efficient, and allows for a plasma concentration of bile acid of less than 0.3 mg/100 ml.

Unabsorbed Sterol.   Fecal excretion of unabsorbed sterol accounts for about 60 percent of the total sterol loss from the body. The sources, named earlier, are dietary, biliary, and cellular. A major portion of the nonabsorbed luminal cholesterol is excreted chemically altered as coprostanol.

BALANCE OF PROCESSES THAT ADD AND REMOVE CHOLESTEROL

Whole-body cholesterol balance is dependent on total sterol addition equaling total sterol removal. Cholesterol absorption by the intestine and biosynthesis by the tissues add cholesterol. Fecal excretion of luminal sources of cholesterol and of bile acids made from cholesterol in the liver remove cholesterol. Each of the body tissues contributes to whole body sterol balance, and each has developed sensitive criteria for regulating the addition and removal of their cholesterol. With regard to cholesterol addition, the cholesterol esters from absorption (luminal, biosynthesized) and from liver biosynthesis are secreted in lipoprotein forms, which are delivered via the plasma to the tissues. Successful addition of cholesterol esters to the tissues from lipoprotein sources requires a specific lipoprotein-apoprotein composition and an ability, which resides with the tissues, to interiorize the cholesterol-ester–containing lipoprotein. This interiorization occurs through cell-surface receptors (high affinity and low affinity) that recognize specific apoproteins on the circulating lipoproteins via receptor-mediated endocytosis. As a consequence of interiorization, the recipient tissues (cells) down-regulate both their biosynthesis of cholesterol and, in many cases, their cell-surface receptors that recognize the cholesterol-ester–carrying lipoproteins. With regard to cholesterol removal, the tissues also have a mechanism for delivering nonmetabolized or excess cholesterol via the plasma lipoprotein(s) to the liver for excretion.[18] The capacity of the cholesterol-accepting lipoprotein(s) is also dependent on the apoprotein composition, and lipoprotein uptake by the liver is largely dependent on specific receptor-mediated endocytosis.

Plasma Lipoproteins That Add Cholesterol

Chylomicrons, VLDL, LDL, and HDL add cholesterol to the tissues. Chylomicrons and $VLDL_{intestinal}$ are the cholesterol-ester–carrying lipoproteins of intestinal origin. In the following discussion, the metabolism of $VLDL_{intestinal}$ is not distinguished from that for chylomicrons.

Prior to delivering their cholesterol esters to the tissues (liver for intestinal lipoproteins), the intestinal lipoproteins undergo essential alterations in the lymph and in the blood (see also Chapter 3). Additional apoproteins are acquired that facilitate removal of most of their triglycerides through the action of lipoprotein lipase. Accompanying the loss of core triglycerides, some surface lipids, some C apoprotein, and most of the A apoproteins are removed to produce remnant particles that are recognized and efficiently removed by the liver. Liver uptake of these remnants occurs primarily through a specific receptor that recognizes only the E apoprotein.[26] The chylomicron pathway is depicted in Fig. 5-7. Alterations and removal are rapid processes that require only a few minutes. To re-emphasize, the cholesterol from intestinal sources is added exclusively to the liver. In the liver, the cholesterol may be removed by excretion in the bile, as described earlier, or may be secreted in lipoprotein form into the blood, as described below, to add cholesterol to the peripheral tissues.

VLDL is a cholesterol-ester–carrying lipoprotein of liver origin. VLDL cholesterol may come from cholesterol of intestinal origin that has entered the liver, from cholesterol biosynthesis in the liver, and, to a large extent, from other plasma lipoproteins, such as HDL (see below). The organization of the synthetic and secretory processes for VLDL in liver duplicate those described earlier for chylomicrons in the intestine. The composition of the nascent liver VLDL differs from that of the intestinal products. The major apoproteins are B_{large} (rather than intestinal B_{small}), Cs, and E. The distinct apoprotein B_{large} is required for VLDL secretion. After secretion and while in the blood, the VLDL acquire additional C apoproteins.[29] This permits removal of triglyceride by the process, and at the sites, described for intestinal lipoproteins. VLDL remnant particles after a few hours lose all their apoproteins except B_{large} and gain cholesterol esters (see Reverse Cholesterol Transport, below). The resulting particles, low-density lipoproteins (LDL),

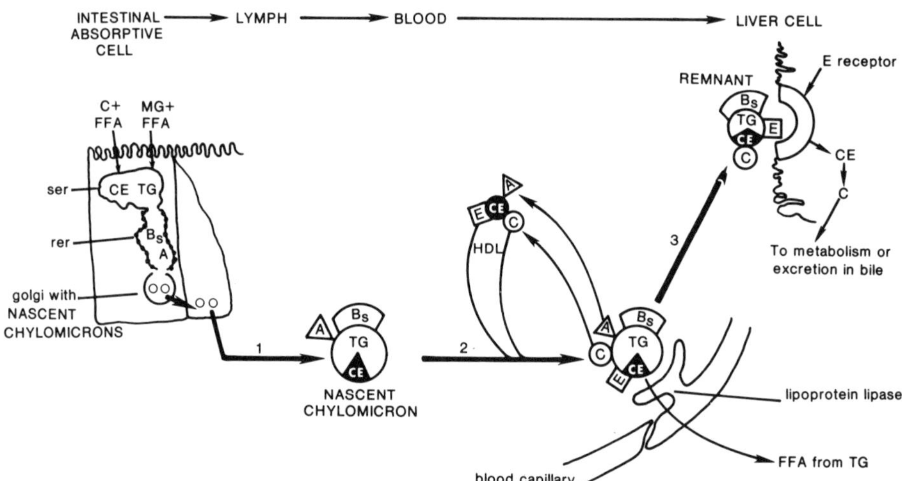

Fig. 5-7. Schematic representation of chylomicron pathway. Abbreviations: CE, cholesterol ester; C, cholesterol; MG, monoglyceride; FFA, free fatty acid; TG, triglyceride; A, A apoproteins; C, C apoproteins; E, E apoproteins; B_s, B_{small}; ser, smooth endoplasmic reticulum; rer, rough endoplasmic reticulum; HDL, high density lipoprotein. See text for explanation of the scheme.

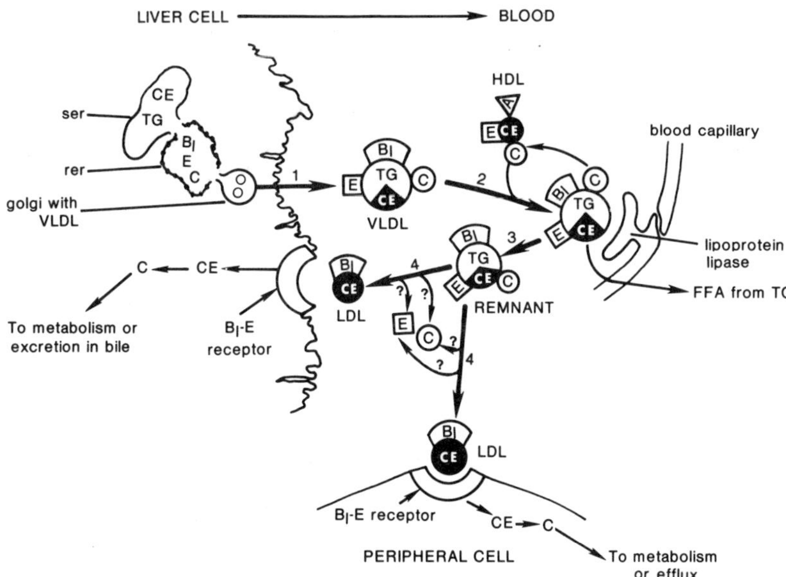

Fig. 5-8.   Schematic representation of VLDL-LDL pathways. Abbreviations: CE, cholesterol ester; C, cholesterol; TG, triglyceride; FFA, free fatty acid; A, A apoproteins; C, C apoproteins; E, E apoproteins; B_L, B_{large}; ser, smooth endoplasmic reticulum; rer, rough endoplasmic reticulum; VLDL, very low density lipoprotein; LDL, low-density lipoprotein; HDL, high-density lipoprotein. See text for explanation of the scheme.

are taken up over a period of days and in about equal amounts by extrahepatic tissues and liver. The uptake occurs through a high affinity receptor that recognizes apoproteins B_{large} and E, through low-affinity LDL receptors, and through pinocytosis.[29] The VLDL-LDL pathways that involve uptake through the high-affinity receptor are depicted in Fig. 5-8.

High-density lipoprotein(s) (HDL) also delivers cholesterol esters to extrahepatic tissues for their utilization and to liver for excretion (see Reverse Cholesterol Transport, below). HDL are biosynthesized in the liver and intestine in a nascent form. The nascent HDL contain a bilayer of phospholipids coated by apoproteins A-I, A-II, and Cs which are secreted or collected from the triglyceride-rich lipoproteins as they undergo catabolism in the plasma (see Chapter 3). The HDL involved in this function contain no apoprotein E and have been termed typical HDL or HDL–without apo-E (a component of the HDL_2 and HDL_3 subclasses).[30] In preparation for delivery of cholesterol esters to extrahepatic tissues that need cholesterol, the typical HDL must acquire excess cholesterol from other extrahepatic tissues. The acquired cholesterol undergoes esterification. The esterification is probably catalyzed by lecithin-cholesterol acyl transferase (LCAT), an enzyme that transfers the fatty acid from HDL phospholipid (lecithin) to HDL cholesterol. The apoprotein A-I that activates this enzyme is a part of HDL. As the content of esterified cholesterol increases, the typical HDL acquire apoprotein E from other plasma lipoproteins and become HDL–with apo-E (called HDL_1 in humans, and HDL_c in several animal species — a component of HDL_2 subclass).[30] Extrahepatic tissues with a need for cholesterol can interiorize the HDL–with apo-E through their B-E receptors, which are expressed under this condition. Extrahepatic tissues with excess cholesterol will have down-regulated their B-E receptors, and they disregard this cholesterol ester source.

Three pathways involving chylomicrons, VLDL, and HDL have been described for adding cholesterol esters to the tissues. As a consequence of such addition, the cholesterol biosynthetic machinery is damped by inhibition of HMG-CoA reductase, and the number of specific receptors on the cell surface is decreased.[31] These are coordinated mechanisms for regulating the cholesterol content of the tissues and maintaining cholesterol balance.

Plasma Lipoproteins That Remove Cholesterol

Reverse Cholesterol Transport.   The usual HDL–without apo-E serve a dual function: they accept cholesterol from some extrahepatic tissues and deliver it to others after becoming HDL–with apo-E.[30] In addition, and perhaps most importantly in terms of cholesterol balance, HDL accept cholesterol from extrahepatic tissues, esterify cholesterol, and participate in reverse cholesterol transport. In this role, the HDL may deliver cholesterol esters directly to the liver or may shuttle them to other lipoproteins that make the liver delivery. In the former case, the HDL–with apo-E are removed through the specfic E-receptor, which recognizes chylomicron remnants, or by the B-E receptor, which recognizes LDL. The cholesterol esters are then hydrolyzed, and the cholesterol can be excreted in the bile as a means of maintaining whole-body sterol balance.

In the latter case, nascent HDL acquire from the plasma additional apoproteins, including A-I, the LCAT activator, LCAT, the cholesterol esterifying enzyme, and apoprotein D, which rapidly transfers cholesterol esters from the HDL subfraction to recipient lipoproteins. This HDL subfraction with all these components has been called the cholesterol transfer complex.[29] The cholesterol for the HDL subfraction comes from the membranes of cells in peripheral tissues and from the surface coat of other lipoproteins. The conversion of free sterol to cholesterol ester, and its transfer to other lipoproteins, creates a gradient that favors continual removal of cellular and lipoprotein cholesterol.[29] The cholesterol-ester recipients are chylomicron remnants and LDL. These particles are cleared by the liver via the E and B-E receptors, respectively, and the cholesterol from their component cholesterol esters may be ultimately excreted in the bile.[29] The quantitative significance of these two potential mechanisms for reverse cholesterol transport to the liver for excretion may depend on the metabolic state, and is very likely to vary from species to species.

EXCESS DIETARY CHOLESTEROL, POSITIVE
CHOLESTEROL BALANCE, AND ATHEROSCLEROSIS

Diets high in cholesterol or in cholesterol and fat regularly cause atherosclerosis in experimental animals including dogs, rabbits, swine, and monkeys. In humans, a decisive effect of dietary cholesterol on plasma cholesterol levels has been demonstrated in a series of controlled experiments.[32] Elevated plasma cholesterol correlates significantly with the incidence of atherosclerosis and heart attack in human population groups (Table 5-1). This correlation and the observed development of atherosclerosis with large dietary intake of cholesterol in the experimental animal, suggest that excessive dietary cholesterol predisposes to atherosclerosis and coronary heart disease. The relationship of dietary cholesterol to incidence of coronary heart disease is shown in Fig. 5-9.

The concept that cholesterol addition to the body or to a particular tissue (such as arterial wall) is balanced by an equal loss seems to fail in the face of a large dietary cholesterol load, that is, addition exceeds removal. In support of this, studies in humans suggest that cholesterol biosynthesis is largely refractory to inhibitory control by increases in dietary cholesterol, and, further, that the fecal excretion of bile acids, cholesterol, and coprostanol fails to increase substantially after the ingestion of increased dietary cholesterol.

Since cholesterol is added to and removed from tissues by lipoproteins, studies have been undertaken to determine how dietary cholesterol alters lipoproteins, both quantitatively and qualitatively, and how these alterations may be atherogenic.

Table 5-1   Total Plasma Cholesterol and Coronary Heart Disease[a]

Plasma Cholesterol (mg/dl)	CHD Events	Group Size	Deaths (%)
<160	10	1,007	1.0
160–179	9	1,157	0.8
180–199	25	1,525	1.6
200–219	32	1,682	1.9
220–239	31	1,480	2.1
240–259	29	1,181	2.5
260–279	29	806	3.6
280–299	26	551	4.7
≥ 300	60	662	9.1

[a]Reproduced with permission, from Blackburn H: Diet-lipid–atherosclerosis relationship: epidemiological evidence and public health implications. In Gotto, AM, Smith LL, Allen B (eds): Atherosclerosis, V. New York, Springer-Verlag, 1980.

Quantitative Changes in Lipoproteins

A relation between dietary cholesterol and increased levels in LDL cholesterol and slight increases in HDL cholesterol has been shown in humans. In one study, 25 subjects who had been consuming a typical American diet high in cholesterol and saturated fat were given cholesterol-free diets for 3 to 4 weeks, and then 1,000 mg of dietary cholesterol (egg yolk) per day for another 3 to 4 weeks in otherwise identical diets. The average plasma cholesterols in all subjects on the cholesterol-free diet was 211 mg/dl and increased to 247 mg/dl on the cholesterol-containing diet. When the dietary cholesterol effect was compared in normal and hypercholesterolemic subjects, the increased plasma cholesterol was mostly in LDL, with a slight increase in HDL (Fig. 5-10).[32]

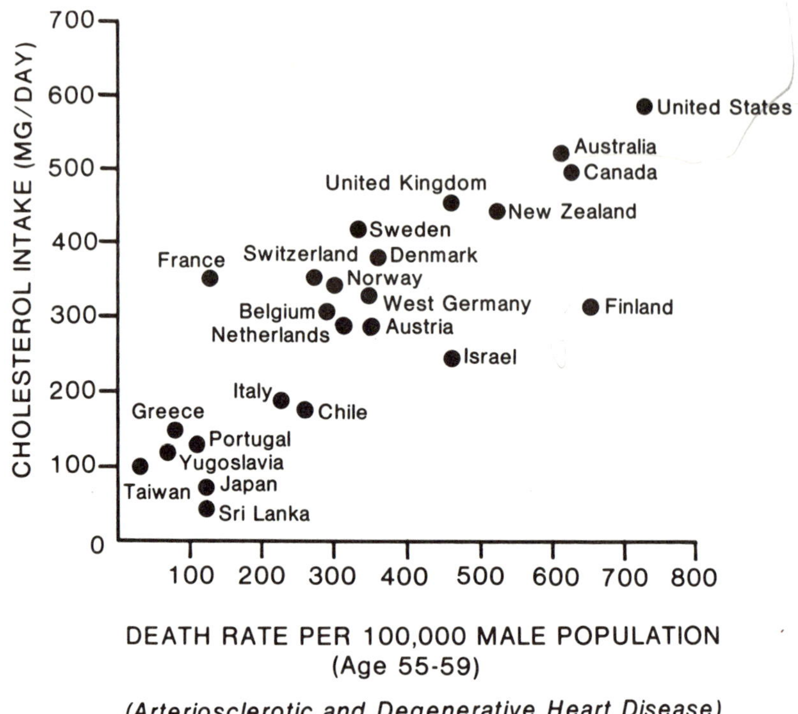

Fig. 5-9.   Relationship between dietary cholesterol and death rate from coronary heart disease. (Reproduced with permission from Connor WE: The relationship of hyperlipoproteinemia to atherosclerosis: the decisive role of dietary cholesterol and fat. In Scanu AM (ed): The Biochemistry of Atherosclerosis. New York, Marcel Dekker Inc. ©1979.)

Qualitative Changes in Lipoproteins

Diets high in cholesterol and fat produce changes in specific lipoproteins in experimental animals and in humans.[30] The changes are similar among the species but may vary in extent. They include the production of a new lipoprotein, called β-VLDL, and alterations in the composition of LDL and HDL (see Chapter 3).

β-VLDL is produced in a variety of animal species and humans fed high-cholesterol or high-cholesterol and high-fat diets. The origin of these particles is uncertain, and may vary with species. It has been suggested that they arise from chylomicron remnants and that they are hepatic in origin. Whatever their origin in the various species, they are physically, chemically, and metabolically similar, are rich in cholesterol ester, and contain apoproteins B_{large} and E.

Similarly, HDL–with apo-E (HDL_c, HDL_1) is increased with cholesterol feeding in all species studied, including humans. While the E increase seen with cholesterol feeding progresses with plasma cholesterol concentration, HDL–with apo-E appears even when cholesterol feeding does not elevate the plasma cholesterol level.[30] The changes in these lipoproteins produced by dietary cholesterol are subtle but may be important over the decades that are required for the development of atherosclerosis in the human.

Studies using experimental animals, in which the progression of atherosclerosis has been accelerated, have led to hypotheses that offer reasonable explanations for how the diet-induced changes in lipoproteins are atherogenic. An early event is the deposition of cholesterol ester.

β-VLDL are atherogenic. β-VLDL can be internalized by the extrahepatic tissues with B-E receptors, including the smooth muscle cells of arterial walls. Historically, these cells have been considered the precursor of the foam cells seen in atherogenesis. However, an accumulation of cholesterol in cultured smooth muscle cells is difficult to demonstrate. While they may behave differently in culture than in vivo, or may behave differently in the atherosclerotic lesion, their failure to become lipid laden (only 2- to 4-fold increases in cholesterol ester, since they apparently down-regulated their B-E receptors), has led to the suggestion that other cell types may be the progenitors of foam cells. In particular, macrophage-monocytes in the arterial wall internalize β-VLDL (not through a B-E receptor) and accumulate tremendous amounts (20 to 160 fold) of cholesterol ester, and then they resemble foam cells.[30] Their receptors for β-VLDL are not down-regulated by cholesterol accumulation. Presently, it is not possible to point to or exclude a particular cell type as having a role in atherogenesis, although the case for the macrophage-monocyte is attractive.

LDL are atherogenic, and this is best demonstrated in the genetic disorder familial hypercholesterolemia (see Chapter 3), in which the B-E receptors are missing on all tissues, LDL cholesterol levels in plasma increase markedly, and homozygotes generally die during the first two decades with severe atherosclerotic disease.[31] Despite much study, the precise mechanism of LDL-colesterol–induced atherosclerosis remains unclear. One postulate is that LDL-cholesterol is taken up

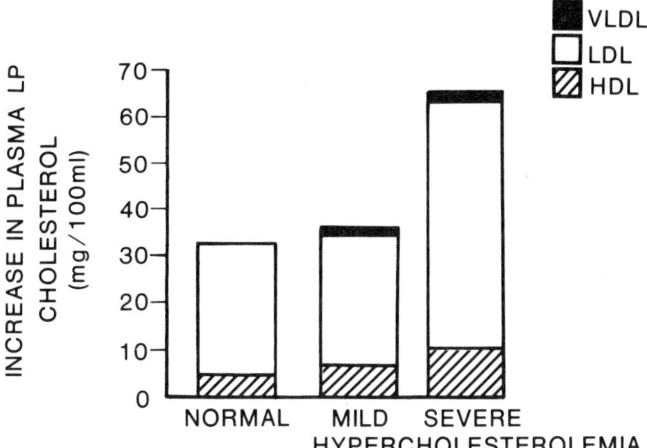

Fig. 5-10.   Changes in VLDL, LDL, and HDL levels with a cholesterol feeding of 1000 mg. (Reproduced with permission from Connor WE, Connor SJ: The dietary treatment of hyperlipidemia. Med Clin North Am. 66(2):490, 1982.)

by scavenger cells in the arterial wall. Another hypothesis is that the increased size of these LDL may promote a greater accumulation of cholesterol in smooth muscle cells than do normal LDL. Also, LDL may undergo some modification in vivo that allows their massive uptake by macrophage-monocytes. Another possible role of LDL found in the atherosclerotic lesions may be stimulation of cell growth and proliferation, characteristics of the atherogenic process. Clearly more study is required to confirm or discard these theories.

HDL are antiatherogenic, with an inverse relationship between HDL levels and coronary artery disease.[33] Typical HDL that accept cholesterol from the tissues become HDL–with apo-E. These are interiorized by the E and B-E receptors of liver, and this process promotes cholesterol excretion, an antiatherogenic event. In the face of a high dietary cholesterol intake and the subsequent excessive delivery of cholesterol to the tissues by the diet-induced β-VLDL and LDL, the ratio of typical HDL to HDL–with apo-E decreases, that is, the availability of the normal acceptor of tissue cholesterol is limited. As the plasma cholesterol increases, the ratio shifts more heavily in the direction of HDL–with apo-E. Thus, these diet-induced changes in lipoproteins appear to favor excessive addition of cholesterol to the tissues (arterial wall) without compensatory removal, and they present a strong case for justifying alterations in the diet that are aimed at lowering the intake of cholesterol and saturated fats.

DIETARY TREATMENT OF HYPERCHOLESTEROLEMIA

The concept has been introduced that a single diet may be used in the treatment of all types of hyperlipidemia and that dietary treatment will almost without exception result in improvement of these disorders,[32] and especially will lower plasma cholesterol (see Chapter 10). This "alternative" diet is low in cholesterol, saturated fat, and total fat, and is high in complex carbohydrates and fiber, compared with the typical American diet. The diet is also lower in calories but is designed to supply the essential micronutrients, that is, vitamins and minerals. The suggested alternative diet and the typical American diet are compared in Table 5-2. The rationale for these dietary changes emerges from studies that demonstrate effects of each dietary component on the quantity or quality of the serum lipoproteins that transport cholesterol.

The effect of lowered intake of dietary cholesterol was presented in the previous section. The effect of dietary fat on the plasma cholesterol level is dependent on the quantity and quality consumed (see Chapter 3). Dietary fat increases cholesterol absorption and plasma cholesterol levels. Saturated fatty acids (no double bonds) increase LDL concentrations and elevate plasma cholesterol, and monounsaturated fatty acids (one double bond) do not alter plasma cholesterol levels; polyunsaturated (essential) fatty acids (two or more double bonds), however, decrease LDL levels and lower plasma cholesterol. A change in diet from saturated to polyunsaturated fat increases the excretion of cholesterol and bile acids in the bile to an extent that accounts for the lowered plasma cholesterol.[32] The alternative

Table 5-2. Chemical Composition of the Present American Diet and the Alternative Diet[a]

Nutrient	American Diet	Alternative Diet (Phase III)
Cholesterol, mg/day	500	100
Fat, percent of total calories	40	20
Saturated fat, percent calories	15	5
Monounsaturated fat, percent calories	16	8
Polyunsaturated fat, percent calories	6	7
P-S value	0.4	1.3
Iodine Number	63	99
Vegetable fat, percent fat	38	75
Animal fat, percent fat	62	25
Protein, percent calories	15	15
Vegetable protein, percent protein	32	56
Animal protein, percent protein	68	44
Carbohydrate, percent calories	45	65
Starch, percent calories	22	40
Sucrose (added to food), percent calories	15	10
Fructose, glucose sucrose, lactose, maltose, percent calories (naturally present in foods)	8	15
Dietary Fiber, g	10–12	48–60
Sodium, mEq	200–300	75–100
Potassium, mEq	30–70	120–150

[a]Reproduced with permission from Connor WE, Connor SJ: The dietary treatment of hyperlipidemia. Med Clin North Am. 66(2):501, 1982.

plasma cholesterol-lowering diet suggests a polyunsaturated to saturated fatty acid ratio (P-S ratio) of 1.3 greater than the P-S ratio of 0.4 in the typical American diet, and less than a P-S ratio of 2.0, which is clearly hypocholesterolemic. Moderation in the use of polyunsaturated fats in the diet is suggested to avoid possible harmful side effects such as gallstone formation, enhanced carcinogenesis and obesity (increased caloric intake), and to avoid increased vitamin E requirements (antioxidant). Overall, the total fat content in the alternative diet is low, 20 percent, with saturated and polyunsaturated fats representing 5 to 6 percent and 6 to 8 percent of the total calories, respectively. This represents a reduction in saturated fat and a small increase in polyunsaturated fat from the typical American diet. Cholesterol is reduced to 100 mg/day. The cholesterol, total fat, and saturated fat content of common foodstuffs are given in Table 5-3. (Further information on fat content of food is provided in Chapter 10).

The carbohydrate content of the alternative diet is increased to 65 percent of total calories (up from 45 percent) to replace the 20 percent loss of calories from fat. Of this carbohydrate, complex carbohydrates (starch) are increased markedly and simple sugars (sucrose) are reduced. Such an increase in the quantity of carbohydrates has minimal effects on the level of plasma lipids and lipoproteins (see Chapter 6).

The dietary changes in protein source (that is, from animal to plant) and fiber content (cellulose, hemicellulose, lignin, and pectin—a 4- to 5-fold increase) are aimed at a lower overall consumption of cholesterol and fat, particularly saturated

Table 5.3. Cholesterol, Total Fat, and Saturated Fat Content of Various Foodstuffs[a]

	Cholesterol (mg/100 g food)	Fat (g/100 g food)	Saturated Fat (g/100 g food)
Visible Fats			
Most vegetable oils	0	100.0	13.0
Soft vegetable margarines	0	81.0	16.0
Soft shortenings	0	100.0	25.8
Butter	227	81.0	49.8
Coconut oil, palm oil, cocoa butter (chocolate)	0	100.0	74.6
Cheeses			
Count-Down, dry-curd cottage cheese, tofu (bean curd), pot cheese, low-fat cottage cheese, St. Otho	6	2.1	0.9
Cottage cheese, Lite-Line, Chef's Delight, Breeze Lite 'n' Lively, part-skim ricotta	29	24.5	4.7
Cheezola, Scandie or Min Chol Hickory Farm Lyte, Pizza Pal, Saffola American[a]	12	7.5	4.6
Green River (lower fat cheddar), part-skim mozarella, Neufchatel (lower fat cream cheese), Keil Kase, Skim American	58	18.2	10.2
Cheddar, roquefort, Swiss, Brie, jack, American cream cheese, Velveeta, cheese spreads (jars)	106	35.0	20.6
Frozen Desserts			
Water ices	0	0	0
Sherbert or frozen yogurt	4	1.2	0.8
Ice milk	14	5.1	3.2
Ice cream, 10 percent fat	40	10.6	6.6
Milk			
Skim milk (0.1 percent fat) or buttermilk	2	0.1	<0.1
1 percent milk	3	1.0	0.6
2 percent milk	6	2.0	1.2
Whole milk (3.5 percent fat)	14	3.5	2.2
Liquid nondairy creamers: store brands Cereal Blend, Coffee Rich	0	11.0	8.5
Liquid nondairy creamers: Mocha Mix, Poly Rich Mello	0	9.8	2.7
Fish			
White fish, clams, scallops, oysters and water-packed tuna	66	0.9	0.2
Shrimp, crab, lobster	112	1.7	0.2
Salmon	75	6.9	1.7
Poultry			
Chicken and turkey, no skin	87	4.9	1.3
Duck and goose, skin	91	33.4	8.0
Veal			
40 percent fat—trimmed roasts and chops, veal cutlets	99	11.4	4.7
15 percent fat—untrimmed loin roasts and chops	99	16.9	7.1
Beef, Pork, and Lamb			
10 percent fat—ground sirloin, trimmed lean beef and lamb	90	10.0	3.7
15 percent fat—ground round, untrimmed lean beef, trimmed pork	90	14.8	5.5
20 percent fat—ground chuck, untrimmed beef and lamb roasts, trimmed fatter beef and lamb	90	19.1	8.3
30 percent fat—ground beef and pork, shortribs, untrimmed, well-marbled steaks, chops (T-bone, etc.), ham	90	30.7	12.9
40 percent fat—spareribs, country-style ribs	90	38.9	10.5

(continued)

Table 5.3.   (*continued*)

	Cholesterol (mg/100 g food)	Fat (g/100 g food)	Saturated Fat (g/100 g food)
Organ Meats	300–2000	4.8	1.6
Eggs			
Whites	0	0	0
Egg substitutes	0	4.2	0
Whole	504	11.5	3.4

[a]Reproduced with permission from Connor WE, Connor SJ: The dietary treatment of hyper-lipidemia. Med Clin North Am. 66(2):506–507, 1982.

[b]Cheeses made with skim milk and vegetable oils

fat. When protein is obtained from plant sources, the associated fat is unsaturated and cholesterol is eliminated. A high fiber intake dictates a higher consumption of plant foods.[32]

It is suggested that the alternative diet be adopted in three phases to avoid abrupt changes in established diets. The phases are summarized in Table 5-4.

PLANT AND MARINE ANIMAL STEROLS: EFFECTS ON CHOLESTEROL ABSORPTION AND METABOLISM

Plant and Marine Animal Sterols

In this discussion, the absorption and metabolism of the plant and marine animal sterols per se are compared conveniently with those of cholesterol. The striking differences detailed below are surprising, considering the minor structural variations in the total group of sterols. Variations in the side-chain of the plant sterols of nutritional significance (campesterol, β-sitosterol, fucosterol, stigmasterol) distinguish them from cholesterol. These variations, respectively, consist of the addition of 24-methyl, 24-ethyl, 24-ethylidine, or 24-ethyl groups plus a double bond between carbons 22 and 23 (Fig. 5-1). Similarly, the major marine sterols (24-methylene cholesterol, 22-dehydrocholesterol, and brassicasterol) differ from cholesterol by a 24-methylidine, a double bond between carbons 22 and

Table 5-4.   Summary of the Three Phases of the Alternative Diet[a]

Phase I:	Avoid foods very high in cholesterol and saturated fat; delete egg yolk, butterfat, lard, and organ meat.
	Substitute soft margarine for butter; vegetable oils and shortening for lard; skim milk for whole milk; egg whites for whole eggs.
Phase II:	A gradual transition from using up to 16 ounces of meat a day to no more than 6 to 8 ounces a day.
	Use less fat and cheese.
	Acquire new recipes using whole grains, beans, and vegetables.
Phase III:	Eat mainly cereals, legumes, fruits, and vegetables.
	Use meat as a condiment.
	Use low-cholesterol cheeses.
	Save these foods for use only on special occasions: extra meats, regular cheese, chocolate, candy, and coconut.

[a]Reproduced with permission from Connor, WE, Connor SJ: The dietary treatment of hyper-lipidemia. Med Clin North Am. 66(2):505, 1982.

23, and the double bond plus a 24-methyl, respectively. (Cholesterol is also a major marine animal sterol.)

In general, the plant and marine animal sterols are poorly absorbed, compared with cholesterol. In the lymph fistula rat administered an acute intragastric test emulsion containing 50 mg of either cholesterol or plant sterol, the absorption of cholesterol was about 43 percent over a 24-hour lymph collection period, while the absorption of β-sitosterol, stigmasterol, and fucosterol did not exceed 5 percent.[35] In humans, the absorption of β-sitosterol is comparable to that reported in the animal studies. Campesterol absorption is equal to or greater than β-sitosterol absorption. Information is limited on the absorption of the other sterols in the human.

Similar systematic absorption studies in experimental animals have not been carried out with the individual marine animal sterols. Available evidence suggests that cholesterol and 22-dehydrocholesterol are absorbed equally well, while brassicasterol and 24-methylene cholesterol are poorly absorbed. With the exception of fucosterol, a substitution in the side chain on the 24 carbon markedly inhibits absorption of plant and marine animal sterols.

The intestinal site(s) of discrimination in the absorption of sterols has not been studied, but among the possibilities for the different sterols are the intestinal lumen, where there may be unequal distribution between the micellar and the oil phases; the intestinal lumen, where the resistance offered by the unstirred water layer, the mucoprotein coat, and/or the cell membrane may vary; inside the cell, where the essential esterification reaction may vary (there is some evidence that esterification is less efficient for the plant sterols). In vitro assays show that cholesterol is the preferred substrate for the mucosal (pancreatic) cholesterol esterase; in vivo studies show that cholesterol accumulating in the intestinal mucosa is 15 to 25 percent esterified, while β-sitosterol is entirely unesterified.[1]

Of the plant and marine animal sterols, only the metabolism of β-sitosterol has been compared with cholesterol in rat and man. Qualitatively, the plant sterol is handled by the same tissues and converted to the same products as cholesterol, but quantitatively there are differences. In the plasma, sitosterol is less esterified and more rapidly cleared; while the two sterols are distributed among the same tissues, the ratios of distribution differ; the adrenal contains and converts both sterols to steroid hormones; both sterols reach equilibrium in the plasma and liver by 9 days after an injected dose; both sterols appear in the bile, for example, 20 percent of the injected β-sitosterol versus 28 percent of the cholesterol by 3 days. A greater percentage of the biliary sitosterol is excreted as neutral sterol rather than as acidic sterols (37.8 percent versus 15 percent of the biliary isotope) relative to cholesterol. Sitosterol is converted in the liver to acidic sterols (bile acids), which are identical to the bile acids produced from cholesterol in man but not identical to the bile acids produced from cholesterol in the rat.[1]

Effects on Serum Cholesterol Levels

The plant sterols campesterol, β-sitosterol, and stigmasterol display hypocholesterolemic effects in experimental animals, including chickens, rats, rabbits, dogs, guinea pigs, gerbils, and nonhuman primates. Generally, when fed in the diet at 0.5 to 1 percent, these plant sterols reduce the cholesterolemia induced by 1 to 5 percent cholesterol feeding and prevent the resultant atherosclerosis. In a critical study, rabbits were fed 1.0 to 1.5 g of cholesterol daily for 2 weeks, which resulted in a 14- to 16-fold increase in plasma cholesterol. As the ratio of β-sitosterol to cholesterol in the diet was varied from 1:1 to 7:1, hypercholesterolemia was progressively reduced. The 7:1 ratio brought the plasma cholesterol to baseline level. With a ratio of 2:1 or larger, there were no aortic lesions, whereas rabbits receiving only the cholesterol had severe lesions. The importance of the ratio has been confirmed in humans. For example, 5 to 45 g/day of plant sterols produce a hypocholesterolemic effect whose magnitude is proportional to the initial level of the serum cholesterol (a reflection of dietary cholesterol level). Numerous other human studies have been reviewed, and these demonstrate that β-sitosterol or phytosterols significantly reduce plasma cholesterol levels.[34] Other factors have been reported to affect the efficiency of plasma cholesterol reduction by β-sitosterol, such as mode of administration (crystalline better than suspension), time of administration (at or before mealtime), age of patient (variable results), extent of hypercholesterolemia (see above), and etiology of the disorder (genetic hypercholesterolemias may or may not respond). The effect of β-sitosterol administration on plasma cholesterol levels can be observed in 2 weeks.

A few other plants and marine animal sterols have been investigated for hypocholesterolemic action. For example, stigmasterol must be administered to humans at 1.5 times the amount of sitosterol to produce a comparable effect.[1] Marine animal sterols, in studies carried out exclusively in experimental animals, vary in their effectiveness to lower plasma cholesterol levels. Mixed sterols from the butter clam and minced oysters or clams (5 to 10 percent of the diet by dry weight) were hypocholesterolemic, while scallop sterols had a marginal lowering effect. Individual marine animal sterols vary similarly. Fucosterol and 24-methylene cholesterol are reported hypocholesterolemic, while brassicasterol is not. The plant and marine animal sterol content in foodstuffs are shown in Tables 5-5 and 5-6.

Effects on Cholesterol Absorption and Metabolism

Those plant sterols that are hypocholesterolemic have been shown in animals and humans to inhibit the intestinal absorption of cholesterol and in some cases to affect cholesterol metabolism. It is logical to suspect that the mechanism of action of the marine animal sterols is identical. Because of the similar physiochemical properties of these sterols and cholesterol, they compete effectively with cholesterol in the luminal, cell-surface, and intracellular phases of the sterol absorption process. The net result is a reduction in cholesterol absorption.

In the lumen, both cholesterol and other sterols are similarly distributed between micellar, oil, and crystalline phases. The latter phase forms after sterol solubility is exceeded in the former phases, and the sterol residing here is considered nonabsorbable. Thus, any sterol that competes with or "pushes cholesterol out" of the oil and micellar phases decreases the amount available for absorption. This explanation is consistent with the relatively large amounts of plant sterols required to inhibit cholesterol absorption.

Table 5-5. Compositions of Sterols in Vegetable Oils[a]

Vegetable oil	Total Sterol g/100 g	Percentage of Total Sterols						
		β-Sitosterol	Stigmasterol	Δ^7 Stigmastenol	Campesterol	Brassicasterol	Fucosterol	Cholesterol
Castor	0.5	44	2	Tr	10	–	21	Tr
Cocoa Butter	0.4	59	26	1	9	Tr	3	2
Coconut	0.4	58	13	6	8	Tr	14	1
Coffee Seed	3.4	54	20	1	19	Tr	6	Tr
Corn	1.3	66	6	1	23	Tr	1	Tr
Cottonseed	0.6	93	1	Tr	4	Tr	2	Tr
Kapok	0.5	86	2	1	9	Tr	2	Tr
Linseed	0.9	46	9	2	29	Tr	13	1
Olive (France)	0.8	91	1	4	2	–	2	–
Olive (Italy)	–	84	1	Tr	3	–	12	–
Palm	0.4	74	8	1	14	Tr	2	1
Peanut	0.4	64	9	3	15	Tr	8	Tr
Rapeseed	0.9	58	Tr	5	25	10	2	Tr
Rice Bran	4.2	49	15	1	28	Tr	5	Tr
Safflower	0.6	52	9	20	13	Tr	1	–
Soybean	0.4	53	20	3	20	Tr	3	Tr
Sunflower	0.7	60	8	15	8	–	4	–
Wheat Germ	3.2	67	Tr	3	22	Tr	6	Tr

[a]Vegetable oils are the only significant source of plant sterols. (Reproduced with permission from Vahouny GV, Kritchevsky D: Plant and marine sterols and cholesterol metabolism. In Spiller G (ed): Nutritional Pharmacology. New York, Alan R. Liss, 1981.)

Table 5-6.   Marine Sterol Content of Foodstuffs[a]

| | | Major Sterol Composition | | | |
Seafoods	Sterol Content (mg/100 g)	Cholesterol (%)	22-Dehydro-cholesterol (%)	Brassicasterol (%)	24—Methylene Cholesterol (%)
Haddock	97	93	–	5	1
Pollok	80	94	–	–	–
Salmon	99	96	–	–	–
Shrimp	209	96	–	–	–
Lobster	171	99	–	1	–
Crab	244	57	4	37	2
Oyster	362	41	3	16	26
Clam	518	37	8	14	20
Scallop	681	26	13	14	20

[a]Modified from Vahouny GV, Kritchevsky D: Plant and marine sterols and cholesterol metabolism. In Spiller G (ed): Nutritional Pharmacology: New York, Alan R Liss, 1981.

Also in the lumen are the cell-surface barriers, which may have a saturation threshold for sterol uptake into the cell. In this case, sterols in similar states of solubility would compete for uptake.

Finally, within the mucosal cell, cholesterol is largely esterified before exit in the transport lipoproteins. The enzyme, mucosal cholesterol esterase, esterifies much or all of absorbed cholesterol. Relative to cholesterol in an in vitro assay, β-sitosterol is esterified to the extent of 35 to 40 percent, and stigmasterol, 15 to 22 percent. Increasing levels of β-sitosterol in the assay progressively decrease cholesterol esterification. These studies suggest that plant and marine sterols compete with cholesterol for the esterifying enzyme, and that this represents a mechanism for their inhibition of cholesterol absorption. The ability of sterols to compete with cholesterol for ACAT, the other cholesterol-esterifying enzyme in intestinal mucosa, has not been tested.

While interference with cholesterol absorption must be a major mechanism for the hypocholesterolemic action of plant and marine animal sterols, it may not account for the total effect. In support of this, it has been observed in humans and chickens that plant sterols are hypocholesterolemic in the absence of dietary cholesterol. Moreover, administration of the plant sterol to rats or chickens by other than oral routes, that is, intraperitoneal or intravenous injection, produces hypocholesterolemic effects. In the rat injected intravenously with β-sitosterol, cholesterogenesis was enhanced. Since the overall effect is a lowering of serum cholesterol, an increased excretion of cholesterol as neutral or sterol or bile acids is implied.

SUMMARY

Cholesterol is added to the body through the diet and biosynthesis in the tissues and removed as either neutral or acidic sterols (bile acids) in the feces. When the addition of cholesterol equals its removal at the tissue or whole-body level, a state of cholesterol balance exists. Upon excessive dietary intake of cholesterol, the plasma cholesterol is elevated. An elevated plasma cholesterol correlates positively with the risk of atherosclerosis. In addition, dietary cholesterol alters its transport lipoproteins in quality and quantity. In the face of these dietary cholesterol-induced changes, cholesterol balance is disrupted. The resulting imbalance leads to cholesterol deposition in the arterial wall, atherosclerosis, and to coronary heart disease.

An elevated plasma cholesterol can be lowered by diets that are low in choleterol and total and saturated fat, high in complex carbohydrates and fiber, and of low caloric density. In many cases plasma cholesterol levels are lowered by plant and marine animal sterols, which are analogs that lower cholesterol absorption.

REFERENCES

1. Vahouny GV, Kritchevsky D: Plant and marine sterols and cholesterol metabolism. In Spiller G (ed): Nutritional Pharmacology: New York, Alan R Liss, 1981.
2. Kudchodkar BJ, Sodhi HS, Horlick L: Absorption of dietary cholesterol in man. Metab 22:155–163, 1973.
3. Green PHR, Glickman RM: Intestinal lipoprotein metabolism. J Lipid Res 22:1153–1173, 1981.
4. Lutton C: The role of the digestive tract in cholesterol metabolism. Digestion 14:342–356, 1976.
5. Treadwell CR, Vahouny GV: Cholesterol absorption. In Code CF (ed): Handbook of Physiology. Baltimore, Waverly Press, 1968.
6. Hofmann AF: Fat digestion: the interaction of lipid digestion products with micellar bile acid solutions. In Rommel K (ed): Lipid Absorption: Biochemical and Clinical Aspects. Baltimore, University Park Press, 1976.
7. Gallo L: Pancreatic sterol ester hydrolase. In Lowenstein JM (ed): Methods in Enzymology, New York, Academic Press, 1982.
8. Hofmann AF, Borgstrom B: The intraluminal phase of fat digestion in man: the lipid content of the micellar and oil phases of intestinal content obtained during fat digestion and absorption. J Clin Invest 43:247–257, 1964.
9. Westergaard H, Dietschy JM: The mechanism whereby bile acid micelles increase the rate of fatty acid and cholesterol uptake into the intestinal mucosal cell. J Clin Invest 58:97–108, 1976.
10. Smithson KW, Millar DB, Jacobs LR, Gray GM: Intestinal diffusion barrier: unstirred water layer or membrane surface mucous coat? Science 214:1241–1244, 1981.
11. Strauss EW: Morphological aspects of triglyceride absorption. In Code CF (ed): Handbook of Physiology. Baltimore, Waverly Press, 1968.
12. Gallo L, Newbill T, Hyun J, Vahouny GV, Treadwell CR: Role of pancreatic cholesterol esterase in the uptake and esterification of cholesterol by isolated intestinal cells. Proc Soc Exp Biol Med 156:277–281, 1977.
13. Gallo L, Chiang Y, Vahouny GV, Treadwell CR: Localization and origin of rat intestinal cholesterol esterase determined by immunocytochemistry. J Lipid Res 21:537–545,1980.
14. Bell CC, Swell L: Effect of total pancreatectomy on cholesterol absorption and the serum cholesterol level in man. Proc Soc Exp Biol Med 128:575–577, 1968.
15. Gallo L, Myers S, Bennett Clark S, Vahouny GV: Rat intestinal ACAT and cholesterol absorption. Fed Proc 41:542, 1982.
16. Gallo L, Myers S, Bennett Clark S, Vahouny GV: Rat intestinal acyl CoA: cholesterol

acyl transferase and cholesterol esterase: roles in cholesterol esterification. Fed Proc 42:1256, 1983.

17. Haugen R, Norum KR: Coenzyme A-dependent esterification of cholesterol in rat intestinal mucosa. Scand J Gastroenterol 11:615–621, 1976.

18. Havel RJ, Goldstein JL, Brown MS: Lipoproteins and lipid transport. In Bondy PK, Rosenberg LE (eds): Metabolic Control and Disease. Philadelphia, WB Saunders, 1980.

19. Cardell RR Jr, Badenhausen S, Porter K: Intestinal triglyceride absorption in the rat. J Cell Biol 34:123–155, 1967.

20. Sabesin SM: Ultrastructural aspects of the intracellular assembly, transport and exocytosis of chylomicrons by rat intestinal absorptive cells. In Rommel K (ed): Lipid Absorption: Biochemical and Clinical Aspects. Baltimore, University Park Press, 1976.

21. Dietschy JM, Wilson JD: Cholesterol synthesis in the squirrel monkey: relative rates of synthesis in various tissues and mechanisms of control. J Clin Invest 47:166–174, 1968.

22. Dietschy JM, Gamel WG: Cholesterol synthesis in the intestine of man: regional differences and control mechanisms. J Clin Invest 50:872–880, 1974.

23. Balasubramanian S, Goldstein JL, Faust JR, Brown MS: Evidence for regulation of 3-hydroxy-3-methyl-glutaryl coenzyme A reductase activity and cholesterol synthesis in non-hepatic tissues of rat. Proc Natl Acad Sci USA 73:2564–2568, 1976.

24. Shefer S, Hauser S, Lapar V: HMGCoA reductase of intestinal mucosa and liver of the rat. J Lipid Res 13:402–412, 1972.

25. McClintock C, Shiau Y: Jejunum is more important than terminal ileum for taurocholate absorption in rats. Am J Physiol, in press.

26. Havel RJ: Approach to the patient with hyperlipidemia. Med Clin North Am. Philadelphia, WB Saunders, 1982.

27. Mahley BW: Atherogenic hyperlipoproteinemia. Med Clin North Am. Philadelphia, WB Saunders, 1982.

28. Goldstein JL, Brown MS: The low-density lipoprotein pathway and its relation to atherosclerosis. In Snell EE (ed): Ann Rev Biochem. Palo Alto, Annual Reviews, Inc, 1977.

29. Connor WE, Connor SJ: Dietary treatment of hyperlipidemia. Med Clin North Am. Philadelphia, WB Saunders, 1982.

30. Eder HA, Gidez LI: The clinical significance of the plasma high density lipoproteins. Med Clin North Am. Philadelphia, WB Saunders, 1982.

31. Goldstein JL, Brown MS: The low-density lipoprotein pathway and its relation to atherosclerosis. In Snell EE (ed): Ann Rev Biochem. Palo Alto, Annual Reviews, Inc, 1977.

32. Connor WE, Connor SJ: Dietary treatment of hyperlipidemia. Med Clin North Am. Philadelphia, WB Saunders, 1982.

33. Eder HA, Gidez LI: The clinical significance of the plasma high density lipoproteins. Med Clin North Am. Philadelphia, WB Saunders, 1982.

34. Pollak OJ, Kritchevsky D: Sitosterol. In Clarkson TB, Kritchevski D, Pollak OJ (eds): Monographs on Atherosclerosis. New York, S Karger, 1981.

35. Vahouny GV, Satchithapandam S, Connor WE, Lin DS, Gallo LL: Comparative lymphatic absorption of β-sitosterol, stigmasterol and fucosterol and differential inhibition of cholesterol absorption. Am J Clin Nutr. in press.

36. Blackburn H: Diet-lipid–atherosclerosis relationship: epidemiological evidence and public health implications. In Gotto AM, Smith LC, Allen B (eds): Atherosclerosis, V. New York, Springer-Verlag, 1980.

6 | Carbohydrate, Fiber, and Heart Disease

Terrence T. Kuske

The changes accompanying the industrial revolution in Western countries brought about dramatic changes in diets. Along with an increase in total caloric intake, principally due to increased ingestion of foods rich in protein and animal fats, came a change in the type of carbohydrate intake of the Western populations. While remaining approximately the same in caloric value, the proportion of carbohydrates consumed as sugar, available readily at cheaper prices, increased dramatically. In addition, the development of high extraction flour milling processes in the latter part of the 19th century made white flour with very low fiber content readily available to the general population, and led to a dramatic decrease in the intake of fiber from flour and milled goods. The resultant effect was an increase in the intake of sugar, and a decrease in the intake of complex carbohydrates and fiber in the Western diet. A number of scientific observers, most prominently Yudkin,[1] as well as Burkitt[2] and Trowell[3] have linked these dietary changes to the development of atherosclerosis in our Western populations. As Great Britain must import its sugar, statistics are available over the past several hundred years for the importation and implied consumption of sugars in the United Kingdom. These appear, in Yudkin's assessment, to be correlated closely to the increasing development and affluence of Britain as well as to the increasing numbers of deaths due to atherosclerotic disease.[4] The availability of sucrose at low cost in the wealthier nations has led to greatly increased use, to the point where currently sucrose is the most common food additive, and the average American consumes 50 kilograms per year.

Yudkin in 1957[5] compared coronary mortality in 14 nations with the intake of proteins, fats, and carbohydrates, and noted a better correlation between the consumption of sucrose and coronary mortality than with other dietary components.

He observed that those individuals demonstrating premature atherosclerosis consumed significantly greater quantities of sugar, especially in coffee or tea, than did healthy controls. He noted the close correlation between consumption of fat and sugar in different nations; he suggested that the reason saturated fat consumption does not correlate well on an individual basis with premature atherosclerotic disease may be because the correlation is better with sugar consumption. His data on a small series tended to confirm that atherosclerotic disease correlated closely with sugar intake, whereas this correlation with disease had not been found in studies of fat intake.

The sugar-atherosclerosis connection may be related to carbohydrate-induced hyperlipidemia. In a study of hypertensive individuals treated with a 100 percent rice diet, Hatch, Abell, and Kendall[6] noted the phenomenon of carbohydrate induction of hypertriglyceridemia. Hypertriglyceridemia was induced in all individuals as long as they were fed this total carbohydrate diet. Individuals with hypertriglyceridemia, however, are more susceptible to dramatic increases in their serum triglycerides than are normal individuals. On diets with lower levels of carbohydrate (high, but less than 80 percent) the individual with hypertriglyceridemia will greatly increase serum triglycerides, whereas the triglycerides will not increase in persons with normal plasma lipid levels. This carbohydrate-induced hypertriglyceridemia was subsequently differentiated from fat-induced, or exogenous, hypertriglyceridemia by Ahrens and collegues in 1961.[7] In a retrospective study of risk factors in young men with coronary heart disease by Hatch and colleagues,[8] endogenous hypertriglyceridemia was shown as a significant risk factor, an observation confirmed by numerous investigators. Subsequently, prospective studies by Carlson and Böttiger demonstrated a linear increase in risk of ischemic heart disease with increase in circulating triglycerides or cholesterol[8] (see Chapters 3 and 5). More recent studies, however, have brought into question the significance of elevated triglycerides as a risk factor. In a review of the various studies of the association between serum triglyceride and coronary artery disease, Hully and colleagues[9] employed bivariate logistic analysis of ischemic heart disease in relation to triglycerides and total cholesterol. They found the standardized odds ratio for cholesterol remained statistically significant, whereas the standardized odds ratio for triglyceride was not statistically significant when cholesterol was considered simultaneously. They suggested that the correlation of triglycerides with ischemic heart disease no longer existed when the data were adjusted for cholesterol correlation, correlation with high-density lipoproteins (HDL), and with total body mass. This statistical assessment, however, is affected considerably by the fact that triglycerides are transported largely as very low density lipoproteins (VLDL), which contain modest amounts of cholesterol and are precursors of low-density lipoproteins (LDL), considered to be the most atherogenic of lipoproteins (Chapter 3). This will be discussed later in this chapter.

Early studies of the effects of the intake of different types of carbohydrates on serum lipids include those of MacDonald and Braithwaite,[10] who assessed the effect of starch or sucrose diets on total lipid levels in normal individuals. They found total lipid increased in individuals ingesting sucrose diets, and decreased in those fed starch diets. This change was interpreted as increase or decrease in triglyceride levels. In long-term studies, Mann and colleagues[11] demonstrated a fall in scrum triglycerides when isocaloric substitution of starch was made for sucrose. Difficulties in maintaining constant weight in these individuals provide some questions in intepretation of this data, as weight reduction results in improvement in serum triglyceride level, and substitution diets frequently are associated with a change in weight. Another study by Grande and colleagues[12] failed to demonstrate a difference in effect on serum lipids in normal individuals fed sucrose or starch.

An additional factor that has not been considered in these theories is the possibility that carbohydrates from starch may not be absorbed completely. The incomplete absorption of carbohydrates from wheat flour may be a possible mechanism for these differential effects.[13]

In individuals with endogenous hypertriglyceridemia (Fredrickson type 4 hyperlipidemia), removal of sucrose from the diet and substitution of starch has been shown in metabolic studies to lead to improvement of hypertriglyceridemia. The diets used for treatment of this disorder restrict sugar intake and substitute other forms of carbohydrates (see Chapter 3).

METABOLIC INTERRELATIONSHIPS OF CARBOHYDRATES AND LIPIDS

The apparently paradoxical effect of high carbohydrate diets in eliciting an increase in total serum lipids, principally as VLDL, can be explained on the basis of an understanding of the interrelationship between carbohydrates and fats in the provision of energy for metabolic processes. Glucose and free fatty acids are metabolic fuels that are interchangeable in most tissues; notable exceptions include the brain, the lens of the eye, and the arterial intima. The storage of glucose, however, is limited to the amount that can be maintained in the form of liver and muscle glycogen, approximately 2000 kilocalories. Storage of free fatty acids takes the form of triglycerides in fat cells, which is limited only by the distensibility of our skin. In the normal, slender male, the amount stored as triglyceride is in excess of 111,000 kilocalories. Further, the storage of energy as triglyceride (9 kcal/g) is more efficient than storage as glycogen (4 kcal/g).

In the fat cell, which is the storage site for this triglyceride, there is a continuing cycle of degradation of triglyceride into free fatty acids and resynthesis of the free fatty acids back into triglycerides. Breakdown occurs through the action of hormone-sensitive lipase, and releases 1 mole of glycerol and 3 moles of free fatty acids per mole of triglyceride. Resynthesis of free fatty acids back into triglycerides, however, requires α-glycerol phosphate, which must come from the degradation of glucose, through the Embden-Meyerhof pathway. The glycerol released during breakdown of triglyceride cannot be directly converted into α-glycerol phosphate in the fat cell, because of the lack of the enzyme glycerylphosphokinase (present in the liver). Therefore, in order to continue synthesis of triglyceride from free fatty acids, the fat cell must have a continuous supply of glucose, which requires insulin. In the absence of insulin, glucose cannot enter the fat cell, and the fatty acids and glycerol that are released from degradation cannot be resynthesized back into triglyceride. They are thus mobilized into the plasma, raising the plasma free fatty acid and glycerol levels. With adequate insulin and glucose, sufficient α-glycerol phosphate is produced intracellularly to re-esterify all free fatty acids produced internally by the catabolism of triglyceride; in addition, the glucose can be converted by the fat cell into acetyl CoA to synthesize new free fatty acids and convert them into triglycerides. Simultaneously, free fatty acids resulting from the breakdown of the triglyceride content of circulating VLDL and chylomicrons by lipoprotein lipase can be taken up by the fat cell and esterified into triglyceride.

This constitutes, then, an elegantly sensitive mechanism for alternate fuel provision. When glucose and insulin are abundant, the free fatty acids in the plasma are taken up by the fat cell and stored, and triglyceride breakdown ceases. When levels of glucose or insulin are low, there is a breakdown in triglyceride stores providing a continuing flow of free fatty acids for fuel. When the quantity of plasma free fatty acids exceeds metabolic demands, the liver removes these free fatty acids and resynthesizes them into triglycerides. This mechanism provides approximately 80 percent of the triglyceride formed in the liver. The other 20 percent is formed by de novo production of free fatty acids from carbohydrate. Through the stimulus of insulin, excess carbohydrate in the diet is converted into free fatty acids by the liver, and thence esterified into triglyceride. These hepatic triglycerides are then transported out of the liver by means of VLDL synthesized for this task. They contain not only these endogenous triglycerides (synthesized in the liver) but also a significant amount of cholesterol, phospholipid, and apolipo-proteins. Upon release from the liver, they are degraded at endothelial surfaces by lipoprotein lipase. This enzyme breaks the triglyceride down once again into free fatty acids, which then can be utilized as fuel by peripheral tissues or taken up by the fat cell for re-esterification into triglyceride. Lipoprotein lipase itself is insulin dependent, in that adequate levels of insulin are required for its continued replen-ishment. Thus, if an individual is deficient in insulin, there is not only increased mobilization of free fatty acids and, thus, increased production of VLDL by the liver, but also decreased removal of VLDL, because of deficient amounts of lipo-protein lipase. As the VLDL are the principal transporters of triglycerides in the plasma in the fasting state, measurement of serum triglycerides when fasting re-flects the levels of VLDL. As noted in Chapter 3, the VLDL then are catabolized to intermediate-density lipoproteins (IDL) and thence to low-density lipoproteins (LDL).

Barter and colleagues[14] studied serum triglyceride, free fatty acids, and in-sulin during a high sucrose diet and noted that triglyceride and free fatty acid levels arose at night and fell during the day, while the insulin levels rose in the daytime and fell at night. They concluded that the highly significant inverse relationship of insulin and triglycerides was related to insulin-mediated increased catabolism of triglycerides. Schlierf and Dorow[15] found that this nocturnal rise in triglycerides during carbohydrate induction of hypertriglyceridemia could be suppressed either by nicotinic acid infusion, which suppresses hydrolysis of fat-cell triglycerides, or by additional nocturnal feedings, both of which resulted in reduction in plasma free fatty acids and triglycerides.

A recent study[16] has demonstrated that continuous insulin infusion in diabetic patients resulted in diminution of both LDL and VLDL, with a concomitant increase in HDL, suggesting once again the importance of continuing levels of insulin in suppressing free fatty acids and maintaining lower levels of endogenous VLDL synthesis.

INDIVIDUAL SUGARS AND HYPERTRIGLYCERIDEMIA

Considerable confusion exists regarding the effects of individual sugars on the induction of hypertriglyceridemia. Much of this may be attributed to the fact that the metabolism of these sugars in the rat differs significantly from that in the human. The rat is a poor model of dietary hyperlipidemia, especially with respect to carbohydrate induction. Fructose appears to induce a significant increase in serum triglycerides in the rat but does not induce hypertriglyceridemia in humans. The substitution of fructose for other sugars in the diet of hypertriglyceridemic men does not increase serum triglycerides in these individuals. Indeed, in diets very high in carbohydrates, fructose has less effect than other carbohydrates, such as dextromaltose.[17] Palumbo and colleagues[18] studied individuals with known coronary artery disease and found that diets containing 4 grams of sucrose or 2 grams of fructose per kilogram of body weight per day produced a significant rise in serum triglycerides in patients with coronary artery disease, compared with healthy control subjects. This suggests that patients with coronary artery disease may be sensitive to this stimulus. There was no correlation, however, with coronary angiograms or severity of disease. Reiser and colleagues[19] in a study of the effects of sucrose on blood lipids in carbohydrate-sensitive individuals demonstrated that triglyceride levels increased significantly as the level of sucrose in the diet increased. Increases in total cholesterol, VLDL cholesterol, and LDL cholesterol were observed as the sucrose content of the diet increased. In reviewing reports of the individual effects of fructose and sucrose versus starch on hypertriglyceridemia, it is apparent that effects in those subjects whose conditions can be categorized as carbohydrate-induced hypertriglyceridemia differ from those in normal individuals. This might explain the different observations of the various investigators (see Chapter 2).

FIBER, CHOLESTEROL, AND ATHEROSCLEROSIS

The development of high extraction "rolling mills" in 1880 has been suggested as the etiologic event in the development, some 40 years later, of an increasing incidence of coronary atherosclerosis, as well as many other diseases. The removal of fiber from wheat flour, with the subsequent ready availability of white flour, coupled with the increased intake of sugar in Western countries correlates at least temporally with the increased incidence of atherosclerotic disease. Whether or not this disease ''epidemic'' relates to specific effects of dietary fiber remains unresolved.

Dietary fiber is defined as the remnants of vegetable cell walls that are not hydrolyzed by alimentary enzymes of humans.[3] Originally determined by acid and alkali extraction of food, producing what is called crude fiber, the unsatisfactory nature of this method has led to more refined techniques.[20] The chemistry has recently been reviewed by Kay.[21] In this chapter, fiber has been subdivided into the classes discussed below.

Polymers of Sugars Forming Cellulose and Fibrils

The first, cellulose, is a compound formed of chains of glucose linked in a beta 1-4 linkage (as opposed to the alpha 1-4 linkage, which is seen in glycogen): therefore, this glucose is unavailable for digestion because the intestinal saccharidases will not attack this linkage. The second group in this category, hemicellulose, is composed of galactose, pentoses, and glucuronic acid in the form of branched polysaccharides. This compound is important in cation exchange, and it binds zinc, calcium, and magnesium. The third, and far more important group under this category with respect to lipid metabolism, is the pectins. Pectins are formed of branched chains of galacturonic acid, galactose, and arabinose; they function as adsorbents for water and entrap bile acids. These fibrils form networks or interstices that sequester sizeable quantities of aqueous solutions and, presumably, micelles as well. In addition, by maintaining increased bulk in the intestinal contents, they reduce the amount of bile salts available at the intestinal mucosal surface for absorption.

Secretory Gums and Mucilage

These compounds have a main chain composed of galactose, glucuronic acids, mannose, galacturonic acid, and rhamnose, and side chains composed of xylose, fucose, and galactose. Gums and mucilages are synthesized by plant secretory cells, with gums being secreted at the site of plant injury by specialized cells. Mucilages prevent desiccation of seed endosperm. Both have extensive use in the food industry as stabilizers. One of the mucilages (guar) has been shown to be of benefit in lowering serum cholesterol[22] (see p. 118).

Lignin

This interesting compound is not a carbohydrate but rather a phenylpropane polymer that provides elasticity to plant structures. It is very complex and cross linked, and resists bacterial degradation in the gut. Lignin is important because of the catalytic surface that it provides within the intestine and because of its water holding capabilities.

The digestibility of these fibers is not known. Considerable bacterial fermentation occurs within the large bowel and contributes, presumably significantly, to breakdown of these compounds. Whether the products released can be absorbed is of some question; however, they do contribute to gas production, forming methane and hydrogen, and may influence absorption of other compounds. Studies in humans using low methoxy pectin and pectin NF showed the digestible energy of these compounds to be 2.86 kcal/g and 3.03 kcal/g, respectively.[23] This study, at least, suggests that there is considerable potential for absorption of the residue after bacterial fermentation of pectin in the gut.

Fiber in general decreases gastrointestinal transit time and has been shown to have beneficial effect in numerous gastrointestinal disorders, as a result of its improvement of intestinal transit time and increased bulk of stool.[24,25] Factors related to lipids and atherosclerosis, however, remain ill defined. Certainly we must consider that the diet high in foods containing large amounts of fiber results in a replacement of fat and sugars in the diet and increases satiety. These effects may lead to weight reduction and decreased serum cholesterol. The question of a specific effect of fiber on reduction in serum cholesterol has been addressed by a number of investigators.

Early studies attempting to induce atherosclerosis in rabbits with saturated fat in a cholesterol-free diet demonstrated that use of commercial rabbit chow prevented significant atherosclerosis despite the addition of sizable quantitites of saturated fat. The feeding of a semipurified diet with saturated fats, however, resulted in rapid development of atherosclerosis.[26] This and other studies led to interest in the effect of dietary fiber on absorption of cholesterol and subsequent demonstration that dietary fiber interacted with bile acids and inhibited their reabsorption. The decrease in transit time of the intestine, along with the increase of bulk in intestinal content, may decrease bile salt reabsorption, or for that matter cholesterol absorption, simply by a physical effect. At the same time, it has been demonstrated that lignin, in vitro, binds bile salts when the acidic groups of those bile salts are blocked. This is felt to be a hydrophobic binding of the bile salts.[27] Studies in humans have shown that citrus pectin is most effective in decreasing serum cholesterol levels, and that diets high in vegetables and fruits are also effective.[28]

The mechanism of reduction of serum cholesterol levels with utilization of fiber has been attributed to the entrapment or binding of bile salts in the intestinal contents. This can be due to a physical entrapment, as suggested with pectins, or physical binding in a hydrophobic state with lignin, or possibly due to the decreased intestinal transit time. In any event, the prevention of reabsorption of bile salts results in a diminution of the total body bile salt pool, with the requirement, thus, that more cholesterol be converted to bile salts to replenish this pool. This effect is similar to, although less effective than, that of the various bile salt binding resins (cholestyramine and colestipol).[29] If this is not compensated for by increased cholesterol synthesis, there is net decrease in the total body cholesterol pool. Simultaneously, the binding and removal of bile acids can conceivably inhibit the formation of micelles, which are essential for the absorption of cholesterol as well as other lipids from dietary and biliary sources (see Chapter 5).

Individual Food Sources and Hypocholesterolemic Effect of Fiber

The individual types of fiber are present in varying quantities in different food stuffs. Therefore, it is of interest to look at the effects of individual food stuffs on the absorption of cholesterol. Studies in rats have demonstrated a significant lowering of serum cholesterol and increase in excretion of bile acids when the animals are fed an alfalfa diet. Studies of this hypocholesterolemic effect of alfalfa have suggested that it is due to the lignin in the alfalfa rather than to the pectins. A similar effect is not observed when animals are fed wheat bran. Use of α-cellulose derived from wood has shown no hypocholesterolemic effect in experimental animals. A study of high fiber diets utilizing powdered cellulose or soy hulls, or both, in comparison with cholestyramine demonstrated that both fiber and resin reduced serum cholesterol, but cholestyramine was far more effective.[29]

In humans, diets high in wheat bran increased serum cholesterol.[28] However, there is evidence that wheat bran from a specific type of grain (hard red spring wheat) results in reduced serum cholesterol.[30] Diets high in oat bran decrease serum cholesterol,[31] as does the addition of guar gum to the diet at levels of 9 grams per day.[22]

Foods particularly high in pectin, and thus presumably more effective in lowering serum cholesterol, are noted in Table 6-1.[32] Citrus fruits are particularly high in pectin, although this may represent primarily the pectin from the white portion of citrus peel rather than the substance of the fruit itself. Squash and carrots are vegetable sources very high in pectins. Legumes demonstrate, in human studies, a hypocholesterolemic effect, and, of grains, rolled oats demonstrate a significant effect to lower serum cholesterol.[31]

In a prospective study evaluating the mortality from coronary heart disease, cancer, and all causes in relation to dietary fiber (the Zutphen study),[33] mortality from coronary heart disease was 4 times higher for men with the lowest level of dietary fiber intake than for those with highest. This relation, however, disappeared after multivariant analyses when the investigators subtracted the effect of

Table 6-1. Pectin Content of Fruits and Vegetables[a]

Plant Variety[b]	Percent of Fresh Weight as Calcium Pectate
Apples	0.71–0.84
Apricots	0.71–1.32
Asparagus	Tr
Bananas	0.59–1.28
Beans	0.27–1.11
Blackberries	0.68–1.19
Carrots	1.17–2.92
Cherries	0.24–0.54
Cucumbers	0.10–0.50
Dewberries	0.51–1.00
Grapes	0.09–0.28
Grapefruits	3.30–4.50
Lemons	2.80–2.99
Loganberries	0.59
Oranges	2.34–2.38
Raisins	0.82–1.04
Raspberries	0.97
Squash	1.00–2.00
Sweet Potatoes	0.78

[a]Reproduced with permission from Campbell LA, Palmer GH. Pectin, In Spiller GA (ed): Topics in Dietary Fiber Research. New York, Plenum Press, 1978, pp 105–115.
[b]Includes peel and/or skin.

other factors. It was noted in this study, however, that there was also a decline in deaths from cancer, particularly lung cancer, and this decline remained significant after multivariant analysis. It was suggested that this may also relate to the high β-carotene intake on a high fiber diet.

Experimental Atherosclerosis

Alfalfa has been shown to reduce serum cholesterol levels and atheroma in rabbits fed atherogenic diets. In monkeys, alfalfa feeding has similarly resulted in significant reduction in serum cholesterol and in atheroma, compared with a diet having a similar cholesterol content without alfalfa. However, alfalfa seeds and sprouts have been shown to induce a systemic lupus erythematosis-like syndrome in monkeys,[34] thought due to the content of L-canavanine. This would suggest that consumption of these alfalfa compounds by humans may be unwise.

Current Dietary Fads

The numerous observations of the beneficial effects of high-fiber diets, as well as low-fat diets, on lipid metabolism have led to the development, by a non-nutritionist, of a diet high in fiber and unrefined carbohydrate and extremely low in fat in an attempt to reduce risk factors for atherosclerosis. This diet combined with an exercise program, is known as the Pritikin Program for Diet and Exercise.[35] This diet is extremely low in fat, with less than 10 percent of dietary calories derived from fat sources, high in carbohydrates, and high in fiber, with no sugars or processed foods. Less than a quarter pound of meat or fish is consumed daily, and the diet is very low in salt as well. Less than 100 milligrams of cholesterol per day is consumed in this diet. The diet is combined with a regular exercise program. It has been suggested by the author of this plan that this regimen is associated with significantly reduced levels of serum cholesterol and blood pressure. While plausible, it remains to be confirmed in the scientific literature. Acceptance of this diet by the patient is complicated by his or her adjustment to this high fiber intake, a problem that includes the change in gut flora and accompanying difficulties with bloating and flatulence. There are also additional difficulties related to the palatability of the diet, as it is such a dramatic change from the usual American diet. While the claims made for the health benefits of this diet remain to be proven, and the extremely low fat intake suggests potential difficulties in absorption of fat soluble vitamins, it is otherwise probably nutritionally sound.

The distressing news that wheat bran not only does not lower serum cholesterol but may raise it, leads to concern over contemporary habits of increasing dietary fiber intake by the addition of miller's bran to the diet. It appears that the principal benefit to be gained is from consuming either oat bran or citrus pectins, neither of which is currently a popular dietary recommendation for increased fiber intake. Perhaps the best solution to the problem is to recommend increased pectin intake, that is, ''an apple a day keeps the doctor away.''

HIGH-FIBER DIETS IN DIABETES

In recent years, considerable interest has developed in the use of high-fiber diets in the management of diabetes. Diets with a high carbohydrate intake that avoid refined sugars have resulted in improvements in glucose tolerance in diabetics; and the more sustained absorption of carbohydrate, with avoidance of peaks of

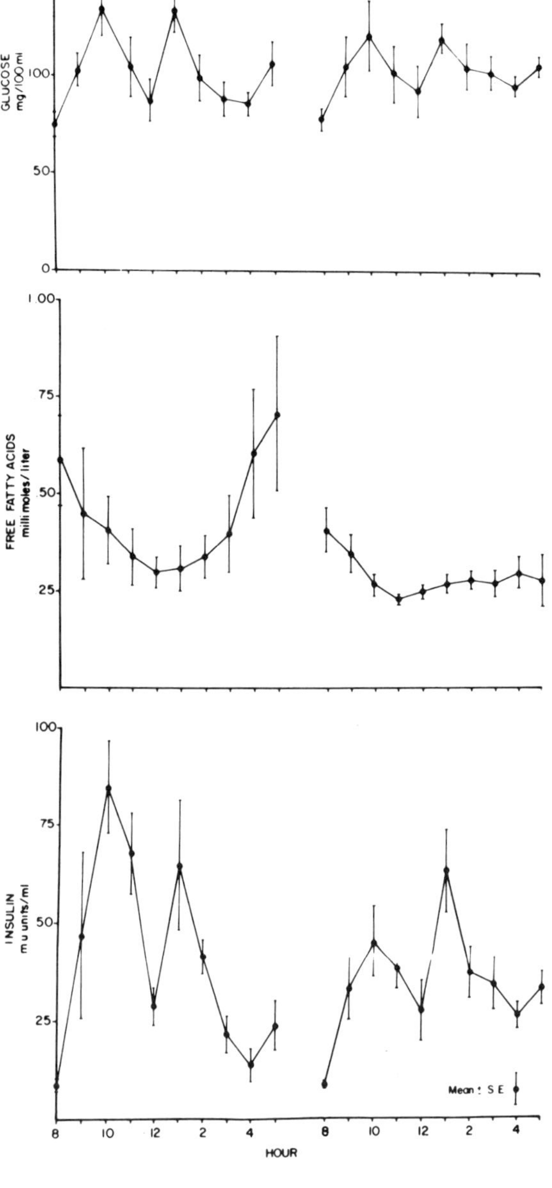

Fig. 6-1. Mean hourly glucose and insulin levels in nine patients, and free fatty acid levels in seven of these patients, ± standard error, on two isocaloric high-carbohydrate diets. Soluble carbohydrates are sugars and highly milled flour; compact carbohydrates are whole grain foods, pasta, and legumes. Values obtained hourly from 8:00 A.M. to 5:00 P.M.; meal times were 8:45 A.M., 12:15 P.M., and 4:45 P.M. (Reproduced with permission from Kuske TT: Carbohydrate nutrition and atherosclerosis. In Feldman EB (ed): Nutrition and Cardiovascular Disease. New York, Appleton-Century-Crofts, 1976.)

carbohydrate absorption, may provide flattened insulin levels, resulting in less mobilization of free fatty acids and thus less production of very low density lipoproteins. The addition of fiber to the diet in the form of guar gum, or the use of diets that are composed of foods naturally high in fiber, have been associated with a significant reduction in insulin requirements, as well as in fasting blood sugars and blood sugar response to diet.[36]

High-carbohydrate, high-fiber diets from natural sources have been associated with significant normalization of values in insulin-dependent diabetics leading to either a decrease in insulin requirements or a cessation of further need for insulin in management of these diabetics. Whether this relates to a specific effect of fiber remains to be demonstrated. Fiber, in the form of bran at least, may reduce intestinal transit time, leading to more absorption of glucose at the more distal portions of the small intestine and thus a reduced rate of absorption. In addition, the interstices formed by fibrils such as those in guar and pectins may inhibit enzymatic cleavage of carbohydrates, may physically retard the access of such enzymes to their substrate, or may reduce accessability of the carbohydrate to intestinal mucosa for absorption. Such delay in absorption of carbohydrate from the gut reduces the rate of glucose infusion from the alimentary tract and thus provides a protracted provision of glucose, resulting in lower levels of insulin that are sustained for longer periods of time. This then results in suppression of plasma free fatty acids for longer periods of time. A study of comparative affects of high carbohydrate diets from refined carbohydrates (soluble), principally sucrose, compared with unrefined carbohydrates or starch (compact) principally from legumes and pasta, is shown in Figure 6-1.[37] While little difference between the diets was noted in serum glucose levels throughout an 8 hour period, insulin levels were significantly lower, with quantitatively less insulin secreted over this period with the unrefined carbohydrate diet. In addition, free fatty acid levels were significantly flattened in this period, suggesting less need for removal of free fatty acids by the liver and reduction of levels of very low density lipoproteins by this mechanism.

SUMMARY AND CLINICAL RECOMMENDATIONS

Though considerable epidemiologic evidence suggests that increasing sugar intake is associated with increasing atherosclerosis, specific etiologic evidence is lacking. Certain individuals, particularly those with endogenous hypertriglyceridemia, respond to high sugar intakes with a marked elevation in serum triglycerides, and thus diets restricted in sugar are used to treat these subjects. Recent analyses of the numerous studies relating elevated serum triglycerides to atherosclerotic risk have suggested that once the effect of serum cholesterol is subtracted, along with that of HDL cholesterol and body mass, there is no longer a significant risk attributable to the triglycerides alone. With these factors in mind, it is difficult to suggest that the entire population eliminate intake of sugar. It would seem advisable, however, to control hypertriglyceridemia by reducing sugar intake.

Certain fibers, especially pectins and guar, assist in lowering serum cholesterol, albeit only a modest amount. Foods high in these fiber sources include citrus fruits and fresh vegetables. Addition of fiber to the diet by means of adding miller's bran is not effective in lowering serum cholesterol and should not be a substitute for increased intake of fiber through consumption of vegetables and fruits. Diabetic patients have been shown to have decreasing insulin requirements when they increase fiber intake in their diets.

It may be appropriate to suggest that modest amounts of sugar in the diet are not harmful to the general population, and that substitution of some of the animal fat in our diet with calories derived from vegetables and fruits would assist in lowering serum cholesterol.

REFERENCES

1. Yudkin J: Dietary fat and dietary sugar in relation to ischemic heart disease and diabetes. Lancet ii:4–5, 1964.
2. Burkett DP, Walker ARP, Painter NS: Dietary fiber and disease. Am J Med 229:1068–1074, 1974.
3. Trowell H: Dietary fibre, ischaemic heart disease and diabetes mellitus. Proc Nutr Soc 32:151–157, 1973.
4. Yudkin J: Sugar and disease. Nature 239:197–199, 1972.
5. Yudkin J: Diet and coronary thrombosis. Lancet ii:155–162, 1957.
6. Hatch FT, Abell LL, Kendall FE: Effects of restriction of dietary fat and cholesterol upon serum lipids and lipoproteins in patients with hypertension. Am J Med 19:48, 1955.
7. Ahrens EH, Hirsch J, Oette K, Farquhar JW, Stein Y: Carbohydrate induced and fat induced lipemia. Trans Assoc Am Physicians 74:134–146, 1961.
8. Carlson LA, Böttiger LE: Ischaemic heart disease in relation to fasting values of plasma triglycerides and cholesterol. Lancet i:865–868, 1972.
9. Hulley SB, Rosenman RH, Bawol RD, Brand RJ: The association between triglyceride and coronary heart disease. N Engl J Med 302:1383–1389, 1980.
10. MacDonald I, Braithwaite DM: The influence of dietary carbohydrate on the lipid pattern in serum and in adipose tissue. Clin Sci, 27:23–30, 1964.
11. Mann JI, Hendricks DA, Truswell AS, Manning E: Effects on serum lipids in normal men of reducing dietary sucrose or starch for five months. Lancet i:870–872, 1970.
12. Grande F, Anderson JT, Keys A: Sucrose and various carbohydrate containing foods and serum lipids in man. Am J Clin Nutr 27:1043–1051, 1974.
13. Anderson IH, Levine AS, and Levitt MD: Incomplete absorption of the carbohydrate in all-purpose wheat flour. N Engl J Med 304:891–892, 1981.
14. Barter PJ, Carrol KF, Nestel PJ: Diurnal fluctuations in triglyceride, free fatty acids, and insulin during sucrose consumption and insulin infusion in man. J Clin Invest 50:583–591, 1971.
15. Schlierf G, Dorow E: Diurnal patterns of triglycerides, free fatty acids, blood sugar, and insulin during carbohydrate induction in man and their modification by nocturnal supression of lipolysis. J Clin Invest 52:732–740, 1973.
16. Dunn FL, Pietri A, Raskin P: Plasma lipid and lipoprotein levels with continuous subcutaneous insulin infusion in type I diabetes mellitus. Ann Int Med 95:426–431, 1981.
17. Turner JL, Bierman EL, Brunzell JD, Chait A: Effect of dietary fructose on triglyceride transport and glucoregulatory hormones in hypertriglyceridemic men. Am J Clin Nutr 32:1043–1050, 1979.

18. Palumbo PJ, Briones ER, Nelson RA, Kottke BA: Sucrose sensitivity of patients with coronary artery disease. Am J Clin Nutr 30:394–401, 1977.

19. Reiser S, Bickard MC, Hallfrisch J, Michaelis OE, Prather ES: Blood lipids and their distribution in lipoproteins in hyperinsulinemic subjects fed three different levels of sucrose. J Nutr III: 1045–1057, 1981.

20. Southgate DAT: Fiber and the other unavailable carbohydrates and their effects on the energy value of the diet. Proc Nutr Soc 32:131–136, 1973.

21. Kay RMcP: Dietary Fiber. J Lipid Res 23:221–242, 1982.

22. Khan AR, Khan GY, Mitchel A, Qadeer MA: Effect of guar gum on blood lipids. Am J Clin Nutr 34:2446–2449, 1981.

23. Palmer GH, Dixon OG: Effect of pectin dose on serum cholesterol levels. Am J Clin Nutr 18:437–442, 1966.

24. Cummings JH: Progress report: dietary fibre. Gut 14:69–81, 1973.

25. Mendeloff AI: Dietary fiber and human health. N Engl J Med 297:811–814, 1977.

26. Kritchevsky D: Experimental atherosclerosis in rabbits fed cholesterol-free diets. J Atheroscler Res 4:103–105, 1964.

27. Eastwood MA, Hamilton D: Studies on the absorption of bile acids to non-absorbed components of diet. Biochin Biophys Acta 152:165–173, 1968.

28. Stasse-Wolthuis M, Albers HFF, vanJeveren JGC, deJong JW, Hautrast JGAJ, Hermus FJJ, Katan MB, Brydon WG, and Eastwood MA: Influence of dietary fiber from vegetables and fruits, bran or citrus pectin on serum lipids, fecal lipids, and colonic function. Am J Clin Nutr 33:1745–1756, 1980.

29. Palumbo PJ, Briones ER, Nelson RA: High fiber diet in hyperlipemia. J Am Med Assoc 240:223–227, 1978.

30. Munoz JM, Sandstead HH, Jacob RA, Logan GM, Reck SJ, Klevay LM, Dintzis FR, Inglett GE, Shuey WC: Effects of some cereal brans and textured vegetable protein on plasma lipids. Am J Clin Nutr 32:580–592, 1979.

31. Kirby RW, Anderson JW, Sieling B, Rees ED, Chen W-JL, Miller RE, Kay RM: Oat bran intake selectively lowers serum low-density lipoprotein cholesterol concentrations of hypercholesterolemic men. Am J Clin Nutr 34:824–829, 1981.

32. Campbell LA, Palmer GH: Pectin. In Spiller GA (ed): Topics in Dietary Fiber Research. New York, Plenum Press, 1978, pp 105–115.

33. Kromhout D, Bosschieter EB, Coulander C: Dietary fibre and 10-year mortality from coronary heart disease, cancer, and all causes. Lancet ii:518–522, 1982.

34. Malinow MR, Bardana EJ, McLaughlin P: Systemic lupus erythematosis-like syndrome in monkeys fed alfalfa sprouts: role of a non-protein amino acid. Science 216, 415–417, 1982.

35. Pritiken N with McGrady PM: The Pritikin Program for Diet and Exercise. Grosset and Dunlap, New York, 1979.

36. Anderson JW, Chen W-JL: Plant fiber. Carbohydrate and lipid metabolism. Am J Clin Nutr 32:346–363, 1979.

37. Kuske TT: Carbohydrate nutrition and atherosclerosis. In Feldman EB (ed); Nutrition and Cardiovascular Disease. New York, Appleton-Century-Crofts, 1976.

7 | Obesity and Heart Disease

R. Joe Teague

"Leave gormandising: Know the grave doth gape for thee thrice wider than for other men."

(Henry IV, V,v,57–58)

The concept that increased morbidity and mortality is associated with obesity is not new. As Framingham, Massachusetts, is far removed from Stratford on Avon, so too contemporary understanding of relative risk is conceptually distant from that so poetically set forth by Shakespeare. Modern knowledge suggests that the "thrice" increased risk reflects poetic license and not fact. The relationship between excess body weight and increased risk of morbidity and mortality of cardiovascular disease is complex, however, and it is clouded by centuries of presupposition and dogma.

Obesity is a disorder that is difficult to study epidemiologically. The variety of etiologies of obesity in animal models suggests that excess body fat is a single physical manifestation of a spectrum of regulatory metabolic abnormalities.[1] To use an analogy, if all instances of fever were considered one entity, there would be a variety of opinions as to the seriousness of fever. Not suprisingly, confusion exists over the risk of excess mortality conferred by excess body fat. Certain degrees of body weight are considered abnormal on the basis of their association with excessive morbidity or mortality.[2] Just as excessive height per se is not considered a disease, excessive fat has few intrinsic pathologic features. The classification of obesity as *pathologic* stems from the increased prevalence of related diseases.

Overweight may be defined as a syndrome characterized by excessive accumulation of body fat as a consequence of an imbalance between energy intake and energy

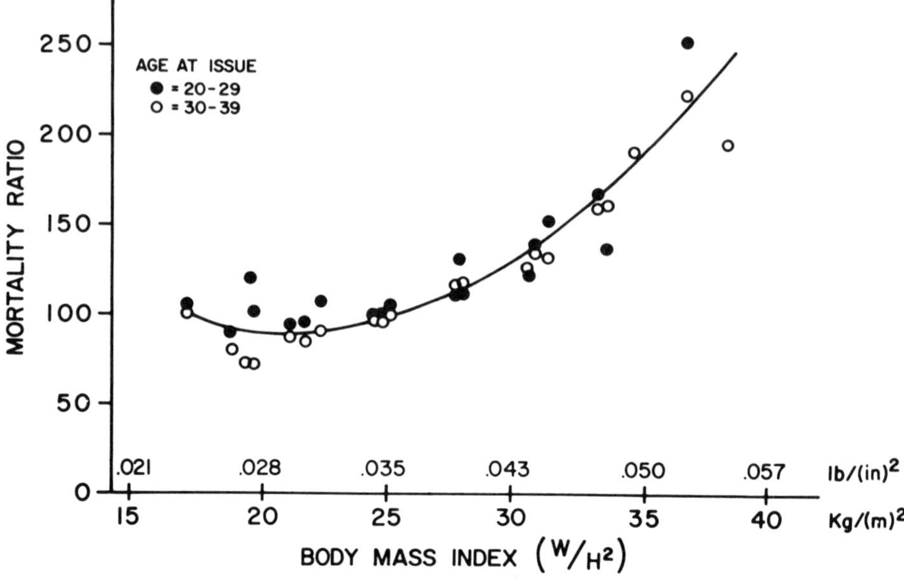

Fig. 7-1.   Body mass index and risk of mortality. (Reproduced with permission from Bray GA: The risks and disadvantages of obesity. In: The Obese Patient. Philadelphia, WB Saunders, 1976.)

expenditure; when overweight leads to morbidity or increased risk or mortality, it becomes *obesity*. Body weight is a continuous distribution rather than a bimodal distribution of normality and obesity. The Build and Blood Pressure Study[3] showed that there was a continuously increasing risk of mortality with increasing body mass index (BMI = Wt (kg)/Ht² (m)) (Fig. 7-1). Risk may differ among different subgroups of the obese, further complicating the operational definition.

In reviewing the data relating obesity to cardiovascular disease, we will deal first with intrinsic effects on the heart followed by influences on the risk of coronary heart disease.

THE EFFECT OF OBESITY ON THE HEART

Nutritionists view the heart as an organ that supplies oxygen to the body for the metabolism of nutrient fuels. Obesity imposes increased demands for oxygen, with subsequent hemodynamic alterations. Changes in the heart itself occur that compensate for the increased demands of peripheral tissues.

Body Size

Among different species as well as within single species, as body weight increases, demand for oxygen increases, thereby increasing basal energy expenditure. As animal species increase in size, metabolic mass increases, which requires more oxygen for survival. Body mass increases proportionately more than surface area. Therefore, when energy expenditure is expressed per unit weight, there is a decrease in calories per unit weight as animal-species size increases, while the energy expenditure per unit surface area remains relatively fixed.[4]

It is difficult to assess whether alterations in oxygen consumption are related to the pathogenesis of obesity. A decrease in energy expenditure and in oxygen consumption would predispose to the development of obesity. Studies in the obese have not identified significant declines in basal metabolic rate but have suggested instead increases in basal metabolic rate similar to those seen as animals species increase in size. Since oxygen consumption is greater in larger subjects, it is difficult to perform simple comparisons of the obese and the lean. This problem has led to attempts to normalize oxygen consumption in the lean and obese, so as to define a change in oxygen consumption independent of the increased body weight. Bray[5] has shown that oxygen consumption of obese patients increases linearly with increasing surface area or increasing body weight. When the obese are compared to the lean by normalizing oxygen consumption per unit weight or per surface area, there is a suggestive decline in oxygen consumption per unit weight and no significant change per unit surface area.[6] Thus, attempts at normalization have not clarified whether changes in oxygen consumption are important in the etiology of obesity. From the standpoint of the heart, however, the demands for oxygen and for cardiac output in an obese subject exceed those of a lean subject of the same height.

Hemodynamics

Hemodynamic studies by several investigators support this concept of a hyperdynamic circulation. Divitiis[7] examined the hemodynamic status of ten obese subjects who showed no stigmata of cardiac or respiratory failure, who had normal electrocardiograms, and who were not hypertensive. Oxygen consumption ($\dot{V}O_2$) was greater than normal and was associated with an increased cardiac output (CO) (Table 7-1). Since the heart rate (HR) was not more rapid than normal, the observed increase in cardiac output could be attributed to a greater stroke volume (SV). The greater stroke volume was secondary to an elevation in preload from the expansion of blood volume. Increased oxygen consumption was not associated with an abnormally widened arterial venous oxygen difference (A-V O_2), but there was a statistically significant correlation between the A-V O_2 difference and body weight. The systemic vascular resistance (SVR) was normal to low, allowing increased cardiac output without the development of hypertension. The elevation in preload, however, led to an elevation of the left ventricular end-diastolic pressure (LVEDP) that was correlated with weight.

The increased LVEDP was transmitted to the pulmonary vasculature as indicated by an elevated pulmonary capillary wedge (PCW) pressure as well as an increased pulmonary artery (PA) pressure. The total pulmonary resistance (TPR) and the arteriolar pulmonary resistance (APR), however, were within normal limits. The elevation of the mean pulmonary artery pressure was also reflected by the fact that the right ventricular end-diastolic pressure (RVEDP) and right atrial (RA) mean pressure were elevated.

Table 7-1. Hemodynamic Effects of Obesity[a]

Hemodynamic Variables	Obese (n = 10) Mean ± SD
VO_2 (ml/min)	311.5 ± 77.1
CO (L/min)	7.56 ± 1.30
HR (beats/min)	84.6 ± 12.97
SV (ml/beat)	91.28 ± 19.40
$A\text{-}VO_2$ (vol %)	4.09 ± 0.63
SVR (dyn-sec-cm^{-5})	1,120.00 ± 234.00
LVEDP (mm Hg)	16.65 ± 6.20
PA wedge Mean (pressure (mm Hg)	16.75 ± 6.20
PA mean pressure (mm Hg)	23.45 ± 6.70
TPR (dyn-sec-cm^{-5})	248.80 ± 63.20
APR (dyn-sec-cm^{-5})	71.60 ± 26.80
RVEDP (mm Hg)	10.70 ± 3.30
RA mean pressure (mm Hg)	9.10 ± 2.82
LVSWI/LVEDP ratio	3.68 ± 1.70
V_{max} (ml/sec)	0.92 ± 0.36

[a]Modified from Divitiis O, Fazio S. Petitto M, et al: Obesity and cardiac function. Circulation 64:477, 1981. By permission of the American Heart Association, Inc.

Examination of the left ventricular function curve, which compares the stroke work index (SWI) with the LVEDP, showed a diminished contractile response that did not allow appropriate systolic work, despite increased ventricular filling pressure. The ratio of SWI to LVEDP, an index of contractile efficiency, was negatively correlated with weight and with the degree of overweight. The contractile element velocity at zero load (V_{max}), which is not highly influenced by preload, also suggested that left ventricular contractility was reduced.

Kaltman and Goldring[8] suggested that similar changes in their obese patients were due primarily to the hypervolemic state and not to impaired left ventricular performance. Their study investigated similar hemodynamic parameters in obese patients at rest, with the legs elevated to increase venous return to the heart, and with exercise. Study of patients at rest to confirm the findings of previous investigators, showed an increased cardiac output achieved by a larger stroke volume at normal heart rate. There was an elevated LVEDP. When the legs of the patients were elevated, increased blood flow to the heart and expansion of central blood volume caused LVEDP to increase significantly, and this effect was further exaggerated by exercise. The central blood volume was expanded out of proportion to the total blood volume. As the distensibility of the central circulation fell, the LVEDP increased. The decrease in distensibility of the central circulation (Δ CBV/ΔP) was related linearly to the increase in total blood volume. These observations suggested that the expansion of blood volume might be the primary adaptive response to the increased demand for cardiac output in the obese. Kaltman and Goldring hypothesized further that the increased total blood volume led to an increased central blood volume and a subsequent increase in LVEDP. The exercise-induced rise in LVEDP caused pulmonary vascular congestion, which contributed to the symptoms of dyspnea on exertion in these patients. Presumably, weight loss and/or diuretics might alleviate these symptoms by reducing blood volume.

The work of other investigators, however, suggests that the hemodynamic changes represent more than a reversible physiologic adaptation to increased cardiac demand imposed by obesity, and are the consequence of intrinsic changes in the myocardium that persist even after weight reduction.[9,10] Alexandar's original study indicated that oxygen consumption and subsequently cardiac output fell with weight loss.[9] Associated with decreased demand for cardiac output was a contraction in blood volume and a concomitant reduction in left ventricular stroke volume and stroke work. Although A-V O_2 differences were at the upper limit of normal before weight loss, these levels declined significantly closer to the mean after weight loss. Although the LVEDP showed some decline toward normal values at rest following weight loss, the elevation in the LVEDP with exercise persisted after weight loss. The continued elevation of the LVEDP with exercise after extreme weight loss and contraction of blood volume suggested that the ventricular dysfunction was attributable to intrinsically reduced ventricular compliance, probably associated with myocardial hypertrophy.

Anatomical data are in accord with this conclusion. Smith reported the linear relation between heart weight and body weight in 1928.[11] Smith found a normal mean ratio of cardiac weight to body weight of .43 percent for men and .40 percent for women. Amad and coworkers[12] later reported data on 12 markedly obese subjects whose heart weight ranged from 400 to greater than 1 kg. Compared with the predicted weight of the heart based on ideal body weight, the hearts of the obese were twice as heavy. Heart weight as a percentage of actual body weight maintained a mean of 0.40 percent, as would be predicted from Smith's study of normals. Although the increase in heart weight in obese subjects follows the normal linear curve of heart weight versus body weight, other anatomic data suggest that these are not normal hearts. In the obese patients, all measurements of the ventricular wall thicknesses were above the highest normal (15 mm).

Right ventricular hypertrophy, by the same criteria of wall thickness, was less consistent. Microscopic examination of the myocardium also suggested that hypertrophy had occurred. Clinically, cardiac hypertrophy can be detected by an increase of 1 mm in cardiac transverse diameter on chest x-ray for every 3 lb increase in body weight between 100 and 200 lbs of excess weight.[13]

Obesity Hypoventilation

The "Pickwickian syndrome," or *obesity hypoventilation*, has important ramifications pertaining to the heart. Burwell characterized the obesity-hypoventilation syndrome as a complex of obesity, hypersomnolence, hypoventilation with periodic breathing, and cor pulmonale.[14] Although right ventricular hypertrophy and congestive heart failure are well-recognized parts of the Pickwickian syndrome, arrhythmias and systemic arterial hypertension have only recently been recognized as a complication of sleep apnea. Tilkian[15] monitored the electrocardiograms of 25 patients with sleep apnea both awake and asleep. All patients had normal sinus rhythm while awake. During sleep, however, nine patients had sinus bradycardia, nine had asystolic intervals of 2.5 to 13.0 seconds, four had second degree AV block, one had atrial tachycardia, and two patients had ventricular tachycardia. Schroeder observed elevation of systolic arterial pressure exceeding 200 mm Hg and diastolic arterial pressure exceeding 120 mm Hg during episodes of sleep apnea.[16] Weight loss may improve Pickwickian syndrome, but some patients with obstructive sleep apnea may require tonsillectomy or tracheostomy. Doxapram and progesterone have been used successfully to stimulate respiration in selected cases; but, like oxygen therapy, these drugs should be administered only with a program of careful monitoring.[17]

OBESITY AND CARDIOVASCULAR DISEASE

Obesity is associated with increased incidence of hyperlipidemia, diabetes mellitus, and hypertension. Obesity has direct impact on the incidence of cardiovascular disease as an independent risk factor, and as an influence on other risk factors.

Hypertriglyceridemia represents the most common form of hyperlipidemia observed in the obese, with hypercholesterolemia found less consistently.[18] High-density lipoprotein (HDL), purportedly inversely correlated with risk of developing cardiovascular disease,[19] is decreased in the obese.[20] Elevations of triglycerides and/or cholesterol may decrease with weight loss; typically, triglycerides decrease, HDL increases, and total cholesterol responds variably.[20] Diabetes is associated so closely with obesity and hypertriglyceridemia that the term *diabesity* has been coined to describe the relationship.[2] Diabesity in the obese may lead to increased cardiovascular risk through altered lipid metabolism or through the angiopathy of diabetes.

Blood Pressure in Obesity

It has been suggested that hypertension alone accounts for the majority of covariant risks in the obese. Keys[21] has pointed out that predictability of coronary heart disease is not improved in some analyses by taking into account the body mass index when other factors such as age, systolic blood pressure, smoking, and cholesterol are considered concomitantly. Before reviewing the epidemiologic studies of indirect blood pressure in the obese, we should examine the accuracy of indirect blood pressure measurements in obese patients. A comparison of direct and indirect measurements of blood pressure do not provide a consistent answer to whether indirect sphygnomanometry is a reliable index of direct blood pressure recordings.[22]

Consistently marked elevations in indirect blood pressure in the obese are not likely to incorrectly diagnose hypertension. An obese arm exerts a complex effect on indirect blood pressure measurement such that the measurement may be more representative of an anthropometric measure (arm circumference) than of the actual blood pressure.

Multiple studies[23–25] demonstrated a decline in the indirect blood pressure reading associated with elongation of the blood pressure cuff bladder or increase of cuff width (usual dimension 12 × 23 cm). In one study,[24] systolic pressure was measured in subjects with arm circumferences exceeding the largest bladder length of 30 cm. Karvonen and associates[26] examined the accuracy of indirect blood pressure readings by obtaining readings with a 14 × 40 cm cuff and the usual 12 ×

23 cm cuff and comparing them direct intrarterial readings. With the larger bladder they observed significantly smaller random errors than with the smaller bladder for both diastolic and systolic blood pressures. The error of the indirect measurements could not be correlated with arm circumference. Since all pataients had an arm circumference less than 32 cm, and the mode of the arm circumference of the patients was only 26 cm, these subjects were not a complete representation of the obese. A subsequent study by Simpson and coworkers[27] showed that widening the cuff from 12 to 14 cm significantly lowered indirect blood pressure readings. The wider cuff did not appreciably alter the large intersubject variability. Lengthening the cuff from 23 to 35 cm and leaving the cuff width at 12 cm yielded lower indirect pressure readings, and also significantly reduced intersubject variation. We can conclude that wider and longer cuffs tend to reduce intersubject variability over a wide range of arm circumference, and tend to reduce the indirect blood pressure reading.

King[28] used a unique approach to examine the effect of obesity on indirect blood pressure readings. He simulated increasing grades of obesity by using a sponge rubber wrapping on the arms of normotensive nonobese subjects. By examining the same subjects, the problems of validating alternate methods of determining "true blood pressure" were obviated and residual variance was minimized. Blood pressure readings progressively increased as arm circumference increased when the 11 cm width cuff was used but did not change significantly with the 15 cm width cuff when both cuffs extended around the arm completely (Fig. 7-2). King subsequently compared the results obtained with combinations of narrow (11 cm) and wide (15 cm) cuff widths and standard (26 cm) and long (42 cm) cuff lengths in the same subjects with the same technique for increasing arm circumference (Fig. 7-3). These observations showed that the wide and long (15 × 42 cm) cuffs produced the most consistent blood pressure reading over wide ranges of arm circumference. King concluded that the accuracy of indirect blood pressure measurement depended on the assumption that the pressure is transmitted equally throughout the tissues enclosed in the cuff; this condition was not met by the shorter cuffs, especially in the obese. He showed that the assymetry of this pressure distribution was greater at higher cuff pressures, which would tend to potentiate the overestimation of blood pressure in the truly hypertensive obese patient.

Thus, use of short of narrow blood pressure cuffs to obtain indirect blood pressure measurements in the obese results in readings that reflect not only the blood pressure, but also contributes an artifactual increase that reflects a complex function of arm circumference. Keys reported that the standard 12 × 23 cm cuff was used irrespective of arm circumference in the Seven Country Study.[29] Thus, Keys' suggestion— that the effect of obesity on the risk of developing coronary heart disease might be totally explained by hypertension[21]—may represent the use of an inappropriately small cuff for the obese subjects, making the resultant reading an anthropometric measure more than one of blood pressure.

It was observed recently that subjects with obesity of the hypercellular type develop disproportionate upper-body obesity compared with lower-body obesity.[30] By influencing the arm circumference, upper-body obesity would lead to inflated indirect blood pressure measurements. Thus, in two obese patients with the same

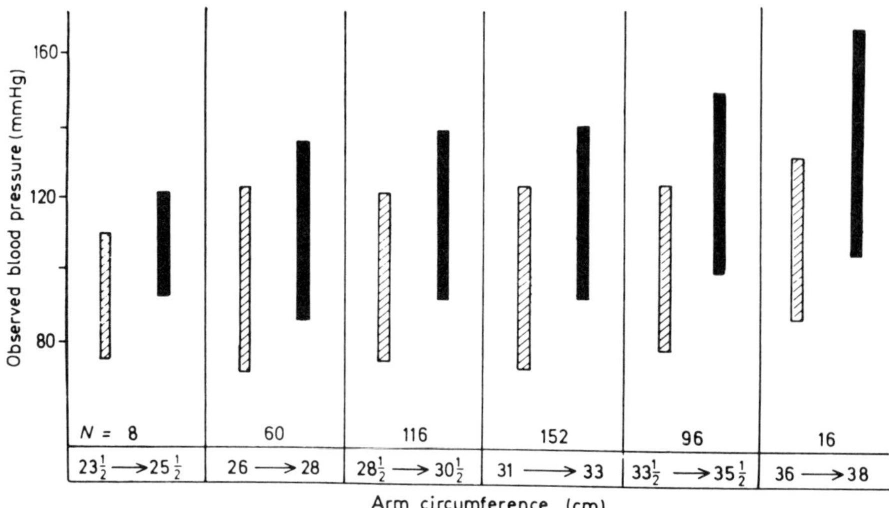

Fig. 7-2. Effect of arm circumference on indirect blood pressure reading taken with a cuff bladder width of 11 cm (black bars) or 15 cm (cross-hatched bars) and 38 cm length. (Reproduced with permission from King GE: Errors in clinical measurement of indirect blood pressure in obesity. Clin Sci 32:223, 1967.)

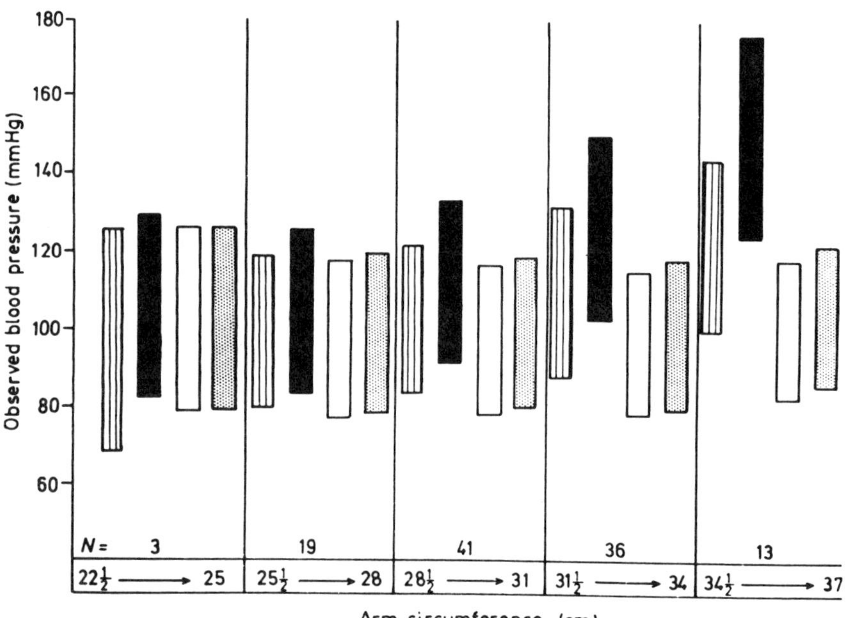

Fig. 7-3. Effect of arm circumference on indirect blood pressure reading taken with cuff bladders of varying widths and lengths. Vertical hatched bars (15 × 26 cm); black bars (11 × 26 cm); open bars (15 × 42 cm); stippled bars (11 × 42 cm). (Reproduced with permission from King GE: Errors in clinical measurement of indirect blood pressure in obesity. Clin Sci 32:223, 1967.)

elevated, the one with the hypercellular upper-body obesity would have the larger arm circumference and potentially a greater artifactual elevation in indirectly measured blood pressure if an inappropriately small cuff were used. An analysis of the HANES-I data found that subscapular skinfold thickness was correlated with blood pressure but triceps skinfold thickness was not. This suggests that, as for diabetes, maturity-onset central obesity carries the highest risk for the development of hypertension; increasing arm circumference (associated with increased triceps skinfold) does not necessarily lead to artifactual increases in blood pressure measured indirectly. The hypercellular type of juvenile-onset obesity may be the common denominator for markedly increased risk of coronary heart disease. Although exactly what the sphygmomanometer measures is unclear, a consistent and marked elevation in this measure of blood pressure probably represents truly elevated intra-arterial pressure. Since this technique was used in predicting cardiovascular risk in the large epidemiological studies, the bias in elevating indirect blood pressure readings introduced by a large arm circumference may represent an important indication of cardiovascular risk, derived from the usual sphygmomanometric measure performed with the small cuff.

Elevated readings are more common in the obese, regardless of the physiologic significance of the indirect blood pressure measurement. The Chicago People's Gas Company Study[31] was a cross-sectional examination of men aged 40 to 59 years, stratified according to the ratio of their observed weight to desirable weight at time of entry. As this ratio increased, there was a stepwise increase in the prevalence of diastolic hypertension when either 95 or 100 mm Hg was used as the cut-off point (Table 7-2). In the CHEC program,[44] which examined more than 1 million subjects, there was a relationship between overweight and hypertension which persisted when age, sex, race, or family history of hypertension were taken into account. A multivariate analysis of the effect of relative weight on blood pressure in more than 13,000 men and women in the Chicago Board of Health Community Survey supported these findings.[33] Relative weight was correlated significantly with diastolic blood pressure after age, heart rate, serum cholesterol, 1-hour postprandial plasma glucose, and hematocrit were taken into account. Thus, a large body of cross-sectional data reveals that blood pressure and weight are correlated significantly (r = 0.2–0.3), suggesting that elevation in indirectly measured blood pressure is prevalent among the overweight.

In longitudinal studies, weight gain is associated with an increased risk of developing hypertension. The People's Gas Company Study[31] suggests that weight

Table 7-2. Hypertension and Body Weight[a]

Relative Weight	Prevalence of Hypertension	
	diastolic BP >95 mm Hg	diastolic BP >100 mm Hg
(wt/desirable wt)	(per 1,000)	
≤ 0.95	61	53
0.95–1.04	68	53
≥ 1.15	143	102
≥ 1.25	178	126

[a]Modified from Stamler J: Lectures on Preventive Cardiology. New York, Grune and Stratton, 1967.

status at an early age and the subsequent rapidity of weight gain are highly corre-lated with the development of hypertension in middle age. The Framingham Study[34] showed that subjects who were 20 percent overweight at time of admission had an 8-times greater risk of developing hypertension at the 12-year point than the group that was 10 percent underweight at the time of admission. Examing the same cohort, Ashley and Kannel[35] reported that for each 10 unit change in relative weight there was a change of 6.6 mm Hg in systolic blood pressure in men and a more modest change of 4.5 mm Hg for women.

Weight loss should have a significant salutary effect on lowering elevated blood pressures. A broad base of evidence supports this concept. When Benedict conducted his classical studies on undernutrition in normal men in 1918,[36] he observed a significant decline in blood pressure in his subjects as they starved. Subsequently, Keys, in the Minnesota experiment in undernutrition,[37] found a mean decrease in blood pressure from 106/69 to 97/64, and also reduction in pulse rate, oxygen consumption, and heart size. These observations suggested that the reduction in blood pressure that occurred in normal-weight individuals with reduc-tion in food intake could be explained by reduced demand on the cardiovascular system to support oxidative metabolism. On a larger scale, Brozek[38] reported observations in the European countries that experienced widespread famine during World War II. There was a reduction in the incidence of hypertension and in hypertensive complications observed clinically and at autopsy. These reports sug-gest that there is a strong relationship between body weight, independent of obesity, and a tendency to hypertension.

Weight reduction in the obese results in a variable but definite decline in indirect blood pressure. A study by Dahl[39] in 1958 hypothesized that the major effect of weight reduction was due to the salt restriction that accompanied caloric restriction. In order to analyze these effects separately, Dahl lowered caloric intake while holding salt intake constant and observed a very minimal decrease in blood pressure. When salt was restricted, but calories were not restricted, there was a marked decrease in blood pressure. Subsequently, Reisin and associates[40] studied 121 obese, hypertensive patients divided into three matched groups. The first group was placed on a weight reduction program and did not receive any antihypertensive drugs; the second group was placed on a weight reduction program and received their regular antihypertensive drugs; the third group was on no dietary program but received their regular antihypertensive drugs. Because of the ethnic kosher diet, it was possible to reduce caloric intake while keeping salt intake at a generous level, though the study did not assess this directly. Both groups on the weight reduction program lost at least 3 kg, with a mean weight loss of 10.5 kg. The blood pressure returned to normal in 75 percent of the first group and 60 percent of the second group. In the third group without a dietary intervention, there was no significant change in weight or blood pressure. These results suggest that caloric restriction and weight loss in the absence of reduction of salt intake can lead to a significant reduction in blood pressure, with or without concomitant antihypertensive medica-tion. There is a definite interrelationship between caloric and salt intake and their ability to modulate the hypertensive response.

Effects of Fasting

Gamble first reported that fasting led to a natriuresis in the early days of a fast.[41] In his classic experiments he showed that the addition of carbohydrate led to the sparing of sodium. Subsequently, several mechanisms have been suggested for the natriuresis of fasting. The suggestion that salt is excreted as the cation of metabolically generated organic anions has the most support,[42] but the antinaturetic effort of insulin may also play a role.[43] Recently DeHaven and coworkers[44] studied obese subjects fed a 400 kcal diet consisting either of 100 percent protein or an isocaloric mixture of 50 percent protein and 50 percent carbohydrate. The total protein diet yielded a significant increase in ketone levels, with concomitant significant increase in sodium excretion. The supine blood pressures in these normotensive patients did not change significantly, but the patients who were on the protein diet had an increased incidence of orthostatic hypotension. There was a 40 percent decline in basal plasma norepinephrine levels and a blunted response of plasma norepinephrine to standing. Had these patients been studied only supine, the investigators would have concluded that there was no significant effect of diet or weight loss on blood pressure; however, standing systolic and diastolic blood pressures declined significantly, especially in the group that had the most markedly negative sodium balance. This study also reveals that there are two components to the hypotensive effect of diet and weight reduction: a volume-dependent, salt-related component and an autonomic component.

Landsburg and Young demonstrated reduction in norepinephrine turnover in tissue of fasted rats compared with rats fed a diet rich in carbohydrate.[45,46] They compared the blood pressure and autonomic response to sodium and high carbohydrate overfeeding in the spontaneously hypertensive rat (SHR) and the normotensive Wistar-Kyoto (WKY) strain. The SHR was more sensitive to diet-induced blood pressure changes than the normotensive WKY. In the SHR, sucrose overfeeding raised blood pressure more than did sodium loading or overfeeding with a high fat diet. Despite differences in the blood pressure response, overfeeding a diet rich in sucrose led to equivalent increases in tissue norepinephrine turnover in both the hypertensive SHR rat and WKY normotensive rats. Jund[47] examined the effect of a low-energy, low-carbohydrate diet on blood pressure, sodium balance, and sympathetic nervous system activity. His patients initially received a high-energy diet containing 40 kcal/kg of desirable body weight and 10 g of fat, 80 g of protein, and 52 mmol of sodium. On this diet, the patients' weights were stable, and there was a net positive sodium balance with a stable blood pressure and urinary 4-hydroxy-3-methoxymandelate (HMMA). Subsequently, the carbohydrate was removed from the diet, reducing it to 9.2 kcal/kg of desirable weight with the same sodium intake. This led to a significant decline in supine blood pressure. Reisen's study,[40] suggests that the decline might have been greater if the blood pressure had been obtained in standing subjects. More importantly, however, there was a decline in plasma norepinephrine and urinary HMMA. Although there was a net decline in the apparent balance of total body sodium on the low-energy diet, the net balance was still positive compared with the prestudy period. In this study carbohydrate mediated autonomic activity appeared to be a more important factor than sodium balance in the hypotensive response to carbohydrate and caloric restriction.

OBESITY AS A RISK FACTOR IN CORONARY HEART DISEASE

Long-term prospective studies since World War II have led to the hypothesis that obesity is a risk factor for the development of coronary heart disease. An analysis of the results of these studies suggests that the relationship is more complex than simple cause and effect. The Build and Blood Pressure Study[3] was the first study to focus on overweight as a risk factor in cardiovascular disease. Marks[48] subsequently reported that when body weight was 30 to 40 percent above the ideal there was an increase in mortality. These early findings were confirmed by the American Cancer Society's study,[49] which showed that the mortality of men and women 30 to 40 percent above the average weight was nearly 50 percent greater than that of subjects of average weight, and was primarily attributable to deaths from coronary heart disease. Death from coronary heart disease was 55 percent higher in subjects who were 30 to 40 percent overweight, and 100 percent higher in subjects greater than 40 percent overweight, compared with normal-weight subjects. Although these studies suggest an increased prevalence of coronary artery disease among the obese, it is much less certain that obesity is either an independent causal factor or even a predictor of cardiovascular disease.

Several lines of evidence have challenged the concept of an increased prevalence of obesity among patients with proven coronary heart disease. Weinsier and coworkers[50] examined the relationship of body fat, measured by tritium dilution, to the prevalence of coronary heart disease, evidenced by overt clinical findings or coronary angiography. Patients with coronary artery disease by clinical assessment or abnormal coronary angiography had no greater percentage of body fat than those without evidence of coronary artery disease. A second study examined over 2,000 men and women referred for coronary angiography.[51] There was no association between obesity and the degree of angiographically proven coronary artery occlusion.

In both studies a selection bias was operative, since the patients were referred because of suspected disease. A second confounding factor may have been the prior effect of diet and weight loss recommended by the referring physician. This is suggested by the fact that the weight of the men and women in the latter study was significantly less than the weight of the average male and female in the comparable local population.[51] Thus, the selection process prior to coronary angiography may preclude determination of the true prevalence of coronary artery disease among the obese.

An alternative means of investigation is to study the degree of coronary atherosclerosis in a large number of accident victims (assuming that accidents occur randomly among the obese as well as among normal-weight individuals). Montenegro and Solberg,[52] as part of the International Atherosclerosis Project, examined in men dying accidentally the interrelation of anthropometric measurements and mean percentage of the intimal surface area of the coronary arteries involved by raised atherosclerotic lesions. The mean surface area involved by raised atherosclerotic lesions in the coronary arteries was analyzed by considering subjects stratified by age and distributed into quartiles of subcutaneous abdominal fat thickness or body weight (Table 7-3). The mean percentage of intimal surface area involved by atherosclerosis was greater in the heavier subjects. Though atherosclerosis was less common in the younger age group, the fractional increase in the surface area involved in the more obese, compared with the less obese, was most marked in the youngest age group. This suggests that obesity in young males is associated with more extensive early coronary atherosclerotic lesions. This study could not demonstrate statistically a consistent relationship between anthropometric measures and coronary atherosclerosis; other necropsy studies also have failed to reach a concensus.[53–55] The presence of more extensive early coronary atherosclerotic lesions in young obese subjects at necropsy is consistent with the finds of large prospective epidemiologic studies that obesity in youth is associated with a higher incidence of coronary events in later life.

In the Manitoba Study[56] in which 4,000 men entered the study at age 30 years and were followed for the next 25 years, body mass index (BMI) was significantly correlated with coronary heart disease endpoints, including sudden death, suspected or definite myocardial infarction, and coronary insufficiency. The association between BMI and the cardiovascular endpoints was not evident until after 16 years of follow-up. At the 18th year of the Framingham Study,[57] the regression coefficient of the incidence of the coronary heart disease on relative weight decreased steadily for men and women with increased age. In the Pooling Project,[58] relative weight correlated with the first major coronary event only in men in the 40 to 44 and 45 to 49 year age groups, while there was no statistical correlation between obesity and first coronary event in the older age groups.

The Harvard and University of Pennsylvania Study[59] examined longitudinally the effect of overweight in adults entering college (Table 7-4). The cardiovascular mortality ratios, as a function of overweight, systolic blood pressure, smoking, and combinations of these factors suggest that overweight is an independent risk factor and also interacts with elevated systolic blood pressure and smoking in predicting development of coronary heart disease. These studies suggest that obesity is a significant independent risk factor in young people, but the impact may not be observed for a protracted period of time. There are two possible explanations for why an effect of obesity on mortality is observed only among those who are obese in their youth. The cumulative pathologic effect of obesity on the development of coronary artery disease may take a long time to develop. Alternatively, obesity in the young may differ intrinsically from obesity in an older age group.

In juvenile-onset obesity, there is higher incidence of hyperplasia of adipocytes.[60] There is an accelerated increase inthe number of adipocytes in obesity that develops at a young age. In comparison, obesity that develops in middle age is usually marked by hypertrophy of the adipocyte.[61] The underlying mechanism leading to hyperplasia, as opposed to hypertrophy of adipocytes, is unknown. Differences in the pathophysiologic processes leading to development of two disparate types of obesity may explain the differences in the incidence and time of

Table 7-3. Coronary Artery Lesions[a]

| Age (years) | Quartile of Body Weight | | | Quartile of Abdominal Fat | | |
| | Lower | Upper | | Lower | Upper | |
	% arterial involvement		% increase in upper quartile[b]	% arterial involvement		% increase in upper quartile[b]
25–34	2.4	5.1	112.5	2.5	5.4	116
35–44	5.9	9.5	61.0	4.6	8.8	91.3
45–54	18.2	18.5	1.6	13.4	15.1	12.7
55-64	18.6	28.7	54.3	19.3	24.8	28.5

[a]Mean percent coronary artery intimal surface involved with raised lesions. Subjects are divided into quartiles of mean body weight (MBW) and quartiles of abdominal fat. (Modified from Metenegro RS and Solberg LA: Obesity, body weight, body length, and atherosclerosis. Lab Invest 18:594, 1968.

[b]($\bar{x}$ upper quartile $-$ $\bar{x}$ lower quartile/$\bar{x}$ lower quartile) $\times$ 100

Table 7-4. Comparison of Effect of Overweight versus Other Risk Factors on Mortality Ratios in Young Men[a]

Risk Factor	Mortality Ratio (Observed/Expected)
Overweight	1.4
Systolic Hypertension	1.6
Smoking	1.6
Overweight plus Smoking	1.9
Systolic Hypertension plus Smoking	2.1
Overweight plus Systolic Hypertension	2.3

[a]Modified from Paffenbarger RS, Notkin J, Krueger DE, et al: Chronic disease in former college students. II, Methods of study and observations on mortality from coronary heart disease. Am J Public Health 56:962, 1966.

development of coronary artery disease. Hypercellular and hypertrophic obesity may represent morphologically different manifestations of one pathophysiologic entity that is expressed in two different ways because of the different periods of development at which it is manifested or the different locations of the fat depot. If this were so, then the different incidences of coronary heart disease could be due to the divergent metabolic effects of hypercellular versus hypertrophic obesity. For instance, the prevalence of hypertriglyceridemia and glucose intolerance is greater in hypertrophic obesity than in hypercellular obesity.[62] Thus, diabetes (of late onset in hypertrophic obesity) and the associated lipid abnormalities may confound the association between obesity and coronary disease in multivariate statistical models. Body weight might then have a negligible association with coronary disease in those patients not classified as diabetic. It is possible that the hypercellular obesity that develops in younger people with a different metabolic abnormality would predispose to the premature development of coronary artery disease, although metabolic derangements have been more common in hypertrophic obesity. A more likely explanation is the progressive nature of juvenile obesity[63] and the correlation between weight gain and risk factors.[35]

SUMMARY AND CONCLUSION

Obesity is a level of overweight associated with an increase in morbidity and mortality largely related to cardiovascular disease. Obesity leads to cardiovascular disease by hemodynamic-induced alterations of the heart, increases in the incidence of hypertension, and as a direct risk factor for coronary heart disease.

Obesity places hemodynamic demands on the heart to supply oxygenated blood to a larger-than-normal metabolic mass. To compensate for this increased demand there is an expansion of blood volume, which leads to ventricular hypertrophy. Anatomic alterations, which result in altered ventricular performance, do not normalize fully even after weight loss.

Indirect blood pressure readings are affected in a complex way by the increased arm circumference of the obese. There is a tendency for an artifactual increase in indirect blood pressure when a narrow or short cuff is used. Although this fact has been ignored generally in studies of the prevalence of hypertension in the obese, there appears to be good collaborative evidence of a increased prevalence of hypertension in the obese. Obesity exerts its effect on blood pressure through a volume-dependent and autonomic-nervous-system–dependent mechanisms. The quantitative significance of these two systems remain to be defined, but both systems respond to reduction in food intake and weight loss.

In addition to the risk attributed to hypertension,the risk of developing coronary artery disease is increased by a small, apparently independent, effect of obesity itself. The effect is most important when obesity develops early in life. The nature of this independent effect or its age predilection for the young remains to be delineated.

The advances of 20th century medicine have substantiated the concept of increased risk of mortality due to overweight, which Shakespeare set forth in the 16th century (see epigraph at the beginning of this chapter). Although the analysis of the cardiovascular risk is more complex today, we may now warn our overweight patients with some certainty that "the grave doth gape for thee . . . wider than for other men."

REFERENCES

1. Bray GA: Experimental and clinical forms of obesity. In: The Obese Patient. Philadelphia, WB Saunders, 1976.
2. Sims EA: Definition, criteria, and prevalence of obesity. In Bray GA (ed): Obesity in America. Washington, US Dept of Health, Education and Welfare, 1979.
3. Build and Blood Pressure Study, vol 1. Chicago, Society of Actuaries, 1959.
4. Bray GA: The risks and disadvantages of obesity. In: The Obese Patient. Philadelphia, WB Saunders, 1976.
5. Bray GA: Energy Expenditure. In: The Obese Patient. Philadelphia, WB Saunders, 1976.
6. Bray GA, Schwartz M, Rozin R, Lister J: Relationships between oxygen consumption and body composition of obese patients. Metabolism 19:418, 1970.
7. Divitiis O, Fazio S. Petitto M, Maddalena G, Contaldo F, Mancini M: Obesity and cardiac function. Circulation 64:477, 1981.
8. Kaltman AJ, Goldring RM: Role of circulatory congestion in the cardiorespiratory failure of obesity. Am J Med 60:645, 1976.
9. Alexander JK, Peterson KL: Cardiovascular effects of weight reduction. Circulation 45:310, 1972.
10. Backman L, Freyschuss V, Hallberg D, Melcher A: Reversibility of cardiovascular changes in extreme obesity. Acta Med Scand 205:367, 1979.
11. Smith HL: Relation of the weight of the heart to the weight of the body and of the weight of the heart to age. Am Heart J 4:79, 1928.
12. Amad KH, Brennan JC, Alexander JK: The cardiac pathology of chronic exogenous obesity. Circulation 32:740, 1965.
13. Alexander JK, Amad KH, Cole VW: Observations on some clinical features of extreme obesity with particular reference to cardiorespiratory effects. Am J Med 32:512, 1962.
14. Burwell G, Robin E, Whaley R, et al: Extreme obesity associated with alveolar hypoventilation: a Pickwickian syndrome. Am J Med 21:811, 1956.

15. Tilkian AG, Motta J, Guilleminault C: Cardiac Arrlaythmias in sleep apnea. In Guilleminault C, Dement WC (eds): Sleep Apnea Snydromes. New York, Alan R Liss, 1978.
16. Schroeder JS, Motta J, Guilleminault C: Hemodynamic studies in sleep apnea. In Guilleminault C, Dement WC (eds): Sleep Apnea Syndromes. New York, Alan R Liss, 1978.
17. Chaudhary BA, Speir WA: Sleep apnea syndromes. Southern Med J 75:39, 1982.
18. Nestel P: Relation of lipoprotein and cholesterol abnormalities to obesity. In Bray GA (ed): Recent Advances in Obesity Research: II. London, Newman Publishing, 1978.
19. Gordon T, Castelli WP, Hjortland MC, Kannel WB, Dawber TR: High density lipoprotein as a protective factor against coronary heart disease. Am J Med 62:707, 1977.
20. Carlsson LA, Ericsson M: Quantitative and qualitative serum lipoprotein analysis. Atherosclerosis 21:417, 1975.
21. Keys A: Overweight and the risk of heart attack and sudden death. In Bray GA (ed): Obesity in Perspective. Washington, US Dept of Health Education and Welfare, 1976.
22. Nielsen PE, Janniche H: The accuracy of auscultatory measurement of arm blood pressure in very obese subjects. Acta Med Scand 195:403, 1974.
23. Smirk FH: High Arterial Pressure. Springfield, Charles C Thomas, 1957.
24. Nukuda A, Nagata H, Kadowaki I, Ishizaki T, Ishibashi M: Cuff size and blood pressure reading. Nishin Igaku 48:186, 1961 (in Japanese). Quoted by Simpson JA, Jamieson G, Pickhaus DW, Grover RF: Effect of size of cuff bladder on accuracy of measurement of indirect blood pressure. Am Heart J 70:208, 1965.
25. Burch GE, Shewey L: Sphygmomanometric cuff size and blood pressure recordings, JAMA 225:1215, 1973.
26. Karvonen MJ, Telivvo LJ, Jarvinen EJK: Sphygmomanometer cuff size and the accuracy of indirect measurement of blood pressure. Am J Cardiol 13:688, 1964.
27. Simpson JA, Jamieson G, Dickhaus DW, Grover RF: Effect of size of cuff bladder on accuracy of measurement of indirect blood pressure. Am Heart J 70:208, 1965.
28. King GE: Errors in clinical measurement of blood pressure in obesity. Clin Sci 32:223, 1967.
29. Keys A, et al: Epidemiological studies related to coronary heart disease: characteristics of men aged 40–59 in seven countries. Seven Countries ACTA Medica Scandinavica, suppl 460, 1966.
30. Kissebah AH, Vydelingum W, Murray R, Evans DJ, Hartz AJ, Kalkhoff RK, Adams PW: Relation of body fat distribution of to metabolic complications of obesity. JCEM 54:254, 1982.
31. Stamler J: Lectures on Preventive Cardiology. New York, Grune and Stratton, 1967.
32. Stamler J Stamler R, Reidlinger WF, Algera G, Roberts RH: Weight and blood pressure. Findings in hypertension screening of 1 million Americans. JAMA 240:1607, 1978.
33. Stamler J, Stamler R, Rhomberg P, Dyer A, Berkson DM, Reedus W, Wannamaker J: Multivariate analysis of the relationship of six variables to blood pressure: Findings from Chicago community surveys, 1965–1971. J Chron Dis 28:499, 1975.
34. Kannel WB, Brand W, Skinner JJ, Dawber TR, McNamara PM: The relation of adiposity to blood pressure and development of hypertension. Ann Intern Med 67:48, 1967.
35. Ashley FW, Kannel WB: Relation of weight change to changes in atherogenic traits: The Framingham Study. J Chron Dis 27:103, 1974.
36. Benedict FG, Roth P: Effect of a prolonged reduction in diet on twenty-five men. Proc Nat Acad Sci 4:149, 1918.

37. Keys A, Henschel A, Taylor H: Size and function of the human heart at rest in semi-starvation and in subsequent rehabilitation. Am J Physiol 150:153, 1947.
38. Brozek J, Chapman CB, Keys A: Drastic food restriction: Effect on cardiovascular dynamics in normotensive and hypertensive conditions. JAMA 137:1569, 1948.
39. Dahl LK, Silver L, Christie RW: Role of salt in the fall of blood pressure accompanying reduction of obesity. N Engl J Med 258:1186, 1968.
40. Reisin E, Abel R, Modan M, Silverberg DS, Eliahou HE, Modan B: Effect of weight loss without salt restriction on the reduction of blood pressure in overweight hypertensive patients. N Engl J Med 298:1, 1968.
41. Gamble JL: Physiological information gained from studies on life raft reation. Harvey Lect 42:247, 1947.
42. Sigler MH: The mechanism of the natriuresis of fasting. J Clin Invest 55:377, 1975.
43. De Fronzo RA: Insulin and renal sodium handling: clinical implications. Int J Obesity 5(suppl 1):93, 1981.
44. De Haven J, Sherwin R, Hendler R, Felig P: Nitrogen and sodium balance and sympathetic-nervous-system activity in obese subjects treated with a low-calorie protein or mixed diet. N Engl J Med 302:477, 1980.
45. Landsberg L, Young JB: Fasting, feeding, and the regulation of sympathetic activity. N Engl J Med 298:1295, 1978.
46. Landsberg L, Young JB: Diet and the sympathetic nervous system: relationship to hypertension. Int J Obesity 5(suppl 1):79, 1981.
47. Jung RT, Shetty PS, Barrand M, Callingham BA, James WPT: Role of catecholamines in hypotensive response to dieting. Br Med J 1:12, 1979.
48. Marks HH: Influence of obesity in morbidity and mortality. NY Acad Sci. 36:296, 1960.
49. Lew EA, Garfinkel L: Variations in mortality by weight among 750,000 men and women. J Chron Dis 32:563, 1979.
50. Weinsier RL, Fuchs RK, Kay TD, Triebwasser JH, Lancaster MC: Body fat: Its relationship to coronary heart disease, blood pressure, lipids and other risk factors measured in a large male population. Am J Med 61:815, 1976.
51. Anderson AJ, Barboriak JJ, Rimm AA: Risk factors and angiographically determined coronary occlusion. Am J Epidemiol 107:8, 1978.
52. Montenegro MR, Solbert LA: Obesity, body weight, body length, and atherosclerosis. Lab Invest 18:594, 1968.
53. Wilens SL: Bearing of general nutritional state on atherosclerosis. Arch Int Med 79:129, 1947.
54. Wilkens RH, Roberts JC, Moses C: Autopsy studies in atherosclerosis in the presence of obesity, hypertension, nephrosclerosis, rheumatic heart disease. Circulation 220:527, 1959.
55. Kannel WB, Gordon T: Obesity and cardiovascular disease: The Framingham Study. In Burland W, Samuel PD, Yudkin J (eds): Obesity. London, Churchill Livingstone, 1974.
56. Rabkin SW, Mathenson FAL, Hsu PH: Relation of body weight to development of ischemic heart disease in a cohort of young North American men after a 25-year observation period: The Manitoba Study. Am J Cardiol 39:452, 1977.
57. Gordon T, Kannel WB: Obesity and cardiovascular disease: the Framingham Study. Clin Endo Metab 5:367, 1976.
58. Pooling Project Research Group: Relationship of blood pressure, serum cholesterol, smoking habit, relative weight and ECG abnormalities to incidence of major coronary events: Final report of the pooling Project. J Chron Dis 31:201, 1978.
59. Paffenbarger RS, Notkin J, Krueger DE, Wolf PA, Thorne MC, Le Baver EJ, Williams

JL: Chronic disease in former college students. II, Methods of study and observations on mortality from coronary heart disease. AM J Public Health 56:962, 1966.
60. Hirsch J, Knittle JL: Cellularity of obese and nonobese human adipose tissue. Fed Proc 29:1516, 1970.
61. Salans LB, Cushman SW, Weismann RE: Studies of human adipose tissue. J Clin Invest 52:929, 1973.
62. Berglund G, Larson B, Anderson O, et al: Body composition and glucose metabolism in hypertensive middle-aged males. Acta Med Scand 200:163, 1976.
63. Krotkiewski M, Sjostrom L, Bjorntorp P, Carlgren G, Smith V: Adipose tissue cellularity in relation to prognosis for weight reduction. Int J Obesity 1:395, 1977.

8 | Alcohol and The Heart

Howard S. Friedman
Charles S. Lieber

Alcohol has marked acute and chronic cardiovascular effects. Even at blood levels that result from the ingestion of only a few cocktails, alcohol will alter cardiac hemodynamics and affect the regional distribution of cardiac output. Chronic alcohol abuse is associated with the development of severe myocardial damage. Although it is widely recognized that ethanol abuse produces a cardiomyopathy, casual alcohol use is generally regarded as having a beneficial effect on the cardiovascular system. Alcohol has, in fact, been suggested for the treatment of angina pectoris for more than 200 years, although evidence supporting this recommendation has not been presented. Epidemiologic surveys have repeatedly shown a lower coronary disease mortality rate in social drinkers when contrasted with teetotalers. This favorable effect has been correlated with dosage, a positive relationship manifested up to the ingestion of 60 ml of ethanol per day, irrespective of the form in which ethanol is ingested. By contrast, epidemiologic studies also suggest a relationship between the level of systemic blood pressure and the use of alcohol. An even stronger relationship has been found between alcohol abuse and hypertension.

The hallmark of alcohol-induced heart muscle disease is a dilated, hypocontractile heart. Such findings are not specific for alcohol, nor does alcohol produce this abnormality experimentally. The diagnosis of alcohol cardiomyopathy is made largely by association with long-standing heavy alcohol abuse and by exclusion of other causes of heart muscle disease. The incidence of alcoholic cardiomyopathy is not known; however, in patient populations in whom substance abuse is common, as in most municipal and federal hospitals, perhaps 10 to 15 percent of patients admitted with congestive heart failure will satisfy the *clinical* criteria for alcohol-induced heart muscle disease. If one considers also alcohol abusers who present with a dilated cardiomyopathy with concomitant valvular, coronary, or hypertensive disease wherein alcohol abuse may be contributing to the heart muscle damage, the incidence of alcohol-induced heart muscle disease may approach 20 to 25 percent of cardiac admissions to these hospitals.

While the hallmark of alcohol heart disease is a cardiomyopathy—a heart muscle disease—alcohol abuse may present primarily as a disturbance of the heart beat or even as an acute myocardial infarction. Paroxysmal and nonparoxysmal sustained atrial and ventricular arrhythmias may occur in the alcoholic, even without the presence of the electrolyte imbalance or an identifiable structural alteration in the heart. Even more intriguing is the occurrence of myocardial infarction—indistinguishable clinically from that occurring with obstructive coronary disease—which has been reported in alcoholics not having coronary artery disease.

An association of alcohol abuse and heart muscle damage has been recognized for more than 100 years. Despite the medical literature being replete with clinical, experimental, and epidemiologic investigations of the acute and chronic effects of alcohol on the heart, the action of alcohol on the cardiovascular system is still controversial, with numerous questions unanswered.

ACUTE CARDIOVASCULAR EFFECTS OF ETHANOL

Hemodynamic Effects

Ethanol is a myocardial depressant. Investigations in isolated atrial[1] and ventricular[2,3] tissue demonstrated reduced contractile function with concentrations of ethanol found with acute alcoholic intoxication. Because of the extracardiac effects of ethanol and its metabolites, studies using intact heart models have yielded conflicting findings. Mierzwiak and coworkers[4] and Wong[5] demonstrated in the dog that with autonomic blockade the cardiac depressant actions of ethanol were accentuated. Such studies suggest that the neurohumoral effects of ethanol on cardiac reflexes obscure the direct myocardial actions of ethanol. Moreover, since ethanol[6] and its metabolites, acetaldehyde[7] and acetate,[8] are vasodilators at concentrations found with alcoholic intoxication, these peripheral effects would also obscure ethanol's direct myocardial actions. By reducing aortic impedance, cardiac "pump" function may appear to be enhanced even though the myocardial contractility is actually depressed. This interpretation is supported by observations of Webb and Degerli,[9] who found in the dog that alcohol increased cardiac output and reduced peripheral resistance, although myocardial dysfunction could be demonstrated by an abnormal response to a volume challenge. Also, Mendoza and coworkers[10] observed that alcohol produced an increase in cardiac output at a time when velocity of contraction of the myocardium was actually reduced. Thus, experimental investigations clearly demonstrate that ethanol is a myocardial depressant; however the peripheral vascular and neurohumoral actions of ethanol and its metabolites may obscure this effect.

Studies in man limited to measurements of cardiac output and pressures and indices derived from these parameters have shown an improvement in cardiac function after ethanol ingestion in healthy subjects. Grollman,[11] Stein and coworkers,[12] and Riff and coworkers[13] demonstrated that ethanol increased cardiac output and reduced peripheral resistance in healthy subjects at ethanol blood levels between 100 and 200 mg/dl. In patients with heart disease, however, either no change[14] or a reduction in cardiac output[15] was observed. By contrast, ethanol depressed left ventricular ejection fraction even in normal subjects at blood ethanol levels averaging less than 150 mg/dl.[16] Similarly, systolic time intervals worsened after alcohol ingestion in normal subjects.[17,18] Thus, studies done in humans and experimental models demonstrate that ethanol is a myocardial depressant at blood ethanol levels found with alcoholic intoxication. In normal subjects, because of ethanol's vascular and neurohumoral effects, cardiac function reflected by cardiac output appears to improve after ethanol ingestion. In patients with left ventricular dysfunction, the myocardial depressant actions of alcohol predominate and cardiac output either does not change or actually declines.

Metabolic Changes

Although alcohol has been shown to produce acute cardiac metabolic changes, the biochemical explanation for the myocardial depressant effects of ethanol is not known. In the liver, acute metabolic effects of ethanol have been related to hepatic oxidation of ethanol.[19] Some of these alterations result from the shift of intracellular NAD-NADH redox potential, which interferes with related metabolic processes. Because the myocardial sarcoplasm lacks alcohol dehydrogenase[20] but not aldehyde dehydrogenase,[21] it is not likely that similar acute effects occur in the heart. Redox changes might occur in an attenuated way in the heart, however, via some reduced metabolite such as lactate that increases in the blood after ethanol ingestion. Increased utilization of lactate by the heart[22] could affect the redox state.

Studies in man[22,23] and in anesthetized dogs[24] demonstrated that ethanol alters lipid metabolism with a reduction in myocardial extraction of fatty acids and an increase in extraction of triglycerides at blood ethanol levels between 100 and 200 mg/dl. Kano and coworkers[25] demonstrated that ethanol reduced free fatty acid oxidation and increased free fatty acid esterification and accumulation of triglycerides in hearts of fasting and fed rats. Also, changes of calcium release and uptake by the sarcoplasmic reticulum[26] and inhibition of $(Na^+ + K^+)$-activated ATPase activity of heart plasma membranes[27] occurred. These findings were observed at ethanol concentrations substantially higher than those found with alcoholic intoxication in man.

Regional Blood Flow

Although ethanol at concentrations associated with alcohol intoxication results in a decline in total peripheral resistance in normal subjects, changes in blood flow measured experimentally were not the same in all regions. Total splanchnic flow,[12,28] and hepatic arterial flow in particular,[29] have generally increased with ethanol; however, not all spanchnic organs responded similarly. At blood levels associated with an increment in hepatic arterial flow, pancreatic flow declined.[29,30] Also, at concentrations of blood alcohol greater than 200 mg/dl, proximal colonic and splenic flow increased. At these levels renal medullary flow declined. In dogs and rats with respiratory rate unchanged or controlled so that hypercarbia would not ensue, brain blood flow declined, at least transiently, most markedly in the cerebellum.[31] While the effects of ethanol on coronary blood flow is controversial, coronary blood flow generally increased in dogs in which cardiac output did not fall concomitantly, ethanol was infused slowly, and in which high blood levels (> 200 mg/dl) were produced. Although the effects of ethanol may be a reflection of increased myocardial oxygen demand,[7] coronary vasodilation may account in part for these changes. Ethanol,[32] acetaldehyde,[33] and acetate[8] are all coronary vasodilators. In the ischemic myocardium in the anesthetized dog,[34,35] however, flow to ischemic myocardium may decline after ethanol administration, even when flow to nonischemic myocardium has increased. This decline in flow may be the result of a "coronary steal;"[35] that is, blood is drawn away from ischemic myocardium by the vasodilation in nonischemic cardiac tissues where resistance falls with alcohol administration. The enhancement of skin blood flow after ethanol ingestion has been appreciated for some time. While these effects of ethanol on regional blood flow may in part reflect the metabolic changes occurring at these sites, studies by Altura and coworkers[36] suggest that some changes may result from direct action of ethanol on the smooth muscle of blood vessels via changes in intracellular transport and the release of calcium.

ALCOHOL-INDUCED HEART DISEASE

Alcohol abuse, even in alcoholics receiving a nutritionally adequate diet, can result in serious cardiovascular abnormalities. The most fulminant manifestation of cardiac injury from alcohol is a congestive, usually dilated, cardiomyopathy. This disorder is distinguished from beriberi heart disease (see Chapter 9), which is characterized by a hyperdynamic circulation, circulatory congestion, and thiamine responsiveness. While these severe forms of cardiac injury are found in relatively few alcoholics, milder abnormalities of cardiac function can be detected even in alcoholics without overt heart disease.[18,37–39] Alcoholics also have increased levels of mitochondrial-derived enzymes on coronary sinus catheterization[40] and small vessel disease at autopsy.[41] Paroxysmal arrhythmias, myocardial infarction without coronary artery obstructions, hypertension, and stroke have also been associated with alcohol abuse.

Alcoholic Cardiomyopathy

Alcoholic cardiomyopathy is a primary disease of heart muscle in which long-standing alcohol abuse is the only apparent cause. The clinical features are indistinguishable from other congestive cardiomyopathies. Congestive heart failure, low cardiac output, cardiac conduction abnormalities, arrhythmias, and thromboembolic complications are the common clinical manifestations.[42–45]

The heart in alcoholic cardiomyopathy is enlarged. There is usually four-chamber cardiac dilatation and ventricular hypertrophy.[44,46] While marked left ventricular hypertrophy may be present,[46] generally the increased left ventricular thickness is not out of proportion to the ventricular dilation. Coronary arteries are usually widely patent, although intramyocardial branches may show varying degrees of vascular and perivascular fibrosis.[41] Myocardial fibrosis with relative sparing of the individual hypertrophy muscle bundles is also visible on light microscopy. Ultrastructural changes include an increase in the number, the swelling, and the altered structure of mitochondria.[47] Sarcoplasmic reticulum swelling, myofibril damage, and increase in glycogen and fat content are also found on electron microscopy.[48,49]

Experimental Effects of Prolonged Alcohol Exposure

Although the hypocontractile, dilated heart of alcoholic cardiomyopathy has not been experimentally replicated in animals, structural, mechanical, and metabolic abnormalities have been demonstrated following chronic administration of alcohol in several animal studies. In rats receiving 25 percent ethanol orally for 4 months, contractile force, blood pressure, and heart rate declined.[50] These changes were not prevented by vitamin supplementation. Burch and colleagues[51] found that mice fed beer or 5 percent and 15 percent ethanol for 6 to 10 weeks developed mitochrondrial, intercalated disc, transverse tubular, and myofibrillar damage, and an accumulation of myocardial fat. Segel and colleagues[52] examined the effects of chronic ethanol consumption in the rat. With a diet containing 25 percent of total calories as ethanol, swelling of mitochondria, transverse tubules, and sarcoplasmic reticulum were observed; there were also dehiscences of the intercalated disc and disintegration of myofibrils. Regan and colleagues[53] found that at 18 months of a diet containing 36 percent of calories as ethanol, dogs had a mucopolysaccharide-like substance in the myocardium, dilatation of the intercalated disc, and electrocardiographic abnormalities. Sarma and colleagues[54] found in dogs after 29 months of ethanol administration abnormalities of muscle mechanics and several metabolic abnormalities. Also, rhesus monkeys receiving 40 percent of total calories as ethanol for 3 months had increased myocardial triglyceride and cholesterol esters, myocardial cell destruction, atrophy of muscle bundles, and fibrosis.[55]

In addition to structural abnormalities, metabolic changes occurred after prolonged administration of ethanol. Lieber and coworkers[56] found that rats receiving 36 percent of total calories as ethanol showed an accumulation of triglycerides that could be reduced if long-chain triglycerides were eliminated from the diet. Mitochondrial function was also disturbed by chronic exposure to ethanol. Pachinger and coworkers[57] and Sarma and coworkers[54] found that with prolonged administration of alcohol the hearts of dogs showed diminished intramitochondrial isocitric dehydrogenase activity and a reduction of myocardial ATP, mitochondrial oxygen consumption, and various respiratory control indices. Sarma and coworkers[54] also found after 20 months of exposure to ethanol that calcium uptake and binding to sarcoplasmic reticulum were reduced and endogenous myocardial calcium was diminished. Thus, chronic alcohol exposure produced myocardial structural changes similar to those found in patients with alcoholic cardiomyopathy, altered myocardial lipid metabolism, inhibited mitochondrial respiration and enzyme activity, and impaired intracellular calcium uptake and binding.

Alcohol-related Heart Disease

The clinical, hemodynamic and pathologic features of alcohol cardiomyopathy can be distinguished from the cardiac findings of three other conditions associated with alcohol abuse: Quebec beer-drinker's cardiomyophathy, cirrhosis, and beriberi heart disease. Quebec beer-drinker's cardiomyopathy appeared as an epidemic in heavy beer drinkers during the mid-1960s[58] (see Chapter 9). This fulminant congestive cardiomyopathy was characterized by polycythemia, cyanosis, large serous cavity effusions, and high mortality. The disease disappeared when cobalt, put in beer to stabilize the foam, was removed. Although cardiomegaly, left ventricular hypertrophy, and perivascular fibrosis may occur in cirrhotics,[41,59,60] concomitant alcohol cardiomyopathy is seen only rarely in such patients. In fact, the circulation in cirrhotic patients is generally hyperdynamic.[61] Even though systolic left ventricular function is enhanced, which is more pronounced in the presence of ascites and hepatic encephalopathy,[61] left ventricular responses to dynamic exercise[62] and afterload stress[22] are abnormal. Whether the findings in cirrhosis are related to increased arteriovenous shunts in this disorder or to a still undefined relationship with intestinal vasoactive hormones is not clear.

Beriberi heart disease, like the cardiac findings in cirrhosis, is characterized by a hyperdynamic circulation. Generally central venous pressure is elevated, cardiac output is increased, and signs of circulatory congestion are present. As the disease progresses a fulminant form, so-called shoshin beriberi, which is characterized by cyanosis, lactic acidosis, and even vascular collapse, may be seen[63] (see Chapter 9). Thiamine deficiency can be demonstrated in such patients by reduced red blood cell transketolase activity, an enzyme in the hexose monophosphate shunt requiring thiaminie pyrophosphate as a cofactor,[64,65] or by hemodynamic responsiveness to thiamine. Cardiac output will decline and total peripheral resistance will increase after administration of thiamine.[65,66] Although a high cardiac output is typical of beriberi, normal and occasionally even reduced cardiac output may be seen when the disease is advanced or when alcohol cardiomyopathy is also present.[64-66] Since thiamine administration increases aortic impedance, in the presence of severe left ventricular dysfunction, cardiac output may fall below normal with thiamine therapy.[66] It is not clear whether primary cardiac muscle dysfunction is present in uncomplicated beriberi heart disease. The pathologic findings are generally not severe or specific, and the hemodynamic abnormalities can be explained by the peripheral vascular effects of thiamine deficiency, that is, low peripheral resistance and increased central venous tone.[65] The cardiac hemodynamic findings moreover are not specific for left ventricular dysfunction. The high ventricular diastolic pressures can be explained by the increased blood volume and high central venoconstriction found in thiamine deficiency. Ejection fraction usually is normal, although it has been suggested that such values are lower than one might expect with a reduced aortic impedance.[65] In any case, just as cirrhosis does not preclude presence of concomitant alcoholic cardiomyopathy, the severe left ventricular dysfunction of alcoholic cardiomyopathy does not preclude a deficiency in thiamine with its attendant hemodynamic effects.

Holiday Heart

Although cardiac arrhythmias would be expected as a complication of alcoholic cardiomyopathy, at times paroxysmal tachycardias may occur in alcoholics without clinical evidence of left ventricular dysfunction. Ettinger and coworkers[67] have termed this disorder *holiday heart* because it generally occurs after episodes of binge drinking. The mechanism for these arrhythmias is not clear. While ethanol produced electrophysiologic changes in the heart,[1,68,69] these observations were made under experimental conditions not relevant to the clinical situation. Greenspon and coworkers,[70] however, observed a prolongation of His-Purkinje conduction and a shortening of corrective sinus recovery times in alcoholics at blood ethanol concentrations of 50 to 100 mg/dl. These investigators also found that arrhythmias could be induced in alcoholics subject to paroxysmal tachycardias by programmed electrical stimulation after ethanol administration.

Acute Myocardial Infarction

Alcohol abuse has been associated with the development of acute myocardial infarction in patients with patent coronary arteries. Regan and coworkers[71,72] believe that this disorder is a toxic cardiomyopathy. They based their conclusion on the presence of increased glycoprotein and perivascular fibrosis in the hearts of patients who succumbed. Such myocardial infarctions in alcoholics were described before the recent reports of rapid, spontaneous dissolution of thrombus in some patients with acute myocardial infarction. Also, the possibility of coronary spasm was not examined. In a recent report, Moreyra and coworkers[73] found acute myocardial infarction after heavy alcohol ingestion in young patients (18 and 22 years old) with patent coronary arteries. This report suggests that ethanol itself might be the provocative substance, with alcohol-induced coronary spasm representing the mechanism. Fernandez and coworkers[74] described a case of Prinzmetal's angina, a disorder produced by coronary spasm, in which an association of ethanol ingestion and angina was found. In dogs, however, H. S. Friedman (unpublished observations) found that ethanol at blood levels greater than 200 mg/dl did not alter the effects of ergonovine (a spasm-producing substance in man) on coronary blood flow.

**EFFECTS OF ETHANOL ON BLOOD LIPIDS:
CHARACTERISTICS AND PATHOGENESIS OF
ALCOHOLIC HYPERLIPIDEMIA***

The initial phase of hepatic lipid deposition after ethanol consumption is accompanied by an increased release of lipoproteins into the blood, tending to counteract lipid accumulation in the liver. The effect is dose dependent, with inhibition after high doses and stimulation after smaller amounts of ethanol.[75] In both humans[76,77] and rats,[78] ethanol in commonly used amounts produces hyperlipidemia, with the most striking changes in the very low density lipoprotein fraction (VLDL). The alcohol-induced hyperlipemia can occur in the fasting state[77] but is markedly

---

*See also Chapter 3.

exaggerated when alcohol is given with a fat-containing diet.[79–81] The effect of alcohol depends not only on the dose but also on the duration of intake. Even moderate but regular use of alcohol raises blood lipids significantly.[82,83] This alcohol effect does not result solely from caloric overload, since no comparable hyperlipidemia was produced by isocaloric amounts of either carbohydrate or lipids.[84]

In both humans and rats, ethanol-induced hyperlipemia results in increased concentrations of various serum lipoprotein fractions, but the major changes occurred in the VLDL. In the postprandial state, this fraction includes VLDL and chylomicrons, and the fatty acids are derived from dietary lipids. In the fasting state, more of the fatty acids are derived from adipose tissue.[85] In patients with alcoholic hyperlipemia, chylomicron-like particles have been observed in the fasting state.[86] In the rat rendered hyperlipemic by ethanol feeding, the lipid-protein ratio of the d < 1.006 lipoproteins approaches that of chylomicrons.[87] The site of origin of these particles cannot be deduced with certainty from physical or chemical characteristics. Studies by Baraona and coworkers[87] indicate that an adequate supply of dietary lipids represents a permissive factor for alcoholic hyperlipemia in the rat. Changes in lymph lipid output do not play a major role in the lipemic effect of ethanol. The site of origin of the increased production of serum lipoprotein is most likely hepatic. The contribution of lymph lipids to the hepatic steatosis also appears to minor.[8]

Altered catabolism of chylomicrons, however, could be contributory to hyperlipemia. Although plasma clearance of chylomicrons to acylglycerol was not significantly affected,[78] that of chylomicron cholesterol ester was impaired suggesting that the accumulation of cholesterol remnants contributes to the hyperlipemia.[89] Lipoprotein lipase of adipose tissue was unaltered under similar conditions.[90] In alcoholic liver disease, accumulation of lipoproteins of intermediate density (considered to be remnants of chylomicrons and VLDL) has been described.[91,92] It is not clear, however, whether such defective catabolism plays a significant role before severe liver disease develops. With significant liver disease higher triglyceridemia ensues secondary to the accumulation of intermediate particles of chylomicron metabolism because of diminished hepatic lipase activity.[93]

Ethanol-induced hyperlipemia is usually moderate. Some alcoholic patients develop marked hyperlipemia, suggesting that factors in addition to ethanol itself contribute. A possible role of postheparin lipolytic activity (PHLA) in alcoholic hyperlipemia has been sugggested on the basis of the finding that six of the eight patients with marked hyperlipemia reported by Losowsky and coworkers[84] had decreased PHLA. Further, a mild decrease in the fractional turnover rate of intravenously injected exogenous triglycerides was reported in alcoholics who develop marked hyperlipemia.[86] In most of the subjects reported by Losowsky and coworkers[84] the PHLA remained low after the hyperlipemia had subsided and after alcohol had been withdrawn for weeks or months. This alteration could not be reproduced either by ethanol in vitro[84] or by administration of ethanol in vivo,[81,94,95] although some inhibition was reported more recently.[96] Thus, one factor in the development of hyperlipemia could be defective removal of serum lipids in some patients. Further, some of the alcoholic patients with marked hyperlipemia had other conditions that contribute to hyperlipemia, such as diabetes[84,95] or pancreatitis.[97] The latter condition was associated with the production of an inhibitor of PHLA.[98] Type IV hyperlipoproteinemia may also predispose to alcoholic hyperlipemia.[99–101] Although alcohol can undoubtedly aggravate type IV hyperlipoproteinemia, many individuals with an unrecognized high alcohol intake may have been misclassified as having type IV hyperlipoproteinemia. Indeed, even moderate alcohol intake in the evening resulted in worse hyperlipemia the next morning in most subjects; in 25 percent of normal individuals there was a sufficient rise to fit the type-IV classification.[83,102]

Another pertinent mechanism involved is an increased capacity to secrete serum lipoproteins upon challenge with alcohol. This may account for the observation that some alcoholic patients have an unusual sensitivity to the hyperlipemic effect of ethanol.[95] Thus, patients with normal PHLA develop hyperlipemia with doses of ethanol (120–160 g/day) that do not produce hyperlipemia in normal subjects nor in individuals with endogenous hypertriglyceridemia (type IV). The mechanism for the increased capacity of these patients to develop alcoholic hyperlipemia remains unknown. Since ethanol consumption results in an increased capacity to secrete lipoproteins[87] the difference in response to ethanol between some alcoholics and some individuals with type IV hyperlipoproteinemia may be secondary to a difference in prior alcohol consumption.

Dietary fat is a striking potentiator of alcoholic hyperlipemia, at least at the fatty liver stage.[103] In patients with alcoholic fatty liver, administration of a high-fat meal, even in the absence of ethanol, produced a striking increase in serum triglycerides (Fig.8-1). This effect tends to disappear with progressive liver damage. The rise in pre-β-lipoproteins, then, also vanishes with other qualitative alterations in lipoproteins (Fig. 8-2). At these later stages, the effects of ethanol may be overshadowed by effects of cholestasis, secondary lecithin-cholesterol acyltransferase (LCAT) deficiency,[92] diminished capacity of the diseased hepatocyte to synthesize and secrete lipoproteins, and possibly endocrine abnormalities (such as hyperestrogenemia) that may alter lipoprotein metabolism. Lipoprotein abnormalities associated with pancreatitis and malnutrition may also complicate the clinical picture.

Usually, alcoholic hyperlipemia is first suspected because of the incidental observation of serum lactescence or of hypercholesterolemia. It is commonly associated with hepatic, gastrointestinal, or pancreatic complications of alcoholism, and on this basis a combination of varying symptoms is seen, including most frequently anorexia, nausea, vomiting, abdominal pain, fever, jaundice, and transient hemolysis. Indeed, transient hemolytic anemia can accompany episodes of hyperlipemia in alcoholics (the so-called Zieve's syndrome).[104] Normally, triglycerides and VLDL predominate, but lipid patterns can vary.[84,105]

The degree of ethanol-induced hyperlipemia varies but is usually moderate. In a few individuals, plasma lactescence can be severe because of potentiating factors such as an underlying abnormality of lipid metabolism (that is, *forme fruste* of essential hyperlipemia), pancreatitis, or diabetes. In addition, striking changes occur with time, as illustrated in Figure 8-3. In this subject, the marked lactescence of the plasma at admission was a result of an increase of triglycerides (approximately 100-fold), phospholipids, and cholesterol. There was also an increase of circulating chylomicrons, not shown on the figure. According to the classification of Fredrickson

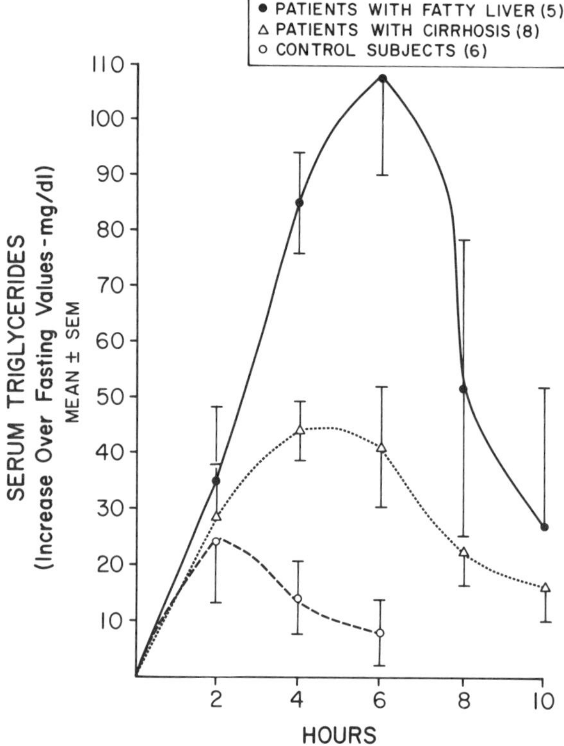

Fig. 8-1. Serum triglyceride response of control subjects and alcoholic patients after a high-fat meal. Note the marked response of patients with fatty liver and the less striking but still significant response in patients with cirrhosis. (Reproduced with permission from Borowsky SA, Perlow W, Barona E, Lieber CS: Relationship of alcoholic hypertriglyceridemia to stage of liver disease and dietary lipid. Dig Dis Sci 25:22–27, 1980. Plenum Publishing Company.)

and coworkers[106] this patient would have fitted the type V phenotype. After a few hours, chylomicrons disappeared; the remaining elevated triglycerides and cholesterol might have been considered typical for type IV hyperlipoproteinemia. After a few days, triglycerides returned to normal, whereas cholesterol remained elevated, a pat-

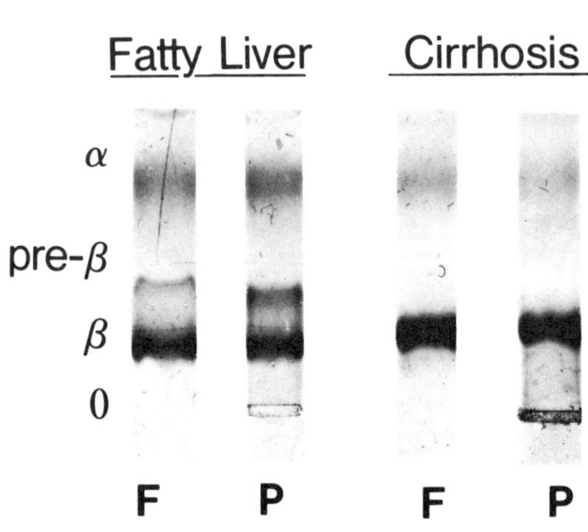

Fig. 8-2. Differences in lipoprotein electrophoretic profile between alcoholics with simple fatty liver and those with cirrhosis (F), and 4 hours after ingestion of a standard fatty meal (P). In contrast with the prominent pre-β band observed in the alcoholic with fatty liver, the patient with cirrhosis has no pre-β lipoproteins, decreased α lipoproteins, increased β-band with slight increase in motility towards the pre-β area, and increased chylomicrons or chylomicron-like particles (P). (Reproduced with permission from Borowsky SA, Perlow W, Barona E, Lieber CS: Relationship of alcoholic hypertriglyceridemia to stage of liver disease and dietary lipid. Dig Dis Sci 25:22–27, 1980. Plenum Publishing Company.)

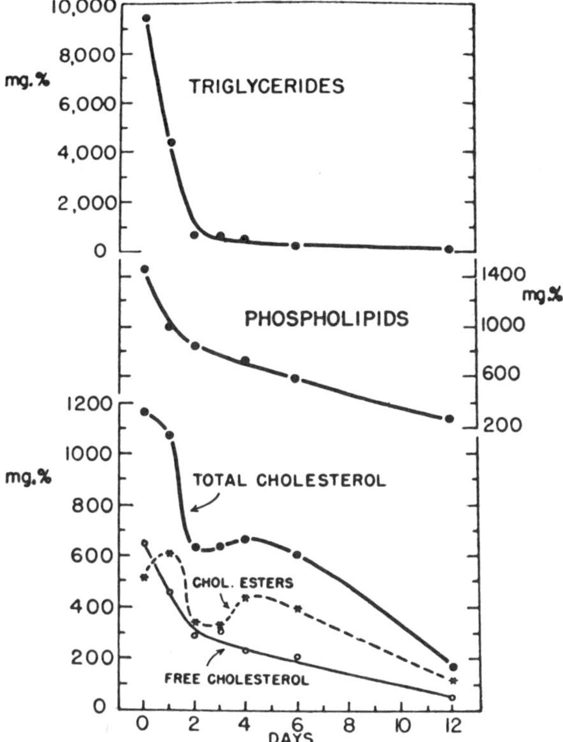

Fig. 8-3. Changes in plasma lipid fractions during recovery from alcoholic hyperlipemia. (Reproduced with permission from Losowsky MS, Jones DP, Davidson CS, Lieber CS: Studies of alcoholic hyperlipemia and its mechanism. Am J Med 35:794–803, 1963.)

tern reminiscent of type II hyperlipoproteinemia. In addition to these temporal changes, liver disease and/or cholestasis complicate the picture, and the replacement of the pre-β band with one of abnormal β mobility may be reminiscent of type III hyperlipoproteinemia. Thus, it is apparent that classification of the hyperlipemia in the alcoholic is fraught with difficulties.

HIGH-DENSITY LIPOPROTEINS, ATHEROSCLEROSIS, AND CORONARY HEART DISEASE*

Since alcohol ingestion has profound effects on lipid and lipoprotein metabolism, a relationship between alcohol use and the development of atherosclerosis would be expected. Uncontrolled pathologic studies have suggested that atherosclerotic disease is less prevalent in patients with Laennec's cirrhosis. Analysis of this apparent negative association has suggested that this is merely a statistical fallacy.[107] When coronary atherosclerotic narrowing was compared in an autopsy population of matched cirrhotics, chronic alcoholics, and accident victims, there was no significant difference in the presence of obstructive coronary disease. When cirrhotics and noncirrhotics were compared, a higher incidence of coronary atherosclerosis was found in the noncirrhotic population. On analyzing this population, the noncirrhotic population had a substantially higher incidence of athe-

---

*See also Chapter 3.

rogenetic risk factors. Specifically, a higher incidence of diabetes mellitus in autopsy populations of noncirrhotics appeared to account for this apparent, but erroneous, negative association of cirrhosis and coronary atherosclerosis. Several epidemiologic studies have shown a favorable influence of alcohol on coronary heart disease. Klatsky and coworkers[108] reviewed the Kaiser-Permanente epidemiologic study of myocardial infarction and found that teetotalers were at greater risk than moderate users of alcohol. Stason and coworkers[109] in the Boston Collaborative Drug Survellance Program found a lower rate of nonfatal myocardial infarction in subjects consuming six or more drinks each day. Similar findings were reported by Yano and coworkers[110] in Japanese men living in Hawaii. These investigators[110] found a negative association between moderate alcohol consumption (up to 60 ml/day) and the risk of nonfatal myocardial infarction and death from coronary artery disease. Henekens and coworkers[111] found that the protective effect of ethanol was related to the amount of alcohol consumption per se (2 ounces daily or less), not to the type of beverage ingested. Yano and coworkers,[110] moreover, have related the reduction in the risk of nonfatal myocardial infarction and death from coronary heart disease to the higher serum levels of HDL cholesterol (see Chapter 3).

A rise in HDL associated with alcohol has been shown both experimentally[78] and in a number of clinical studies.[112,113] This alcohol-induced increase of HDL may be particularly significant, in view of the negative correlation between HDL blood levels and the development of coronary heart disease,[114,115] either because HDL promotes the transport of cholesterol out of the cell or because HDL competes with LDL for uptake, thereby suppressing the increment in cell sterol content induced by LDL.[116]

It is not clear whether the increased HDL after ethanol reflects enhanced peripheral mobilization of cholesterol rather than decreased removal by the liver. Indeed, in the rat, ethanol increases cholesterogenesis in the liver[117] and in the small intestine.[118] Further, ethanol feeding decreases degradation of cholesterol to bile acids[117] and excretion of bile acid,[117] although the opposite was observed after cessation of ethanol administration.[119] In the presence of alcohol, however, biliary secretion of bile acids was depressed.[120–122] The reduction of bile acid excretion could be secondary to a diminution in cholesterol 7-α-hydroxylase activity.[123] Alcohol favors cholesterol ester accumulation not only in the liver[117] but also in the aorta.[124]

Whatever the mechanism whereby ethanol affects HDL and atherosclerosis, the "protective" action was observed in a population comprised of moderate rather than heavy drinkers.[110,125,126] Even in moderate drinkers, there may not be an overall decreased mortality associated with the alcohol intake, despite the reduced incidence of coronary heart disease. As discussed below, alcohol may also promote hypertension.[127] Thus, alcohol appears to affect cardiovascular mortality rates in a bimodal fashion. Both the teetotaler and the alcohol abuser appear to be at higher risk of coronary heart disease than occasional or moderate users of alcoholic beverages.

Despite the evidence that ethanol may exert a beneficial effect on the development of coronary atherosclerosis, there is no evidence that ethanol has a place in the treatment of an acute anginal episode. Experimental studies[34,35] have demonstrated that alcohol reduces blood flow to ischemic myocardium. Moreover, patients with coronary heart disease perform worse on dynamic stress testing after ethanol ingestion.[128,129] Also, ethanol does not have a beneficial effect in preventing episodes of angina pectoris in patients with established coronary heart disease.

HYPERTENSION

Since hypertension is a leading risk factor for stroke and coronary heart disease, the effect of alcohol on blood pressure is important. Epidemiologic studies[130,131] have identified an association of alcohol abuse with systemic hypertension. Also, similar studies[132–34] have demonstrated relationships between alcohol consumption and average systemic blood pressure. The correlation is strongest with systolic pressure, and this relationship tends to be linear in men.[134] In women, however, a U-shaped relationship has been found.[132,135] Women who use alcohol have *lower* mean systolic blood pressures than women teetotalers. Average systemic blood pressure in women correlated inversely with alcohol consumption up to 20 g/day[135]; however, women who consumed more than 30 g of alcohol daily had higher average systolic blood pressures than teetotalers or women who used lesser amounts.

More than 50 percent of alcoholics consuming more than 80 g of alcohol daily had blood pressures exceeding 140/90 during detoxification from alcohol.[136] Clark and Friedman[137] found that 33 percent of alcoholics admitted for detoxification but not having delirium tremens had blood pressures of 160/95 or greater on admission or within the first 72 hours of admission. Hypertension associated with alcohol abuse is generally transitory. Blood pressure returns to normal in more than 70 percent of these alcoholics[137] and stays normal if patients remain abstinent.[136] In less than 10 percent of alcoholics hypertension persists even with abstinence. Since this percentage is consistent with the prevalence of hypertension in the general population, the group with sustained elevated blood pressure may coincidentally have had essential hypertension. Saunders and coworkers[136] correlated the hypertension of alcoholics both with daily alcohol consumption during the 3 months preceding detoxification and with the severity of withdrawal symptoms. Clark and Friedman,[137] however, found no relationship of hypertension to withdrawal symptoms, estimated recent alcohol use, or blood alcohol level measured on admission. Although average basal plasma renin activity is elevated in alcoholics,[138] alcoholics with hypertension do not have significantly higher levels of this enzyme than normotensive alcoholics.[137] Similarly, serum magnesium, glutamic oxaloacetic transaminase (SGOT), and creatinine levels in alcoholics with hypertension do not differ from those in normotensive alcoholics.[137]

Alcohol-induced hypertension is not benign. The risk of stroke in alcoholics has been related to their higher blood pressure.[139] Clark and Friedman[137] found that left atrial enlargement and left ventricular hypertrophy were more common in alcoholics with alcohol-induced hypertension than in alcoholics without hypertension and than in alcoholics with sustained (essential) hypertension. Although the mechanism of alcohol-induced elevation of blood pressure is not clear, there is considerable evidence that regular use of alcohol in men elevates blood pressure, and that hypertension in alcoholics may contribute to the increased cardiovascular complications of problem drinkers.

CONCLUSION

Given the widespread use of alcoholic beverages, it would be reassuring if alcohol had a beneficial effect on the heart. Such a view would not be a new one. Heberden[140] suggested that alcohol be used for the treatment and prevention of angina pectoris. At least some uncontrolled pathologic studies have suggested a favorable effect of alcohol on reducing atherosclerosis. More recently, epidemiologic studies have shown that users of alcohol have fewer coronary events than teetotalers, an effect that appeared dose dependent but not related to the type of alcoholic beverage.

Alcohol abuse is associated with a severe form of heart muscle disease. It has also been related to acute myocardial infarction in young patients with patent coronary arteries. In some people, alcohol provokes cardiac arrhythmias. Epidemiologic studies also have shown a relation between alcohol abuse and hypertension and an increased incidence of coronary events. Clinical and experimental studies have also demonstrated that alcohol depresses cardiac function (especially in hearts with already reduced cardiac performance), exerts an unfavorable effect on blood flow in ischemic hearts, and reduces blood flow to the brain. From the standpoint of its cardiovascular effects, alcohol should be used only in moderation, and patients with known heart disease should perhaps abstain from it entirely.

REFERENCES

1. Gimeno AL, Gimeno MF, Webb LJ: Effects of ethanol on cellular membrane potentials and contractility of isolated rat atrium. Am J Physiol 203:194–196, 1962.
2. Spann JF, Mason DT, Beiser GD, Gold HK: Actions of ethanol on the contractile state of the normal and failing cat papillary muscle. Clin Res 16:249 (abstract), 1968.
3. Nakano J, Moore SE: Effects of different alcohols on the contractile force of the isolated guinea-pig myocardium. Eur J Pharmacol 20:266–270, 1972.
4. Mierzwiak DS, Wildenthal K, Mitchell JH: Acute effects of ethanol on the left ventricle in dog. Arc Int Pharmacodyn 199:43–52, 1972.
5. Wong M: Depression of cardiac performance by ethanol unmasked during autonomic blockade. Amer Heart J 86:508–515, 1973.
5. Altura BM, Ogunkowa A, Gebrewold A, Altura BT: Effects of ethanol on terminal arterioles and muscular venules: Direct observations of the microcirculation. J Cardiovasc Pharmacol 1:97–113, 1979.
7. Friedman HS, Matusuzaki S, Choe S, Fernando HA, Celis A, Zaman Q, Lieber CS: Demonstration of dissimilar acute hemodynamic effects of ethanol and acetaldehyde. Cardiovasc Res 13:480–491, 1979.
8. Liang CS, Lowenstein JM: Metabolic control of the circulation: Effects of acetate and pyruvate. J Clin Invest 62:1029–1038, 1978.
9. Webb WR, Degril IU: Ethyl alcohol and the cardiovascular system: Effects on coronary blood flow. JAMA 191:77–80, 1965.
10. Mendoza LC, Hellberg K, Rickart A, Tillich G, Bing RJ: The effect of intravenous ethyl alcohol on the coronary circulation and myocardial contractility of the human and canine heart. J Clin Pharmacol 7:165–176, 1971.
11. Grollman A: The influence of alcohol on the circulation. Quart J Stud 3:5–14, 1942.

12. Stein SW, Lieber CS, Leevy CM, Cherrick GR, Abelman WH: The effect of ethanol upon systemic and hepatic blood flow in man. Am J Clin Nutr 13:68–74, 1963.

13. Riff DP, Jain AC, Doyle JT: Acute hemodynamic effects of ethanol on normal human volunteers. Am Heart J 78:592–597, 1969.

14. Greenberg BH, Schutz R, Grunkemeier GL, Griswold HE: Acute effects of alcohol in patients with congestive heart failure. Ann Intern Med 87:171–175, 1982.

14. Gould L, Zahir M, DeMartino A, Gomprecht RF: Cardiac effects of a cocktail. JAMA 218:1799–1802, 1971.

16. Delgado CE, Fortuin NJ, Ross RS: Acute effects of low doses of alcohol on left ventricular function by echocardiography. Circulation 51:535–540, 1975.

17. Ahmed SS, Levinson GE, Regan TJ: Depression of myocardial contractility with low doses of ethanol in normal man. Circulation 48:378–385, 1973.

18. Timmins GC, Ramos RC, Gordon S, Gangadharan V: The basis for differences in ethanol-induced myocardial depression in normal subjects. Circulation 51:1144–1148.

19. Lieber CS: Interference of ethanol in hepatic cellular metabolism. Ann NY Acd Sci 252:24–50, 1975.

20. Cherrick GR, Leevy CM: The effect of ethanol-metabolism on levels of oxidized and reduced nicotinamide-adenine dinucletide in liver, kidney, and heart. Biochem Biophys Acta 107:29–37, 1965.

21. Forsyth GW, Nagawawa HT, Alexander CS: Acetaldehyde metabolism by the rat heart. Proc Soc Exper 144:498–500, 1973.

22. Regan TJ, Levinson GE, Oldewurtel HA, Frank MJ, Weisse AB, Moschos CB: Ventricular function in noncardiacs with alcoholic fatty liver: Role of ethanol in the production of cardiomyopathy. J Clin Invest 48:397–407, 1969.

23. Wendt VE, Ajluni R, Bruce TA, Prasad AS, Bing RJ: Acute effects of alcohol on the human myocardium. Am J Cardiol 17:804–812, 1966.

24. Regan TJ, Koroxenidis G, Moschos CB, Oldewurtel HA, Lehan PH, Hellems HK: The acute metabolic and hemodynamic responses of the left ventricle to ethanol. J Clin Invest 45:270–280, 1966.

25. Kano KJ, Liu MS, Thornton MJ: Changes in fatty acid composition of myocardial triglyceride following a single administration of ethanol to rabbits: J Mol Cell Cardiol 5:473–489, 1973.

26. Swartz MH, Repeke DI, Katz AM, Rubin E: Effects of ethanol on calcium binding and calcium uptake by cardiac microsomes. Biochem Pharmacol 23:2369–2376, 1974.

27. Williams JW, Tada M, Katz AM, Rubin E: Effects of ethanol and acetaldehyde on the $(Na^+ + K^+)$-activated adenosine triphosphatase activity of cardiac plasma membranes. Biochem Pharmacol 24:27–32, 1975.

28. Shaw S, Heller EA, Friedman HS, Baraona E, Lieber CS: Increased hepatic oxygenation following ethanol administration in the baboon: Proc Soc Exper Bio Med 156:509–513, 1977.

29. Friedman HS, Lowery JR, Scorza J: Is acute pancreatitis caused by a "splanchnic steal"? Clin Res 30:282A (abstract), 1982.

30. Horwitz LD, Meyers JH: Ethanol-induced alterations in pancreatic blood flow in conscious dogs: Circulation Res 50:250–256, 1982.

31. Friedman HS, Lowrey R, Archer M, Scorza J: The effects of ethanol on brain blood flow in awake dogs: Clin Res 29:192A, 1981.

32. Abel FL: Direct effects of ethanol on myocardial performance and coronary resistance: J Pharmacol Exp Ther 212:28–33, 1980.

33. Gailis L; Verdy M: The effect of ethanol and acetaldehyde on the metabolism and vascular resistance of perfused heart. Can J Biochem 49:227–233, 1971.

34. Leighninger DA, Reuger R, Beck CS: Effects of pentaerythritol tetranitrate, amyl nitrite and alcohol on arterial blood supply to ischemic myocardium: Am J Cardiol 7:533–537, 1961.

35. Friedman HS; Acute effects of ethanol on myocardial blood flow in the nonischemic and ischemic heart: Amer J Cardiol 47:61–67, 1981.

36. Altura BM, Altura BT: Microvascular and vascular smooth muscle actions of ethanol, acetaldehyde and acetate: Fed Proc 41:2447–2451, 1982.

37. Spodick DH, Pigott VM, Chirife R: Preclinical cardiac malfunction in chronic alcoholism: Comparison with matched normal controls and with alcoholic cardiomyopathy. New Engl J Med 287:677–680, 1972.

38. Wu CF, Sudhakar M, Jaferi G, Ahmed SS, Regan TJ: Preclinical cardiomyopathy in chronic alcoholics: A sex difference. Am Heart J 91:281–286, 1976.

39. Matthews EC, Gardin JM, Henry WL, DelNegro AA, Fletcher RD, Snow JA, Epstein SE: Echocardiographic abnormalities in chronic alcoholics with and without overt congestive heart failure. Am J Cardiol 47:507–578, 1981.

40. Wendt VE, Wu C, Balcon R, Doty G, Bing RJ: Hemodynamic and metabolic effects of chronic alcoholism in man. Am J Cardiol 15:175–184, 1965.

41. Factor SM: Intramyocardial small-vessel disease in chronic alcoholism. Amer Heart J 92:561–575, 1976.

42. Evans W: Alcoholic cardiomyopathy. Am Heart J 61:556–567, 1961.

43. Bridgen W: Alcoholic heart disease. Brit Med J 21:1283–1289, 1964.

44. Alexander CS: Idiopathic heart disease. Am J Med 41:213–228, 1966.

45. Burch GE, DePasquale: Alcoholic cardiomyopathy. Cardiologia 52:48–56, 1968.

46. Massumi RA, Rios JC, Gooch AS, Nutter D, Devita VT, Datlow DW: Primary myocardial disease: Report of fifty cases and review of the subject. Circulation 31:19–41, 1965.

47. Alexander CS: Idiopathic heart: Electron microscopic examination of myocardial biopsy specimens in alcoholic heart disease. Am J Med 41:229–234, 1966.

48. Alexander CS: Electron microscopic observations in alcoholic heart disease. Brit Heart J 29:200–206, 1967.

49. Hibbs RG, Ferrans VJ, Black WC, Weilbaecher DG, Walsh JJ, Burch GE: Alcoholic cardiomyopathy: An electron microscopic study. Am Heart J 69:766–779, 1965.

50. Maines JE, Aldinger EE: Myocardial depression accompanying chronic consumption of alcohol. Am Heart J 73:55–63, 1967.

51. Burch GE, Colcolough HL, Harb JM, Tsu CY: The effect of ingestion of ethyl alcohol, wine and beer on the myocardium of mice. Am J Cardiol 27:522–528, 1971.

52. Segel LD, Rendig SV, Choquet Y, Chacko K, Amsterdam EA, Mason DT: Effects of chronic graded ethanol consumption on the metabolism, ultrastructure, and mechanical function of the rat heart. Cardiovasc Res 9:649–663, 1975.

53. Regan TJ, Khan MI, Ettinger PO, Haider B, Lyons MM, Oldewurtel HA: Myocardial function and lipid metabolism in the chronic alcoholic animal. J Clin Invest 54:740–752, 1974.

54. Sarma JSM, Ikeda S, Fischer R, Maruyama Y, Weishaar R, Bind RJ: Biochemical and contractile properties of heart muscle after prolonged alcohol administration. J Mol Cell Cardiol 8:951–972, 1976.

55. Vasdev SC, Chakravarti RN, Subrahamanyam D, Jain AC, Wahi PL: Myocardial lesions induced by prolonged alcohol feeding in rhesus monkeys. Cardiovasc Res 9:134–140, 1975.

56. Lieber CS, Spritz N, DeCarli LM: Accumulation of triglycerides in heart and kidney after alcohol ingestion. J Clin Invest 45:1041 (abstract), 1966.

57. Pachinger OM, Tillmanns H, Mao JC, Fauvel JM, Bing RJ: The effect of prolonged

administration of ethanol on cardiac metabolism and performance in the dog. J Clin Invest 52:2690–2696, 1973.

58. Morin YL, Foley AR, Martineau G, Roussel J: Quebec beer-drinkers' cardiomyopathy, forty eight cases. Canada Med Ass J 97:883–904, 1967.

59. Lunseth JH, Olmstead EG, Forks G, Abboud F: A study of heart disease in one hundred and eight hospitalized patients dying with portal cirrhosis. Arch Intern Med 102:405–413, 1958.

60. Hognestad J, Teisberg T: Heart pathology in chronic alcoholism. Acta Path Microbid Scand (section A) 81:315–322, 1973.

61. Fernando HA, Friedman HS: Demonstration of the hyperdynamic heart of cirrhosis by echocardiography. Clin Res 24:613A (abstract), 1976.

62. Gould L, Shariff M, Zahir M, Dilieto M: Cardiac hemodynamics in alcoholic patients with chronic liver disease and a presystolic gallop. J Clin Invest 48:860–868, 1969.

63. Attas M, Hanley HG, Stultz D, Jones MR, McAllister RG: Fulminant beriberi heart disease with lactic acidosis: Presentation of a case with evaluation of left ventricular function and review of pathophysiologic mechanisms. Circulation 58:566–572, 1978.

64. McIntyre N, Stanley N: Cardiac beriberi: Two modes of presentation. Brit Med J 3:567–569, 1971.

65. Ikram H, Maslowski AH, Smith BL, Nicholls MG: The hemodynamic histopathological and hormonal features of alcoholic cardiac beriberi. Q J Med 200:359–375, 1981.

66. Robin E, Goldschlager N: Persistence of low cardiac output after relief of high output by thiamine in a case of alcoholic beriberi and cardiac myopathy. Am Heart J, 80:103–108, 1970.

67. Ettinger PO, Wu CF, De la Cruz C, Weisse AB, Ahmed SS, Regan TJ: Arrhythmias and the "holiday heart": Alcohol associated cardiac rhythm disorders. Am Heart J 95:555–562, 1978.

68. Goodkind JM, Gerber NH, Mellen JR, Kostis JB: Altered intracardiac conduction after acute administration of ethanol in the dog. J Pharmacol Exp Ther 194:633–638, 1975.

69. Snoy FJ, Harker RJ, Thies W, Greenspan K: Ethanol-induced electrophysiological alterations in canine cardiac purkinje fibers. Journal of Studies on Alcohol 41:1023–1030, 1980.

70. Greenspon AJ, Leier CV, Sachaal SF: Acute ethanol effects, cardiac arrhythmias and conduction in man. Clin Res 29:200A (abstract), 1981.

71. Regan TJ, Wu CF, Weiss AB, Moschos CB, Ahmed SS, Lyons MM: Acute myocardial infarction in toxic cardiomyopathy without coronary obstruction. Circulation 51:453–461, 1974.

72. Regan TJ, Wu CF, Weiss AB, Moschos CB, Ahmed SS, Lyons MM: Acute myocardial infarction in toxic cardiomyopathy without coronary obstruction. Circulation 51:453–461, 1975.

73. Moreyra AE, Kostis JB, Passannante AJ, Kuo PT: Acute myocardial infarction in patients with normal coronary arteries after acute ethanol intoxication. Clin Cardiol 5:425–430, 1982.

74. Fernandez D, Rosenthal JE, Cohen LS, Hammond G, Wolfson S: Alcohol-induced prinzmetal variant angina. Am J Cardiol 32:238–239, 1973.

75. Estler CJ, Ammon HPT: The influence of beta adrenergic blockade on the ethanol-induced derangement of lipid transport. Arch Int Pharmacodyn 166:333–341, 1967.

76. Lieber CS, Jones DP, Mendelson J, DeCarli LM: Fatty liver, hyperlipemia and hyper-uricemia produced by prolonged alcohol consumption, despite adequate dietary intake. Trans Assoc Amer Physicians 76:289–300, 1963.

77. Jones DP, Losowsky MS, Davidson CS, Lieber CS: Effects of ethanol on plasma lipids

in man. J Lab Clin Med 62:675–682, 1963.

78. Baraona E, Lieber CS: Effects of chronic ethanol feeding on serum lipoprotein metabolism in the rat. J Clin Invest 49:769–778, 1970.

79. Brewster AC, Lankford HG, Schwartz MG, Sullivan JF: Ethanol and alimentary lipemia. Am J Clin Nutr 19:255–259, 1966.

80. Barboriak JJ, Meade RC: Enhancement of alimentary lipemia by preprandial alcohol. Am J Med Sci 255:245–251, 1968.

81. Wilson DW, Schreibman PH, Brewster AC, Araky RA: The enhancement of alimentary lipemia by ethanol in man. J Lab Clin Med 75:264–274, 1970.

82. Ostrander LD, Lamphiear DE, Block WD, et al: Relationship of serum lipid concentrations to alcohol consumption. Arch Intern Med 134:451–456, 1974.

83. Barboriak JJ, Hogan WJ: Preprandial drinking and plasma lipids in man. Atherosclerosis 4:323–325, 1976.

84. Losowsky MS, Jones DP, Davidson CS, Lieber CS: Studies of alcoholic hyperlipemia and its mechanism. Am J Med 35:794–803, 1963.

85. Schubotz R, Muhlfellner G, Schneider J, et al: Verhalten der Triglycerid-fettsauren bei fastenden und isokalorisch emahrten Versuchspersonen unter akuter Athanolbelastung. Einfuss der Lipolysehemmung durch Nikotinsaure and Glucose. Res Exper Med 167, 139–148, 1976.

86. Chait A, February AE, Mancini M, Lewis BL: Clinical and metabolic study of alcoholic hyperlipidaemia. Lancet 2:62–64, 1972.

87. Baraona E, Pirola RC, Lieber CS: The pathogenesis of postprandial hyperlipemia in rats fed ethanol containing diets. J Clin Invest 53:296–303, 1973.

88. Ockner RK, Mistilis SP, Poppenhausen RB, Stiehl AF: Ethanol induced fatty liver: Effect of intestinal lymph fistula. Gastroenterology 64:603–609, 1973.

89. Redgrave TG, Martin G: Effects of chronic ethanol consumption on the catabolism of chylomicron triacylglycerol and cholesteryl ester in the rat. Atherosclerosis 28:69–80, 1977.

90. Johnson O, Hernell O: Effects of ethanol on the activity of lipoprotein lipase in adipose tissue of male and female rats. Nutr Metabol 19:41–44, 1975.

91. Avogaro P: Changes in the composition and physiochemical characteristics of serum lipoproteins during ethanol-induced lipaemia in alcoholic subjects. Metabolism, 24:1231–1232, 1975.

92. Sabesin SM, Hawkins HL, Kuiken L, Ragland JB: Abnormal plasma lipoproteins and lecithin-cholesterol acyltransferase deficiency in alcoholic liver disease. Gastroenterology 72:510–518, 1977.

93. Miller P, Fellin R, Lambrecht J, et al: Hypertriglyceridemia secondary to liver disease. Europ J Clin Invest 4:419–428, 1974.

94. Verdy M, Gattereau A: Ethanol, lipase activity, and serum-lipid level. Am J Clin Nutr 20:997–1004, 1967.

95. Kudzma DJ, Schonfeld G: Alcoholic hyperlipidemia: Induction by alcohol but not by carbohydrate. J Lab Clin Med 77:384–395, 1971.

96. Nikkila EA, Taskinen MR, Huttunen JK: Effect of acute ethanol load on postheparin plasma lipoproteinlipase and hepatic lipase activities and intravenous fat tolerance. Horm Metab Res 10:220–223, 1978.

97. Albrink MJ, Klatskin G: Lactescence of serum following episodes of acute alcoholism and its probable relationship to acute pancreatitis. Am J Med 23:26–33, 1957.

98. Kessler JI, Kniffen JC, Janowitz HD: Lipoprotein lipase inhibition in the hyperlipemia of acute alcoholic pancreatitis. N Engl J Med 269:943–948, 1963.

99. Mendelson JH, Mello NK: Alcohol-induced hyperlipidemia and beta lipoproteins. Science 180:1372–1374, 1973.

100. Ginsberg H, Olefsky J, Farquhar JW, Reaven GW: Moderate ethanol ingestion and plasma triglyceride levels. Ann Intern Med 80:143–149, 1974.

101. Derby G, Mejean L, Max J, et al: Effects of alcohol intake on several metabolic parameters in primary hyperlipoproteinemias. In: Avogaro P, Sirtori CR, Tremoli F (eds): Metabolic Effects of Alcohol. Elsevier/North Holland Biomedical Press, 227–234, 1979.

102. Taskinen MR, Nikkila EA: Nocturnal hypertriglyceridemia and hyperinsulinemia following moderate evening intake of alcohol. Act Med Scand 202:173–177, 1977.

103. Borowsky SA, Perlow W, Baraona E, Lieber CS: Relationship of alcoholic hypertriglyceridemia to stage of liver disease and dietary lipid. Dig Dis Sci 25:22–27, 1980.

104. Zieve L: Jaundice, hyperlipemia, and hemolytic anemia: A heretofore unrecognized syndrome associated with alcoholic fatty liver and cirrhosis. Ann Intern Med 48:471–496, 1958.

105. Baraona E, Leiber CS: Alcoholic hyperlipemia. In: Schettler G, Greten H, Schlierf G, Seidel D, (eds): Handbuch der Inneren Medizin Band VII/4 Fettstoffwechsel. Berlin, Heidelberg, Springer-Verlag, 1976.

106. Fredrickson DS, Leevy RI, Lees RS: Fat transport in lipoprotein. An investigated approach to mechanisms and disorders. N Engl J Med, 276:32–44, 94–103, 148–156, 1967.

107. Parrish HM, Eberly AL: Negative association of coronary atherosclerosis with liver cirrhosis and chronic alcoholism—statistical fallacy. Journal Indiana State Med Assoc 54:341–347, 1961.

108. Klatsky AL, Friedman GD, Siegelaub AB: Alcohol consumption before myocardial infarction: Results from the Kaiser-Permanente Epidemiologic study of myocardial infarction. Am Int Med 81:294–301, 1974.

109. Stason WB, Neff RK, Miettinen OS, Jick H: Alcohol consumption and nonfatal myocardial infarction. Am J Epidemiol 104:603–608, 1976.

110. Yano K, Rhoads GG, Kagan A: Coffee, alcohol, and risk of coronary heart disease among Japanese men living in Hawaii. N Engl J Med 297:405–409, 1977.

111. Hennekens CH, Willett W, Rosner B, Cole DS, Mayrent SL: Effects of beer, wine and liquor in coronary deaths. JAMA 242:1973–1974, 1979.

112. Johansson BC, Medhus A: Increase in plasma A-lipoproteins in chronic alcoholics after acute abuse. Acta Med Scand 195:273–277, 1974.

113. Castelli WP, Gordon T, Hjorland MC, et al: Alcohol and blood lipids. Lancet 2:153–155, 1977.

114. Miller GJ, Miller NE: Plasma high-density-lipoprotein concentration and development of ischemic heart-disease. Lancet 1:16–19, 1975.

115. Miller NE, Forde OH, Thelle DS, Mjos OD: The Tromso heart study. High-density lipoprotein and coronary heart disease: A prospective case-control study. Lancet 1:965–967, 1977.

116. Carew TW, Koschinsky T, Hayes SB, Steinberg D: A mechanism by which high-density lipoproteins may slow the atherogenic process. Lancet 1:1315–1317, 1976.

117. Lefevre AF, DeCarli LM, Lieber CS: Effect of ethanol on cholesterol and bile acid metabolism. J Lipid Res 13:48–55, 1972.

118. Middleton WRJ, Carter EA, Drummey GD, Isselbacher KJ: Effect of oral ethanol administration on intestinal cholesterogenesis in the rat. Gastroenterology 60:880–887, 1971.

119. Boyer JL: Effect of chronic ethanol feeding on the bile formation and secretion of lipids in the rat. Gastroenterology 62:294–301, 1972.
120. Maddrey WC, Boyer JL: The acute and chronic effects of ethanol administration on bile secretion in the rat. J Lab Clin Med 82:215–225, 1973.
121. Marin GA, Karajoo M, Ward N, Rosato E: Effects of alcohol on biliary lipids in the presence of a chronic biliary fistula. Surg Gynecol Obstet 141:352–356, 1975.
122. Ideo G, Bellobuono A, Bellati G, et al: Bilirubin excretion in bile decreased by large amount of ethanol in isolated and perfused rat liver. Biomedicine 29:225–227, 1978.
123. Lakshmanan MR, Veech RL: Short- and long-term effects of ethanol administration in vivo on rat liver HMG-CoA reductase and cholesterol 7 A-hydroxylase activities. J Lipid Res 18:325, 1977.
124. Subbiah MTR: Ethanol and atherosclerosis: Effect of chronic ethanol ingestion on plasma cholesterol, cholesterol excretion, and aortic cholesterol accumulation in spontaneously atherosclerosis-susceptible pigeons. Artery 3:495–506, 1977.
125. Hennekens CH, Rosner B, Cole DS: Daily alcohol consumption and fatal coronary heart disease. Am J Epidemiol 107:196–200, 1978.
126. Barboriak JJ, Anderson AJ, Rimm AA, Tristani FE: Alcohol and coronary arteries. Alcoholism. Clin Exp Res 3:29–32, 1979.
127. Klatsky AL, Friedman GD, Siegelaub AB: Alcohol use, myocardial infarction, sudden cardiac death, and hypertension. Alcoholism. Clin Exper Res 3:33–39, 1979.
128. Russek HI, Naegele CF, Regan FD: Alcohol in the treatment of angina pectoris. JAMA 143:355–357, 1950.
129. Orlando J, Aronow WS, Cassidy J, Prakash R: Effect of ethanol on angina pectoris. Ann Intern Med 84:562–656, 1976.
130. Wilhelmsen L, Hans W, Gosta T: Multivariate analysis of risk factors for coronary heart disease. Circulation 48:950–958, 1973.
131. Dyer AR, Stamler J, Paul O, Berkson DM, Lepper NH, McKean H, Shekelle RB, Lindberg HA, Garside D: Alcohol consumption, cardiovascular risk factors and mortality in two Chicago epidemiologic studies. Circulation 56:1067–1074, 1977.
132. Klatsky AL, Friedman GD, Siegelaub AB, Gerard MJ: Alcohol consumption and blood pressure Kaiser-Permanente multiphasic heath examination data. N Engl J Med 296:1194–1200, 1977.
133. Harburg E, Ozgoren F, Hawthorne VM, Schork MA: Community norms of alcohol usage and blood pressure: Tecumseh, Michigan. Am J Public Health: 70:813–820, 1980.
134. Arkwright PD, Beilin LJ, Rouse I, Armstrong KB, Phil D, Vandongen R: Effects of alcohol use and other aspects of lifestyle on blood pressure levels and prevalence of hypertension in a working population. Circulation 66:60–66, 1982.
135. Wallace RB, Lynch CF, Pomrehn PR, Criqui MH, Heiss G: Alcohol and hypertension: Epidemiologic and experimental considerations. Circulation 64:41–47, 1981.
136. Saunders JB, Beevers DG, Paton A: Alcohol-induced hypertension. Lancet 2:653–656, 1981.
137. Clark LT, Friedman HS: Alcohol-induced hypertension: Assessment of mechanisms and complications. Clin Res 30:692A (abstract), 1982.
138. Linkola J, Fyhrquist F, Ylikahri R: Renin, aldosterone and coritsol during ethanol intoxication and hangover. Acta Physiol Scand 106:75–82, 1979.
139. Kozararevic JJ, Vojvodic N, Dawber T, McGee D, Racic Z, Gordon T, Zxkel W: Frequency of alcohol consumption and morbidity and mortality. Lancet 1:613–616, 1980.
140. Heberden W: Some account of a disorder of the breast. M Trans Coll Phys (London) 2:59–67, 1772.

9 | Vitamins and Minerals in Heart Disease

Henry K. J. Hahn
Robert E. Burch

A chapter on vitamins and minerals in heart disease is appropriate in view of the vast literature on the role of nutrition in cardiovascular disease. Unfortunately, this is a confusing subject. For example, the role of trace elements in human cardiovascular disease is obscured by variations in results due to methodologic problems, conflicting data, and the fact that many of the studies in humans are epidemiologic. Thus, it is difficult to draw firm conclusions.

Vitamins are vital organic dietary substances that cannot be synthesized in the body or, as with vitamins D, K, or niacin, cannot be synthesized in adequate amounts. Vitamins are utilized in small amounts to maintain normal metabolism. Minerals are inorganic elements widely distributed in nature; many also have vital roles in metabolic processes. Vitamins and minerals ordinarily must be supplied in food; minerals may also be supplied from the environment. Vitamins and minerals are noncalorigenic substances that are required in minute quantities, and they may be intimately associated. For example, zinc is intimately involved with vitamin A transport and metabolism. Cobalt, by contrast, is an integral component of vitamin B_{12}. Selenium is an antioxidant and functions synergistically with vitamin E. In spite of these and other relationships, the majority of experimental studies have been conducted with either vitamin deficiency or mineral deficiency. Vitamin and mineral deficiencies, acting in concert, have not been studied routinely. Further, whether the myocardial effects of vitamin deficiency or mineral deficiency are

This work was supported by the Veterans Administration Research Service.

caused by a direct effect of the deficiency, per se, or are secondary to some other mediated disturbances, has usually not been questioned.

Deficiency of any mineral results in a characteristic deficiency syndrome in a manner analogous to a specific vitamin deficiency. The deficiency syndrome is associated with specific structural, functional, biochemical or physiologic abnormalities. These abnormalities, in turn, are prevented or reversed after administration of the deficient vitamin or mineral. Similarly, toxicity may result from excesses of these minerals, just as in the case of vitamins A or D. It does not follow that if a little is good, then more should be better.

NOMENCLATURE

Mineral nomenclature deserves some explanation. Minerals are classified according to the quantity present in living tissues. If the concentration of an element can be expressed in milligrams, then one of the terms macromineral, macroelement, or macronutrient is used. Those elements present in microgram quantities or less are designated as microelements or micronutrients. Early workers used the adjective *trace* for those elements present in such small amounts in living tissues that they could not be quantified with the available methods. This term has remained in popular usage, despite the fact that virtually all the trace elements can now be estimated with great accuracy and precision. The term *trace elements* is retained here because it is brief and it has historical associations. Of the minerals appearing in the body, seven elements (Ca, Mg, Na, K, P, S, and Cl) have been designed "essential" as macronutrients and ten elements (Fe, Cu, Zn, Mn, Co, I, Se, Mo, Cr, and F) have been designed as "essential" trace elements. Four other elements (Ni, V, Si, and Sn) are currently viewed as essential trace elements, but their exact function is not yet established. An element is considered essential when a deficiency of that element induces identical, reproducible structural and physiologic abnormalities and addition of that particular element prevents or reverses the abnormalities. There are also four toxic, nonessential elements (Cd, As, Pb, and Hg) that accumulate with aging. However, all essential trace elements, if given in large enough doses, can be toxic.

The term *interaction* has appeared frequently in recent years. This term does not imply that two elements interact chemically, although chemical reaction between two metals is possible by changing the oxidation state. Rather, the term means an influence of one mineral in the presence of another.

THIAMINE (VITAMIN B₁)

Thiamine deficiency produces the clinical condition known as beriberi, an ancient nutritional disorder formerly widespread in the Orient.[1,2] This disease is caused by inadequate dietary intake of thiamine in countries where polished rice is the major carbohydrate in the diet. The incidence of beriberi in certain areas of Asia could also be augmented by antithiamine factors present in the diet (tea leaves, herring, shell fish, and raw carp).[2] If the rice were parboiled before milling (which conserves the vitamin B complex), beriberi could be prevented. Although beriberi may be associated with a refined rice diet, the disease has also occurred among groups who consumed excessive amounts of highly milled wheat.[3,4] These are classic examples of how manufacturing practices can influence nutrition and induce disease. In the United States today, the excessive ingestion of ethanol is the most common entity associated with thiamine deficiency (Chapter 8).

On the basis of the most prominent presenting clinical features, beriberi has been divided into two syndromes[5,6]: dry beriberi (polyneuropathy) and wet beriberi (congestive heart failure). Dry or neuritic beriberi is the most frequent syndrome occurring with thiamine deficiency and is associated with symptoms and signs related to the neuromuscular system. This type of beriberi is found frequently in older adults. Individuals subsisting on a diet that contains 0.2 to 0.3 mg thiamine/1,000 kcal (this is slightly less than the thiamine requirement) will slowly become depleted of thiamine and will develop peripheral neuropathy. The muscles become progressively more wasted and weaker. If the deficiency continues, walking finally becomes impossible. Parallel with the motor impairment, sensory changes occur. Other changes affect the spinal cord and the brain stem. The neuritis is seldom the cause of death, which occurs primarily due to heart failure.

The most acute type of thiamine deficiency is Wernicke's encephalopathy,[7,8] which occurs primarily in alcoholics but is not restricted to these patients. Thus, low thiamine intake associated with food faddism, social isolation, poverty, and the like may be associated with Wernicke's encephalopathy. Manifestations of this entity range from mild confusion to full-blown coma. Wernicke's encephalopathy is clincally characterized by ophthalmoplegia, polyneuropathy, ataxia, and mental confusion. Early recognition and therapy with thiamine is imperative, since Wernicke's encephalopathy may result in damage to the cerebral cortex and result in the development of Korsakoff's psychosis. Korsakoff's psychosis is usually associated with severe impairment of retentive memory and cognitive function. Because of the disordered memory function, some patients are only capable of performing the simplest of tasks. A retrograde amnesia covering a variable time period is quite common, and these patients tend to confabulate.

The neuropathy of beriberi, as noted above, is sensory and motor in nature. The deep tendon reflexes, which are usually increased initially, may be absent as the deficiency continues. Similarly, foot and wrist drop may occur. Sensory abnormalities are usually striking. Patients may experience hypoesthesia, hyperesthesia, and dysesthesia, and deep pressure or light touch may be quite unpleasant to the patient. In some instances thiamine deficiency may result in cranial nerve involvement, with vertigo, deafness, amblyopia, hoarseness, and dysphagia.

Wet or cardiac beriberi (see Chapter 8) is a more severe form of thiamine deficiency. If an individual is consuming a diet containing less than 0.2 mg of thiamine per 1,000 kcal, then, in addition to the neuropathic signs and symptoms, the patient will develop fluid retention, which results in edema formation. With progression, the heart becomes enlarged. The cardiac involvement is primarily right sided.[5,9] As congestive heart failure increases, venous pressure progressively increases and edema progresses. Venous engorgement ensues, and may be associated with anasarca, ascites, hydrothorax, hydropericardium, and hepatic engorgement. Gastrointestinal disturbances such as anorexia, nausea, vomiting, and constipation may occur along with oliguria. Although venous pressure is elevated in these patients, the circulation time may be shortened or normal. This is attributed to arteriovenous shunting, which occurs with thiamine deficiency and results in high output congestive heart failure. Acceleration of the circulation and enlargement of the right side of the heart, predominating features in this form of heart failure, are not sufficiently characteristic to confirm a diagnosis of thiamine deficiency. With progression of the cardiovascular phenomena of thiamine deficiency, the neurologic symptomatology becomes more and more apparent.

A more acute fulminant form of cardiac beriberi has been designated Shoshin beriberi. This name derives from the province in China where this syndrome was studied extensively. This form of cardiac failure is also primarily right sided, but, rather than being chronically progressive, it is characterized by acute cardiovascular collapse.[10,11] Patients with Shoshin beriberi rapidly succomb with cardiac failure. Systolic hypotension, venous distention, and peripheral cyanosis are usually prominent.

An infantile form of beriberi is nearly always acute and may be rapidly fatal.[12] This form of the deficiency occurs almost exclusively in infants who have been breast fed by mothers subsisting on a thiamine-deficient diet. These infants become ill between the 1st and 4th month of life. The major manifestations in these infants are constipation, diminished volume of urine, weakeness, rigidity, irritability, edema, and tachycardia. These infants may acutely develop cardiac failure. In others, symptomatology may be neurologic, with aphonia and meningismus. In some children, symptomatology may progress rapidly and end in death; in others, findings may wax and wane. Thiamine therapy promptly relieves the cardiovascular abnormalities. As in the adult, neurologic involvement usually improves slowly, and long-term treatment may be necessary.

Some of the clinical manifestations of thiamine deficiency can be related to the biochemical functions of this vitamin. Thiamine deficiency results in impairment of anerobic glycolysis (decreased conversion of pyruvate to acetyl CoA) and aerobic glycolysis (decreased conversion of α-ketoglutarate to succinyl CoA). Impairment of these two reactions results in reduced oxidative phosphorylation. Thus, there is diminished availability of high energy phosphate bonds to carry out metabolic functions.

The clinical manifestations of beriberi depend, to some extent, on the age of the patient, as well as on the duration and the severity of the deficiency. In the United States, thiamine deficiency is fairly common among alcoholic patients. Usually these patients manifest their deficiency as a neuropathy that may progress to Wernicke's disease or Korsakoff's syndrome. Rarely do these patients develop severe congestive heart failure on the basis of thiamine deficiency. Although the alcoholic may be consuming a large number of calories, these calories are primarily in the form of ethanol. The thiamine content of this diet is low. Further, these patients have impaired absorption of thiamine in the presence of continuing ethanol ingestion.

ASCORBIC ACID (VITAMIN C)

Ascorbic acid may play a role in the pathogenesis of atherosclerosis and progression of coronary artery disease. This concept is supported by many experimental and epidemiologic studies showing a relationship between vitamin C and cholesterol metabolism.[13,14] Plasma vitamin C levels of humans were low in smokers, hyperlipidemic patients, and patients with acute myocardial infarction.[15,16] Dietary supplements of ascorbic acid have been shown to decrease serum cholesterol concentrations in normal people under 25 years of age,[17] hyperlipidemic subjects,[18] and myocardial infarction patients.[19] These findings have been disputed by others.[20,21] Discrepancies are probably due to selection criteria of patients and body stores of the vitamin, since vitamin C treatment is probably only effective in hypercholesterolemic people whose initial ascorbic acid status is low.[21] The marked decline in coronary mortality rate has also been attributed to higher intake of synthetic ascorbic acid.[21]

There have been a considerable number of studies in recent years evaluating the cholesterol content of the high-density lipoprotein (HDL) fraction of plasma. It has been shown that low concentration of cholesterol in the serum HDL fraction is associated with an increased incidence of ischemic heart disease, and that this may function as a predictor of cardiovascular disease in man (see Chapter 5). A positive correlation between HDL cholesterol and plasma ascorbic acid has also been observed in ischemic heart disease.[23–25] It has been hypothesized that plasma HDL retards the progression of atherosclerosis by transporting cholesterol out of the arterial wall. A second possible mechanism for the antiatherogenic effect of high-density lipoprotein is that HDL inhibits the uptake of the cholesterol-rich, low-density lipoprotein by arterial smooth muscle.

Clinical studies have suggested that serum cholesterol could be lowered in hypercholesterolemic patients by the administration of ascorbic acid.[25] It has also been observed that daily administration of ascorbic acid was associated with a significant rise in HDL cholesterol. This could protect against the earlier development of ischemic heart disease. The possible role of ascorbic acid in the prevention of human coronary artery disease needs further investigation.

Convincing evidence, in experimental animals, has been presented to illustrate the relationship between vitamin C status, hypercholesterolemia, and atheromatous changes in the vascular system. Guinea pigs fed a scorbutogenic diet for 14 days were maintained on subnormal intake of vitamin C (0.5 mg/kg/day). The chronic and latent vitamin C deficiency lasted for more than 3 months. These animals developed marked atheromatous lesions in their vascular system, largely involving the coronary arteries.[14] The development of atheroma was directly related to vitamin C status (intake). The animals on the lowest intake had the most advanced lesions. These animals also had 50 percent increase in circulating cholesterol, and the liver had increased cholesterol content. HDL cannot be studied in normal guinea pigs because they have no detectable lipoproteins with alpha mobility.

In addition to the induction of hypercholesterolemia and hypertriglyceridemia, ascorbic acid deficiency also results in abnormal connective tissue formation in the blood vessel walls. The biochemical role of ascorbic acid in collagen synthesis is well known. Ascorbic acid is essential for the enzymes prolyl hydroxylase and lysyl hydroxylase. These enzymes are involved in hydroxylation of proline and lysine after their incorporation into a polypeptide chain. The lack of hydroxylation results in abnormal collagen and weak elastic tissue, and it is believed that vitamin C deficiency results in decreased hydroxylation of proline and lysine via decreased enzyme activity. Disorders of collagen biosynthesis have shown marked improvement with administration of pharmacologic doses of vitamin C. One patient with lysyl hydroxylase deficiency showed improved muscle strength and wound healing capacity after receiving 4 g of ascorbic acid per day.[26] Another patient who had osteogenesis imperfecta showed some improvement after administration of 25 to 50 mg vitamin C/kg/day.[27]

In spite of the extensive studies, there is no unified hypothesis regarding the role of vitamin C in the pathogenesis of atherosclerosis. One of the main problems is in the choice of different experimental animals. Some of these animals synthesize ascorbate (rat, rabbit, chicken and pig) and some do not synthesize ascorbate (guinea pigs, bats, monkeys and man). Another obvious factor is severity of onset of the vitamin C deficiency.

SPECULATIVE VITAMINS

Niacin (nicotinic acid) has frequently been employed in the past for the treatment of hyperlipidemias (see Chapter 3). The rationale was that pharmacologic doses of nicotinic acid reduced the circulating levels of cholesterol, triglycerides, and β–lipoproteins.[28] However, there are many undesirable side effects with its use.[29] Recent studies have indicated that evidence of efficacy of niacin in coronary heart disease is lacking.[30] Niacin is an effective hypolipidemic agent when administered in large doses exceeding its requirements as a vitamin. Niacin has an inhibitory effect on lipolysis of adipose tissue and very low density lipoprotein synthesis. It results in a decrease in free fatty acid, plasma cholesterol, and triglyceride levels. The reduction in very low density lipoprotein levels leads to a subsequent decrease in low-density lipoproteins. Therefore, niacin is a very useful drug in the treatment of hyperlipidemia, especially types II, IV, and V. However, large doses (3 to 10 g/day) of niacin may cause toxic effects, such as liver disease and hyperuricemia.

Studies in infants and children have indicated, that there was a great occurrence of congestive heart failure among riboflavin-deficient children.[31] The probable mechanism was a poor dietary intake combined with gastrointestinal malabsorption similar to the complication of heart disease which occurred in folic acid deficiency.[32,33]

Vitamin B_6 is believed to be associated with the development of atherosclerosis. Feeding a pyridoxine-deficient diet to monkeys successfully produces atherosclerosis similar to that in humans.[34] A greater degree of cholesterolemia is present in the pyridoxine-deficient monkey receiving low cholesterol than in the normal animal that receives considerably higher quantities of cholesterol. The arteriosclerotic changes in the vitamin B_6-deficient monkey may link the vitamin to cholesterol metabolism, possibly through its association with esential fatty acid metabolism. Vitamin B_6 lowers the requirement for essential fatty acids to some extent. Vitamin B_6 functions in the conversion of linoleic acid to arachidonic acid.[35] It is still uncertain what role vitamin B_6 plays in fat metabolism.[36]

Vitamin E has been studied extensively to determine its efficacy for heart disease, arteriosclerosis, progressive muscular dystrophy, and sterility in the male.[37–39] However, evidence linking vitamin E and cardiovascular disease is not available.[39] Similarly, evidence linking vitamin E to human muscular dystrophy and sterility in the male is also lacking. Vitamin E has been found to be a potent biological antioxidant. The range of activity of these biologic antioxidants is broad. Vitamin E participates is specific enzymatic systems and promotes fertility in experimental animals. However, its precise function in humans is still unknown.

MACROMINERALS, HYPERTENSION, AND CARDIOVASCULAR DISEASES

It is well known that calcium (Ca^{2+}) is essential for excitation-contraction process of muscles, but significant advances in cardiovascular pharmacology have been achieved only within the past 10 years. Unlike skeletal muscle cells, myocardial cells primarily depend on the influx of extracellular Ca^{2+} in excitation-contraction coupling. Electrical depolarization of cardiac muscle is initiated with rapid influx of Na^+. Tension developed by the heart muscle in response to electrical stimulation depends on the ratio of extracellular ($Ca^{2+}/[Na^+)^2]$. Mycardial contractility is dependent on the environmental Ca^{2+} because heart muscle cells have limited intracellular calcium stores. Variations in the extracellular calcium concentration profoundly affect the myocardial contractility by affecting the transmembrane supply of Ca^{2+} for contraction.

Consistently higher myocardial calcium concentrations have been observed in patients with ischemic heart disease.[40,41] Indeed, there is a rapid uptake of calcium into myocardial tissue following a period of transient ischemia.[42] Calcium antagonists are new pharmacologic agents used in the treatment of ischemic heart disease.[43] They are also known as calcium channel blocking agents, calcium entry blockers, and slow channel calcium blockers. The three most important calcium antagonists are verapamil, nifedipine, and diltizem.[44] Despite the structural heterogenecity, all three compounds depress the slow channel in cardiac muscle. The inhibitory effects on Ca^{2+} transport are restricted to the sarcolemma.[44,45] Thus far, numerous clinical trials of calcium antagonists have shown them to be very effective in the treatment of coronary vasopasm,[46,47] angina pectoris,[48] and in the reduction of myocardial infarct size.[49]

Epidemiologic studies associating water hardness and mortality rates from cardiovascular diseases have generated tremendous interest and controversy. These studies presented very convincing evidence that the death rate from ischemic heart disease was increased in areas with soft drinking water in the United States, [50–52] the United Kingdom, [53,54] and Canada.[55,56] The causes of increased cardiovascular death have been attributed to a deficiency of magnesium and/or calcium rather than to an excess of one or more of the minerals studied. The hardness of drinking water is determined by its calcium and magnesium content and is a crude measurement of these substances. Drinking water can be viewed as an end result of the cycling process of minerals into and through living systems, particularly from soil to plants to animals and back to soil. This cycling process makes it difficult to establish normal values for water hardness. Nevertheless, these studies have shown an inverse correlation between hardness of water and cardiovascular death rates.

There is a small but significant decrease in the magnesium concentration of normal heart muscle from individuals in soft water areas, compared with hard water areas.[40] In contrast, significantly increased concentrations of myocardial magnesium were found in individuals residing in soft water areas.[57] Similarly, those dying from ischemic heart disease have been shown to have low myocardial magnesium concentrations.[40–41] A stronger correlation exists between sudden death from ischemic heart disease and low myocardial magnesium.[58] There have been numerous studies on serum magnesium levels in myocardial infarction, but a variety of nonspecific causes unrelated to heart disease can alter total serum magnesium concentrations, such as prolonged diarrhea or vomiting, protein-calorie malnutrition, and disease characterized by intestinal malabsorption. For reasons of convenience, it is often attempted to diagnose the mineral status of an individual by analysis of serum. The serum magnesium level does not necessarily reflect dietary intake or heart magnesium content, since magnesium is an intracellular element. Thus, the interpretation of these results is difficult.

The studies relating cardiovascular disease and water hardness were conducted without consideration of the dietary habits of the population. Average intake of calcium (1,000 to 1,400 mg/day in western countries and 200 to 500 mg/day in developing countries)[50] and magnesium (200 to 400 mg/day)[60] from food is adequate to meet the requirement of the recommendated daily dietary allowances (RDA).[61] Thus, individuals from soft water areas could ingest large amounts of calcium and magnesium.

To illustrate the effect of limited intake of calcium and magnesium on heart, an experiment was conducted to study heart tissue mineral composition. One group of animals was fed *ad libitum* and the dietary intake of the other group was restricted to 50 percent *ad libitum* fed levels. Pups (Fisher 344) were weaned at 21 days and placed in individual stainless steel cages until sacrificed. The purified diet (AIN-76) was chosen to eliminate mineral variations in commercial diets. Diets contained 5,200 mg Ca/kg, 500 mg Mg/kg, and adequate trace elements and vitamins to meet the nutrient requirement of the rat.[62] Food consumption and body weight were measured daily. Rats were given deionized water *ad libitum*.

The effect of this restricted diet on calcium concentration in male rat hearts is shown in Fig. 9-1. It can be seen that there were no differences between the two dietary groups. In fact, the 50 percent *ad libitum* fed rats had a tendency for higher calcium concentrations than *ad libitum* rats, but these differences are not statistically significant. The effect of diet restriction on magnesium content is shown in Fig. 9-2. Similar results were obtained. However, the magnesium content of heart from both dietary groups tended to decrease at 24 months of age. These studies illustrate that calcium and magnesium content of heart did not change even with severe restriction for a long

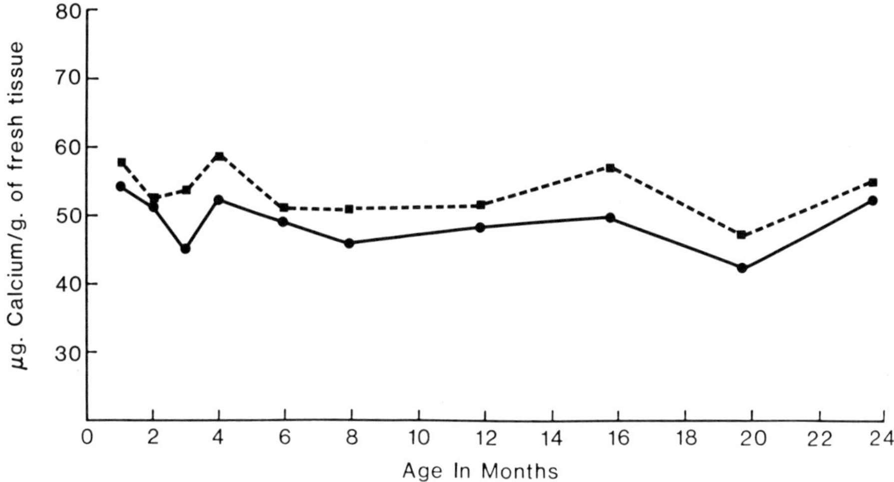

Fig. 9-1. The effect of restricted diet on calcium concentration in male rat hearts (---- 50 percent *ad libitum*; _________ *ad libitum*).

period of time. Thus, it is difficult to imagine that the softness of drinking water could cause a deficiency, since very hard water probably contributes not more than 20 percent of mineral intake.[63] On the other hand, these studies measured total cardiac content of magnesium and calcium. Intracellular composition of these two elements was not measured.

Good and consistent correlations have been reported between dietary sodium intake and the incidence of hypertension. A progressive increase in hypertension can be ob-

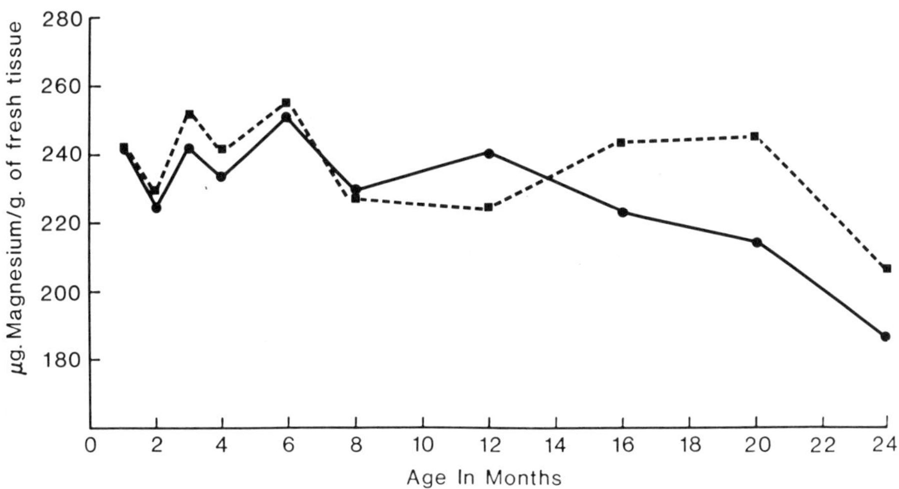

Fig. 9-2. The effect of restricted diet on magnesium concentration in male rat hearts (---- 50 percent *ad libitum*; _________ *ad libitum*).

served when sodium intake is plotted against prevalence of hypertension.[64] The highest incidence of hypertension (30 to 40 percent) is observed among patients with sodium intakes exceeding 435 mEq/day. Hypertension was practically nonexistent in populations on a salt-free diet.[65,66] An increase in incidence of hypertension is observed in a primitive population after the introduction of salt to their diet.[67] Several epidemiologic studies support the correlation between high salt intake and hypertension.

The role of sodium in the pathogenesis of hypertension is not clear. It is known that the concentration of salt ingested is proportional to the extracellular fluid volume. An increase in salt intake will increase the circulating blood volume, which in turn may raise the blood pressure. It appears that genetic factors may be involved, since renal inability to handle a high sodium load is prevalent within the families of hypertensives.[64] Despite the lack of firm data, it is clear that 20 percent or more of the children in industrialized countries are currently destined to become hypertensive adults; therefore, restriction of sodium intake may be beneficial in the prevention of hypertension. However, prolonged severe sodium restriction should be avoided, since hyponatremia may result in a more complex disorder. A reduction in the serum sodium level is frequently associated with congestive heart failure and is not corrected by hypertonic saline.[68]

It is common knowledge that an abnormal level of sodium may adversely affect the function of heart muscle, but it is less profound than cardiac muscle dysfunction due to hypokalemia. Even small variations in serum potassium concentration are reflected in electrocardiographic changes, and hypokalemia may result in cardiac arrest. Indeed, a recent study has shown that the prevalence of hypertension is inversely proportional to the serum potassium level.[69] This study suggests that there are significant interactions between calcium, magnesium, sodium, and potassium in the etiology of hypertension.

TRACE ELEMENTS

There is abundant evidence for the relationship between trace elements and cardiovascular disease; however, the only source of trace elements considered in these studies was the drinking water.[40,50,51,54] Trace elements in water are probably not of major concern, since food is the major source of trace elements ingested by humans. Further, none of the trace elements studied is closely associated with hardness of water. It is more appropriate to reveiw the direct clinical and experimental evidence on the relationship of trace elements to cardiovascular disease.

Hypertension can be induced in rats by cadmium, and this was first reported by Schroeder.[70] The effect of cadmium on the development of arterial hypertension in humans is controversial.[71–73] Correlation between cadmium levels and blood pressure is not a universal finding. The influence of smoking habits, however, gives more positive results.[72–74] Cigarette smoking is often a common airborne source of cadmium.[72]. The hypothesis that cadmium is related to hypertension in humans is supported by the clinical observation that the metal is present in high concentration in the kidneys and urine of hypertensive patients.[51,75] Cadmium is always present in human kidneys, and relatively higher concentrations occur in the kidney than any other organ.[76] Cadmium is one of the few metals that exhibit organ specificity. Conceivably, the observed hypertension may be the secondary result of kidney damage due to long-term exposure; however, cadmium workers exposed to cadmium over a long period of time do not show a high incidence of hypertensive disease.[77] Thus, the role of cadmium in the development of hypertension is unknown.

Myocardial damage has been reported with ingestion of beer containing excessive amounts of cobalt.[78–79] Clinical manifestations of "beer drinkers' cardiomyopathy" or "cobalt cardiomyopathy" are similar to beriberi heart disease. However, difficulty was encountered in inducing beer drinkers' cardiomyopathy in experimental animals by the simple addition of cobalt to the diet. Similarly, the synergistic effect of alcohol, cobalt, and thiamine deficiency could not reproduce the syndrome.[80] It is unknown how cobalt induced cardiomyopathy in humans. Nonetheless, this syndrome disappeared after manufacturers removed cobalt from beer.

It has been postulated that an imbalance of the zinc-copper ratio is a major factor in the etiology of coronary heart disease.[81–82] In rats, a high ratio of dietary zinc to copper resulting from low dietary intake of copper and a relative copper deficiency is associated with hypercholesterolemia.[83] In contrast, other studies have failed to show any relationship between zinc-copper ratios and serum cholesterol levels in rats [84,85] and humans.[86,87] It has long been known that high levels of dietary zinc can interfere with copper absorption.[88,89] It has recently been found that hypocupremia can be induced in adult patients with sickle cell anemia treated with 10 times the recommended daily dietary allowances (RDA) of zinc.[90] Hy pocupremia also can occur in rats, but 67 times the zinc requirement is needed.[91] Thus, it is not the zinc-copper ratio but the actual concentrations of these trace elements in the diet that is critical.

Most studies on zinc and copper interactions have been conducted with weanling rats. The dietary interactions of zinc and copper in adult rats must be studied, since grown rats are not experiencing the same rapid changes as weanling rats. Further, in those weanling rats studied, the copper content in the diet was too low to meet this nutrient's requirement. The hypothesis should be tested in the presence of adequate copper nutrition. Cholesterol should also be included in the diet so that it would resemble our dietary habits. Further studies are needed to ascertain the basic mechanism involved in the development of hypocholesterolemia in copper deficiency. Similarly, the administration of excess zinc must be done in the presence of adequate dietary copper. At the present time, there is insufficient evidence to support the zinc-copper hypothesis in coronary heart disease.

Trace element deficiency can occur in humans. In general, trace element deficiency can result from inadequate dietary intake, impaired intestinal absorption, excessive excretion, and certain inherited disease states. Copper deficiency has been reported in premature infants fed copper deficient formulas, in severely malnourished infants with chronic diarrhea, in untreated malnourished infants, and in severe chronic malabsorption resulting from disaccharidase deficiency. Copper, zinc, and selenium deficiency have occurred in infants, children, and adults receiving total parenteral nutrition. A classical example of human copper defiiciency is

Menkes' kinky hair syndrome. This syndrome is characterized by kinky hair, convulsions, mental retardation, abnormalities of the metaphyses of long bone, abnormal elastic tissue in arteries, tortuosity of cerebral vessels, aneurysms, and hypothermia. Aneurysms occur secondary to defective collagen cross-linkage due to decreased activity of lysyl oxidase, a copper metalloezyme. This is a genetically determined defect in copper absorption and utilization.

Selenium was initially known for its toxic effects on livestock, resulting in diseases such as "blind staggers" and "alkali disease." Attention is now being focused on the beneficial role of selenium, because selenium deficiencies are known to cause white-muscle disease, nutritional muscular dystrophy, and Zenker's disease.[76] Whether or not a selenium deficiency causes heart disease in humans is not proven; however, it has been found that selenium deficiency appears to increase man's susceptibility to heart disease. Epidemiologic studies have shown that there is an inverse relationship in mortality and selenium bioavailability.[92,93] Death rate, due to various heart disease (coronary, hypertension, cardiovascular-renal, and cerebrovascular disease) is increased 25 percent or more from high to low selenium areas.[92] Recently, selenium deficiencies in humans have been reported.[94,95] One of the symptoms of selenium deficiency associated with the administration of total parenteral nutrition was marked muscle weakness, which responded to selenium therapy.[94] A report from China presents the most significant evidence that selenium is essential to normal heart function.[95] A form of heart disease of unknown cause called "Keshan's disease" is prevalent in low-selenium areas of China, and was successfully treated with sodium selenite. Untreated patients developed heart failure, and at least half of them died. The people most susceptible to this disease were children and women of child-bearing age. This disease resembles the "mulberry heart disease" found in selenium-deficient swine. The lower selenium contents of whole blood and hair, and the activity of glutathione peroxidase, indicate selenium deficiency in these patients. Vitamin E and selenium act together in many physiologic processes, but there was no evidence of vitamin E deficiency in Keshan's disease. Therefore, the cardiomyopathy associated with Keshan's disease is most likely due to selenium deficiency alone.

SUMMARY

Over the past decade, coronary mortality rates have been steadily declining. This decline may be due to many factors, such as a more nutritious diet (decreased consumption of cholesterol and saturated fats, and an increased consumption of polyunsaturated fats and vitamins), better control of hypertension, improved coronary care units, and exercise programs. Classic vitamin deficiency diseases are rare, but marginal vitamin deficiency, without clinical symptoms, may occur, since marginal vitamin intake in school children is more common than anticipated. Milk formulas have an insufficient quantity of vitamins and trace elements. Therefore, infants consuming infant formulas may be prime subjects of marginal vitamin deficiency. Marginal vitamin deficiency is an important area of research in view of experimental animal studies. For example, a chronic marginal ascorbate deficiency in guinea pigs produces hypercholesterolemia and hypertriglyceridemia.

Vitamin C and the B vitamins, in general, are relatively nontoxic substances when given in large quantities. They are simply catabolized and excreted without additional benefit or harm. However, repeated intake of pharmacologic doses or megadoses of vitamins may result in undesirable side effects. One should be especially cautious about administering large doses to pregnant mothers and children.

It is well established that essential minerals play an important role in a number of biologic processes and in the maintenance of normal physiologic functions. Therefore, it is reasonable to assume that these minerals would also exert an action on cardiovascular function. There is no clear evidence of any interaction between cardiovascular disease and macromineral deficiency. The findings of epidemiologic studies on water hardness are inconsistent.

Whether excess salt intake induces hypertension is controversial, but it is agreed that moderate restriction of sodium intake in hypertensive patients is beneficial. Calcium antagonists as cardiovascular therapeutic agents are rapidly gaining a wider spectrum of utility. These agents could allow us to examine some of the membrane biophysical and electrophysical phenomena of cardiac tissue and the basic physiologic process of excitation-contraction with transmembrane movements of Na, K, and Ca ions. Among the trace elements, copper and selenium deficiencies have been associated with heart disease.

REFERENCES

1. Takaki B: The preservation of health amongst the personnel of the Japanese Navy and Army. Lancet I:1369, 1451, 1520, 1906.
2. Tanphaichitr V: Thiamine. In: Present Knowledge in Nutrition. Washington, The Nutrition Foundation, Inc. 1976, pp 141–147.
3. Aykroyd WR: Beriberi and other food-deficiency diseases in Newfoundland and Labrador. J Hyg 30:357, 1930.
4. Hehir P: Effects of chronic starvation during the siege of Kut. Br Med J 2:865, 1922.
5. Weiss S: Occidental beriberi with cardiovascular manifestations: Its relation to thiamine deficiency. JAMA 115:832, 1940.
6. Platt BS: Beriberi—clinical features of endemic beriberi. Fed Proc 17 (suppl 2):8, 1958.
7. Victor M, Adams RD: On the etiology of alcohol neurologic diseases with special reference to the role of nutrition. Am J Clin Nutr 9:379, 1961.
8. Cole M, Turner A, Frank O, et al: Extraocular palsy and thiamine therapy in Wernickes' encephalopathy. Am J Clin Nutr 22:44, 1969.
9. Blankenhorn MA: Occidental beriberi heart disease. JAMA 131: 717, 1946.
10. Wolf PL, Levin MB: Shoshin beriberi. N Engl J Med 262:1302, 1960.
11. Sambrook PN, Dalton WR: Shoshin beriberi. Aust NZJ Med 11: 190, 1981.
12. Van Gelder DW, Darby FU: Congenital and infantile beriberi. J Pediatr 25:226, 1944.
13. Turley SD, West CE, Horton BJ: The role of ascorbic acid in the regulation of cholesterol metabolism and the pathogenesis of atherosclerosis. Atherosclerosis 24:1, 1978.
14. Ginter E: Marginal vitamin C deficiency, lipid metabolism and Atherogenesis. Adv Lipid Rec 16:167, 1978.

15. Pelletier O. Vitamin C and cigarette smokers. Ann NY Acad Sci 258:156, 1975.
16. Ramirez J, Flowers NC: Leukocyte ascorbic acid and its relationship to coronary artery disease in man. Am. J. Clin Nutr 33:2079, 1980.
17. Spittle CR: Atheroselerosis and vitamin C. Lancet 2:1280, 1971.
18. Ginter E: Vitamin C and plasma lipids N Engl J Med 294:559, 1976.
19. Bordia AK: The effect of vitamin C on blood lipids, fibrinolytic activity and platelet adhesives in patients with coronary artery disease. Atherosclerosis 35:181, 1980.
20. Peterson VE, Phyllis BP, Cropo PA, et al: Quantitation of plasma cholesterol and triglyceride levels in hypercholesterolemic subjects receiving ascorbic acid supplements. Am J Clin Nutr 28:584, 1975.
21. Ginter E, Kayaba I, Nizer O: The effect of ascorbic acid on cholesterolaemia in healthy subjects with seasonal deficiency of vitamin C. Nutr Metab 12:76, 1970.
22. Ginter E: Decline of coronary mortality in United States and vitamin C. Am J Clin Nutr 32:511, 1979.
23. Gordon T, Castelli WP, Hjortland MC, et al: High density lipoprotein as a protective factor against coronary heart disease. Am J Med 62:707, 1977.
24. Bates CJ, Mandal AR, Cole TJ: HDL cholesterol and vitamin C status. Lancet 2:611, 1977.
25. Horsey J, Livesley B, Dickerson JWT. Ischaemic heart disease and aged patients: Effects of ascorbic acid on lipoproteins. J Human Nutr 35:53, 1981.
26. Elsas LJ, Miller RL, Pennell SR: Inherited collagen lysyl hydroxylase deficiency: Ascorbic acid response. J Pediatr 92:378, 1978.
27. Kurz D, Eyring EJ: Effects of vitamin C on osteogenesis imperfecta. Pediatrics 54:56, 1974.
28. Parsons WB, Jr: Treatment of hypercholesteremia by nicotinic acid. Arch Int Med 107:639, 1961.
29. Mosher LR: Nicotinic acid side effects and toxicity. A Review. Am J Psychiatry 126:129, 1970.
30. The Coronary Drug Project Research Group: Clofibrate and niacin in coronary heart disease. JAMA 231:360, 1975.
31. Steier M, Lopez R, Cooperman JM: Riboflavin deficiency in infants and children with heart disease. Am Heart J 92:139, 1976.
32. Brody JI, Soltys HD, Zinsser HF: Folic acid deficiency in congestive heart failure. Br Heart J 31:741, 1969.
33. Rook GD, Loped R, Shimiza N, et al: Folic acid deficiency in infants and children with heart disease. Br Heart J 35:87, 1973.
34. Rinehart JF, Greenberg LD: Pathogenesis of experimental artheriosclerosis in pyridoxine deficiency. Arch Pathol 51:12, 1951.
35. Ross Pediatric Research Conference: The role of vitamin B_6 in the metabolism of fatty acid. In: Vitamin B_6 In Human Nutrition. Reports of the Ross Pediatric Research Conference. 10:28, 1953.
36. Mueller JF: Vitamin B_6 in fat metabolism. Vitam Horm 22:787, 1964.
37. DiPalma JR, Ritchie DM: Vitamin toxicity. Ann Rev Pharmacol Toxicol 17:133, 1977.
38. Hodges RE: Vitamin E and coronary heart disease. J Am Diet Assoc 62:638, 1973.
39. Olson RE: Vitamin E and its relation to heart disease. Circulation 48:179, 1973.
40. Anderson TW, Neri LS, Shreiber GB, et al: Ischaemic heart disease, water hardness and myocardial magnesium. Can Med Assoc J. 113:199, 1975.
41. Chipperfield B, Chipperfield JR: Difference in metal content of heart muscle from ischaemic heart disease. Am Heart J 95:732, 1978.

Shen AC, Jennings RB: Myocardium calcium and magnesium in acute ischaemic injury. Am J Path 67:417, 1972.

Fleckstein A: Specific inhibitors and promoters of calcium action in the excitation-contraction coupling of heart muscle. In Harris P, Opiz L. (eds): Calcium and the Heart. New York, Academic Press, 1971, pp 135–188.

Millard RW, Lathrop DA, Grupp G, et al: Differential cardiovascular effects of calcium channel blocking agents: potential mechanisms. Am J Card 49:499, 1982.

Nayler WG, Grinwald P: Calcium entry blockers and myocardial function. Fed Proc 40:2855, 1981.

Endo M, Kanda I, Hosoda S, et al: Prinzmetal's variant form of angina pectoria: re-evaluation of mechanisms. Circulation 52:33, 1975.

Mueller JE, Gunter SJ: Nifedipine therapy for prinzmetal's agina. Circulation 57:137, 1978.

Antman E, Mueller J, Goldberg S, et al: Nifedipine therapy for coronary artery spasm. N Engl J Med 302:1269, 1980.

Meils CM, Grass GJ, Brooks HL, et al: Reduction of myocardial infarct size by the calcium antagonist FR 7534. Cardiology 68:146, 1981.

Voors AW: Minerals in the municipal water and other atherosclerotic heart death. Am J Epidemiol 93:259, 1971.

Shroeder HA, Kraemer LA: Cardiovascular mortality, municipal water and corrosion. Arch Environ Health 28:303, 1974.

Dudley EF, Beldin RA, Johnson BC: Climate water hardness and coronary heart disease. J Chron Dis 22:25, 1969.

Crawford MD, Gardner MJ, Morries JN: Cardiovascular disease and the mineral content of drinking water. Br Med Bull 27:21, 1971.

Elwood PC, Albernethy M, Morton M: Mortality in adults and trace elements in water. Lancet 2:1470, 1974.

Neri LC, Mandel JS, Hewitt D: Relationship between mortality and water hardness in Canada. Lancet 1:931, 1972.

Anderson TW, LeRiche WH, MacKay JS. Sudden death and ischaemic heart disease. Correlation with hardness of local water supply. N Engl J Med 280:805, 1969.

Chipperfield B, Chipperfield JR, Behr G, et al: Magnesium and potassium content of normal heart muscle in areas of hard and soft water. Lancet 1:121, 1976.

Behr G. Burton P: Heart muscle magnesium. Lancet 2:450, 1973.

FAO/WHO Expert Group: Calcium requirements. WHO Technical Report Series No. 230, 1962, p. 42.

Seelig MS: The requirement of magnesium by normal adult. Am J Clin Nutr 14:342, 1964.

Food and Nutrition Board: Recommended Dietary Allowance. Washington, National Academy of Science, 1974.

AIN Ad Hoc Committee on Standard for Nutritional Studies: J Nutr 107:1350, 1977.

Sharret AR: Water hardness and cardiovascular disease-elements in water and human tissues. Sci Total Environ 7:47, 1977.

Fries ED: Salt, volume and the prevention of hypertension. Circulation 53:589, 1976.

Sasaki N: The relationship of salt intake to hypertension in the Japanese. Geriatrics 19:735, 1964.

Oliver WJ, Cohen EL, Neel JV: Blood pressure and sodium intake and sodium related hormones in the Yanomamo Indians: a "no salt" culture. Circulation 52:146, 1975.

Lowenstein TW: Blood pressure in relation to age and sex in the tropics and subtropics.

A review of the literature and an investigation in two tribes of Brazil Indians. Lancet 1:389, 1961.

68. Elkinton JR, Squires RD, Bluemle JN: The distribution of body fluids in congestive heart failure. Circulation 5:58, 1952.

69. Ueshima H, Tangigaki M, Iida M, et al: Hypertension, salt, and potassium. Lancet 1:504, 1981.

70. Schroeder HA, Venton WH: Hypertension induced in rats by small doses of cadmium. Am J Physiol 202:515, 1962.

71. Glauser SC, Bello CT, Glauser EM: Blood-cadmium levels in normotensive and untreated hypertensive humans. Lancet 1:717, 1976.

72. Beevers DG, Campbell BC, Goldberg A, et al: Blood cadmium in hypertensives and normotensives. Lancet 2:1222, 1976.

73. Manthey J, Stoypher M, Morgenstern W, et al: Magnesium and trace metals: Risk factors for coronary heart disease? Associations between blood levels and angiographic findings. Circulation 64:722, 1981.

74. Nandi M, Stone D, Tick H, et al: Cadmium content of cigarettes. Lancet 1:1329, 1969.

75. Axelson O, Piscator M: Renal damage after prolonged exposure to cadmium, Arch Environ Health 12:360, 1966.

76. Underwood EJ: Cadmium. In: Trace Elements in Human and Animal Nutrition. New York, Academic Press, 1971, p 267.

77. Flick DF, Kraybill HF, Dimitroff JM: Toxic effects of cadmium, A review. Environ Res 4:71, 1971.

78. McDermott PH, Delaney RL, Egan JD, Sullivan JF. Myocardosis and cardiac heart failure in man. JAMA 198:252, 1966.

79. Sullivan JF, Egan JD, George RP: A distinctive myocardiopathy occurring in Omaha, Nebraska: Clinical aspects. Ann NY Acad Sci 156:526, 1969.

80. Burch RE, Williams RV, Sullivan JF: Effects of cobalt, beer and thiamine-deficient diets in pigs. Am J Clin Nutr 26:403, 1973.

81. Klevay LM: Coronary heart disease: The zinc/copper hypothesis. Am J Clin Nutr 28:764, 1975.

82. Petering HG, Murthy L, O'Flaherty E: Influence of dietary copper and zinc on rat lipid metabolism. J Agri Food Chem 25:1105, 1977.

83. Allen KGD, Klevay LM: Copper deficiency and cholesterol metabolism in the rat. Atherosclerosis 31:259, 1978.

84. Fischer PWF, Giroux A, L'Abbe MR: The effect of dietary zinc on intestinal copper absorption. Am J Clin Nutr 34:1670, 1981.

85. Caster WO, Doster JM: Effect of the dietary zinc/copper ratio on plasma cholesterol levels. Nutr Rep Int 19:773, 1979.

86. Genders JM: Relationship between zinc and copper nutrition status and risk factors associated with cardiovascular disease. Fed Proc 38:5524A, 1979.

87. Fischer PWF, Collins MW: Relationship between serum zinc and copper and risk factors associated with cardiovascular disease. Am J Clin Nutr 34:595, 1981.

88. Van Campen DR, Scaife PU: Zinc intereference with copper absorption in rats. J Nutr 91:473, 1967.

89. Whanger PD, Weswig PH: Effect of some copper antagonists on induction of ceruloplasmin in the rat. J Nutr 100:341, 1970.

90. Prasad AD, Brewer GJ, Schoomaker EB, et al: Hypocupremia induced by zinc therapy in adults. JAMA 240:2166, 1978.

91. Whanger PD, Weswig PH. Effect of supplementary zinc on the intracellular distribution of hepatic copper in rats. J Nutr 101:1093, 1971.

92. Shamberger RJ, Tytko SA, Willis CE: Selenium and Heart disease. In: Trace Substances in Environmental Health IX, 15. Columbia, Mo, 1975.
93. Frost DV, Lish PM: Selenium in biology. Ann Rev Pharmacol 15:259, 1975.
94. Van Rij AM, Thomson CD, McKenzie JM, Robinson MF: Selenium deficiency in total parenteral nutrition. Am J Clin Nutr 32:2076, 1979.
95. Keshan Disease Research Group of the Chinese Academy of Medical Science: Observation on Effect of Sodium Selenite in Prevention of Keshan Disease. Chinese Med J 92:471, 477, 1979.

10 | Variations on the Prudent Diet

Lynne W. Scott
John P. Foreyt
Antonio M. Gotto

About 80 percent of patients who die from or are disabled by cardiovascular disease have one or more primary risk factors: hypercholesterolemia, hypertension, or cigarette smoking. Diabetes is important, probably next in order after the primary factors. Obesity, although not an independent risk factor, significantly influences hyperlipidemia, hypertension, and diabetes. This chapter will discuss ways that the diet-related risk factors, hyperlipidemia, hypertension, and obesity may be affected favorably through use of the Prudent Diet and its variations. We also describe the use of the diet for pregnant and lactating women, and for children and adolescents at high risk.

THE PRUDENT DIET DEFINED

The Prudent Diet is designed as a preventive and therapeutic diet. It provides no more than 300 mg cholesterol per day, with 50 percent of the calories from carbohydrates, 20 percent from protein, and the remaining 30 percent from fat,

This work was supported by grant HL 17269 from the National Heart, Lung, and Blood Institute for the National Research and Demonstration Center, Baylor College of Medicine, and The Methodist Hospital, Houston, Texas.

including less than 10 percent from saturated fat, up to 10 percent from polyunsaturated fat and the remainder from monounsaturated fat sources. The Prudent Diet may be used for control of weight in obese individuals with hypertriglyceridemia, diabetes, or hypertension. Restricting sodium is important for normalizing blood pressure in hypertensives.

CONTROL OF HYPERLIPIDEMIA

Few disorders depend as much on dietary intervention as the hyperlipidemias.[1] In some cases, diet alone can normalize elevated plasma lipid levels (see Chapters 3 and 5 for normal levels). The five major families of lipoproteins are characterized in Chapter 3. The dietary treatment of hyperlipoproteinemia is discussed in Chapter 3.

There is wide consensus supporting the view that elevated plasma cholesterol and elevation of LDL are important risk factors for the development of coronary heart disease (CHD), with a strong inverse correlation between HDL and risk of CHD (see also Chapter 5). There is less strong evidence supporting elevated triglyceride as a risk factor for coronary disease. Hypertriglyceridemia is a risk factor in diabetics and in patients with chronic renal disease. Elevated triglycerides may be the result of a treatable medical cause, such as alcohol, estrogen therapy, or uncontrolled diabetes. If there is no medical cause for the elevated triglyceride levels but the individual has a family history of premature CHD, dietary treatment should be initiated. Weight reduction and moderate alcohol intake control triglycerides in most patients. Carbohydrate restriction extends only to simple sugars, primarily sucrose. Exercise also helps lower triglycerides. As weight reduction occurs, triglycerides are usually lowered, and a reduction in cholesterol may also occur as well. Reducing triglycerides often results in a concomitant rise in HDL. Thiazide drugs and oral contraceptives also increase triglyceride levels (see Chapters 3 and 6).

Dietary factors affecting plasma concentrations of lipids and lipoproteins include total calories, intake of sterol, particularly cholesterol, content of triglyceride, ratio of polyunsaturated fat to saturated fat (P/S ratio), consumption of sugar and alcohol, and the proportion of total calories derived from fat, carbohydrate, and protein. Excessive or unbalanced intake of one or more of these components could perturb lipoprotein metabolism and lead to changes in concentrations of the plasma lipids and lipoproteins.

HDL can be raised by running, by other high levels of aerobic activity, by estrogen, and by alcohol (see Chapter 3, Table 3-6). VLDL can be decreased by weight loss, reduction or elimination of alcohol, decreased intake of concentrated carbohydrates, limiting the proportion of calories from fat to 30 percent or less, and limiting dietary cholesterol to 300 mg or less. Dietary saturated fat tends to raise the cholesterol and LDL concentrations, whereas polyunsaturated fat tends to lower them.

CONTROL OF CHOLESTEROL

The Prudent Diet is recommended for persons who wish to maintain normal values of lipids, blood pressure, and body weight. It can be adapted for the treatment of mild hyperlipidemia, and may be used initially for persons with severe elevations of plasma cholesterol or triglyceride (Step 1). If this diet does not normalize the lipids, the fat and cholesterol content can be reduced to 25 percent fat and 250 mg cholesterol (Step 2), or to 20 percent and 100 mg, respectively (Step 3). This stepwise progressive approach to treating patients means more gradual diet changes (see Chapter 5, Table 5-3). Abrupt changes in dietary habits are very difficult and often undesirable. Patients with elevated triglycerides and/or chylomicrons are advised to follow the Prudent Diet for Control of Weight. The number of servings from each food group (Table 10-1) can be used as a guideline for the Prudent Diet for Control of Cholesterol. Food groups without fat do not need to be limited except to control body weight.

The Prudent Diet is well-balanced and contains foods from the meat, poultry and seafood group; eggs; the dairy products group; the fat group; the bread, cereal, and grains group; and the fruits and vegetable group (Appendix). Dietary fat plays an especially important role in all food groups because of its effect on plasma lipids. The plasma cholesterol concentration rises in proportion to calories derived from saturated fat. Monounsaturated fat has no effect on plasma cholesterol (see Chapters 3 and 5). Fat is present in all the food groups, either naturally or as an addition (for example, vegetables prepared with margarine). Thus, the emphasis in initial nutrition counseling sessions is on recognizing fat sources and then replacing them with lower-fat foods.

Meat, Poultry, and Seafood Group (Appendix A, B)

Meat, poultry, and seafood contain protein needed for growth and maintenance and repair of cells and tissues. Protein is also necessary for the formation of hormones, antibodies, and enzymes. The amount of protein required to maintain normal body processes varies with age and sex. The average adult needs 0.8 g of protein per kg of body weight daily. For a man weighing 80 kg (176 lbs), 64 g of protein are needed daily; a 60 kg (132 lb) woman requires 48 g of protein. Pregnant and lactating women require an additional 30 g and 20 g of protein, respectively. One ounce of lean meat, poultry, or seafood provides an average of 8 g of protein. The meat group is not the only good source of protein: dairy products also contain about 8 g of protein per serving, and bread, cereal, and grain products contain 2 g per serving.

Care should be exercised in selecting meat, poultry, and fish, which account for about 41 percent of fat in the average diet.[2] Some meat has a very high fat content and is often prepared with additional fat. Protein foods of animal origin (meat, eggs, and dairy products) provide saturated fat and cholesterol, while most of the plant-origin protein foods have none (see Chapter 5, Tables 5-2, 5-4, 5-5). Since saturated fat and cholesterol tend to increase serum cholesterol, the Prudent

Table 10-1.   Number of Exchanges (Servings) from Each Food Group for Specific Calorie Levels

Food Group	1,200 kcal	1,500 kcal	2,000 kcal	2,500 kcal
Meat, poultry, seafood[a]	6 oz	6 oz	6 oz	6 oz
Egg Yolks[a]	2 per week	2 per week	2 per week	2 per week
Dairy products[a]	2	2	2	2
Bread, cereal and grain	3	6	12	15
Fat[a]	5	7	10	14
Fruit	3	3	3	4
Vegetables	ad lib	ad lib	ad lib	ad lib
Extras (alcoholic beverages, sweets)	1	1	1	1
Percent calories protein	24	21	19	17
Percent calories fat	30	30	28	30
Percent calories carbohydrate	40	45	51	53
P/S ratio	1.1	1.3	1.5	1.7

[a]Foods containing fat and cholesterol, which need to be limited on the Prudent Diet for Control of Cholesterol

Diet recommends no more than 6 oz of meat, poultry, or seafood daily. "Lean" meat contains no more than 10 percent fat after cooking.

Seafood.   Seafood, including shellfish, and finfish, is an excellent source of protein in the Prudent Diet. The fat content of shellfish is between 1 and 3 percent. For finfish, the fat is between 1 and 20 percent, depending on the species. There is also some variation seasonally for some species. The most common fatty acid in seafood is palmitic acid (C16:0). Oleic acid (C18:1) is the most commonly occurring monounsaturated fatty acid. Seafood contains several polyunsaturated fatty acids not found in significant amounts in other foods; docosahexaenoic acid (C22:6) and eicosapentaenoic acid (C20:5) are the most common, composing up to 45 percent in some species, such as scallops and Atlantic cod.[3,4] (see Chapter 4).

Poultry.   Poultry is also low in saturated fat. Removing the skin on chicken before cooking reduces its fat even more, since fat stored beneath the skin penetrates the lean tissue when cooked. When eating fried chicken, removing the skin and batter reduces its fat and calorie content. For turkey, the skin need not be removed prior to cooking, since the fat does not seem to penetrate the lean meat of this fowl.

Veal and Calf.   Veal and calf, young forms of beef, contain less fat than older animals. Veal refers to milk-fed beef slaughtered between the ages of 3 weeks and 3 months. Calf refers to an animal between 14 and 52 weeks old. Lean veal has about 2 percent fat. Cuts of veal which have not had the fat removed are lower in fat than comparable trimmed cuts of beef.[5]

Beef.   The fat content of beef ranges from 8 to 45 percent after the fat has been trimmed. The degree of marbling in some cuts of meat is very high. Usually the fat content is higher in older animals. Fatty acids in beef are primarily saturated and monounsaturated. The fatty acid composition for separable lean and separable fat of beef are similar. Beef is classified according to fat content, that is, prime, choice, good, standard, and utility. Beef with no more than 10 percent fat is allowed on the Prudent Diet. "Regular" hamburger meat may have a lot of fat added to it and may contain up to 30 percent fat. Many types of sausage and luncheon meat contain approximately 30 percent fat (Table 10-2); however, their fat content goes up to 46 percent in some varieties, such as pepperoni.[6] Cooking lowers the fat content of beef. Methods that allow the fat to drip away from the meat during cooking are preferable. The best example is broiling on a rack. There is no significant difference in fatty acid composition whether dry or moist heat methods are used.[7]

Pork. Pork contains about 25 mg of cholesterol per ounce and has more monounsaturated than saturated or polyunsaturated fatty acids. A common misconception is that pork is higher in cholesterol than beef (which has 27 mg/ounce). Pork cuts, however, are often higher in fat than comparable cuts of beef (Chapter 5, Table 5-2).

Lamb. Lamb cuts that are very lean are included on the Prudent Diet. Oleic acid (C18:1), a monounsaturated fatty acid, is the major fatty acid; palmitic acid (C16:0) is the major saturated fatty acid.[5]

Game. Game such as deer, rabbit, dove, quail, squirrel, duck, and goose can be low fat selections for the Prudent Diet, if care is taken to remove the fat. Wild varieties of duck and goose have lower fat content than domesticated varieties and are preferable.[8]

Organ Meats. Organ meats include brains, heart, liver, and kidney. Beef and pork organ meats differ in fatty acid composition from skeletal muscle and adipose tissue, with a higher percentage of polyunsaturated fatty acids and more cholesterol. The cholesterol content of beef, pork, lamb, and chicken liver varies. In 1 oz cooked portions, beef liver has 86 mg cholesterol; chicken liver, 177 mg; lamb liver, 86 mg; pork liver, 86 mg; and turkey liver, 175 mg.

Meat Portions. All meat, poultry, and seafood portion sizes should be determined after cooking (with any remaining fat and bone removed). Meat loses moisture and some fat during the cooking process. Lean meats lose about 25 percent of their weight between the raw and cooked state. Fatty meats, such as ground beef and pork, may lose up to 50 percent of their raw weight. Guidelines for estimating 3 oz meat portions appear in the Appendix B. The most accurate method, of course, is to weigh the meat.

Meat Extenders and Replacers. Meat extenders and replacers, such as the grain products, provide a good source of protein with less fat and cholesterol than

Table 10-2.   Fat Content of Sausages and Luncheon Meats[a]

Sausages	Sources of Fat	Fat (g) in 100 g
Bockwurst	pork, veal, eggs, milk	30.0
Chorizos	pork, beef	38.3
Italian brand sausage	pork, beef	28.8
Luncheon meat	pork, beef	32.1
Pepperoni	pork, beef	45.5
Salami, dry (hard)	pork, beef	33.3
Summer sausage, semi-dry (soft)	pork, beef	29.2

[a]Modified from Anderson BA: Comprehensive evaluation of fatty acids in foods: XIII. Sausages and luncheon meats. J Am Diet Assoc 72:48, 1978. Copyright the American Dietetic Association.

in meat, eggs, and dairy products (Table 10-3, also Chapter 5, Table 5-2). Grain products can be used alone or mixed with meat as a means of extending without decreasing protein content. Soybeans are the most complete protein of all plant products. Since soybeans are very bland, they combine well with other foods, usually taking on their flavor. They can absorb and hold more than their weight in moisture. Textured vegetable protein (TVP) can be added to meat to extend it; however, if fatty ground beef is used, the fat will be absorbed and will not cook out. As the sole source of protein, soy protein produces a lowering of serum cholesterol and in animal studies retards the development of atherosclerosis (see Chapters 2, 3, and 5). Casein and meat proteins raise serum cholesterol and accelerate atherosclerosis. The cholesterol-lowering mechanism, discrepancies between effects of "textured" protein and "isolated" soy protein, and the importance of the ratio of the amino acids lysine to arginine, are discussed in Chapter 2.

Eggs (Appendix C)

Egg yolk is a concentrated source of cholesterol and is also high in phospholipids, especially lecithin. All of the fat and cholesterol in egg is in the yolk, with larger eggs having more fat per egg. Duck, goose, quail, and turkey eggs are similar in lipid content to chicken eggs.[9] Egg whites, which are without cholesterol and are low in calories, are allowed ad lib on the Prudent Diet. The protein content of the white and yolk is similar, 3.4 and 2.8 g respectively. One egg yolk contains 274 mg of cholesterol. The Prudent Diet recommends no more than three egg yolks per week. Unless eggs are added to a diet in which there is no cholesterol, very little change occurs in the plasma cholesterol. Egg consumption may raise a subfraction of HDL cholesterol and perhaps also LDL.

Fat Group (Appendix D)

The Prudent Diet recommends that no more than 30 percent of calories come from fat. The Nationwide Food Consumption Survey showed that Americans con-

Table 10-3.   Comparison of Calories, Protein, Fat and Cholesterol for Selected Meats and Beans[a]

Food	Amount	Calories (kcal)	Protein (g)	Fat (g)	Cholesterol (mg)
Beef, lean round steak	2 oz	107	18	3	52
Pork, lean picnic ham	2 oz	120	16	6	50
Chicken, light meat without skin	2 oz	94	18	2	44
Cod, canned, drained	2 oz	48	11	trace	28
[b]Great Northern beans	1 cup	212	14	1	0
[b]Kidney beans	1 cup	218	14	1	0
[b]Lentils	1 cup	212	16	trace	0
[b]Soybeans, cooked	1 cup	234	20	10	0

[a]Modified from Adams CF: Nutritive Value of American Foods in Common Units. Handbook 456. Washington, Agricultural Research Service, US Dept of Agriculture, 1975.

[b]Beans are higher in calories than *lean* beef, pork, or chicken for comparable protein, because of their carbohydrate content.

Table 10-4.   Comparison of Calories and Percent Calories from Fat for Selected Foods[a]

	Amount	Weight (g)	Calories (kcal)	Percent Calories From Fat
Bologna	1 slice	28	86	82
Chocolate cake with chocolate icing	1/12 of cake	99	365	40
Chocolate chip cookies	4 cookies	40	206	52
Frankfurters	1 frankfurter	45	139	80
Doughnut, yeast	1 whole	42	176	58
Fried chicken	1/2 breast	94	160	29
French fried potatoes	10 strips	78	214	43
Ice cream, 16% fat	1 cup	148	329	65
Milk chocolate candy	1 bar	56	294	56
Pecan Pie	1/8 of pie	103	431	49
Potato chips	10 chips	20	114	63
Pound cake	1 slice	30	142	56

[a]Modified from Adams CF: Nutritive Value of American Foods in Common Units. Handbook 456. Washington, Agricultural Research Service, US Dept of Agriculture, 1975.

sume about 43 percent of their calories as fat: about 15 percent saturated, and 6 percent polyunsaturated, with a P/S ratio of 0.4[10] (Chapter 5, Table 5-1). The Prudent Diet recommends that less than 10 percent of calories come from saturated fat, up to 10 percent from polyunsaturated, and the remainder from monounsaturated. The degree of unsaturation affects the chemical properties and reactivity of a fatty acid. At room temperature, all of the common unsaturated fatty acids are liquid. Because of the double bonds, these fatty acids exist as cis-trans isomers. Most naturally occurring unsaturated fatty acids occur in the cis form, with trans isomers found in small quantities. Relatively large quantities of fatty acids are converted from the cis to the trans form as a result of heating or hydrogenation, as in the preparation of some shortenings and margarines (see also Chapter 2). Fat is the most concentrated source of calories, with twice as many calories per unit as carbohydrate or protein, 9, 4, and 4 cal/g respectively. Alcohol has 7 cal/g. Polyunsaturated, monounsaturated, and saturated fats have comparable caloric values.

Much of the fat in food is "hidden" and not readily recognized as such. All fried foods are high in fat, as are most processed, prepared, and baked goods in which fat comprises most of the calories (Table 10-4). Some general guidelines for determining the amount of fat in prepared foods are shown in Table 10-5.

Saturated Fats.   Saturated fats, usually solid at room temperature, occur naturally in all foods of animal origin and in a few vegetable products. Meat, butter, cream, and whole milk are foods with a high percentage of saturated fat, although large amounts of oleic acid, a monounsaturated fat, are also present. Dairy products, such as cheese, also contain saturated fat. Vegetable fat sources of saturated fat include coconut, palm, and palm kernel oil, which are frequently used in commercial products because of their long shelf life. Common retail market food items containing these products are nondairy creamers, nondairy whipped toppings, crackers, and bakery products. Cocoa butter, the fat in chocolate, is another saturated fat of vegetable origin. All varieties of chocolate—semisweet baking chocolate, German chocolate, chocolate chips, and most chocolate candy—are

Table 10-5.   Fat Content of Prepared Foods

Pan fried meat	½ teaspoon fat per ounce of meat
Breaded and fried meat	1 teaspoon fat per ounce of meat
Vegetables seasoned with fat	½ teaspoon fat per ½ cup vegetables
Breaded and fried vegetables	1 teaspoon fat per ½ cup vegetables
Stir fried vegetables	½ teaspoon fat per ½ cup vegetables
Fried eggs	1 teaspoon fat per egg
Potato salad	1 tablespoon fat per ½ cup salad
Gravy and sauce	1 teaspoon fat per 2 tablespoons gravy or sauce

high in saturated fat. Cocoa powder is a form of chocolate that is not saturated, since most of the fat is removed.

Polyunsaturated Fats.   Polyunsaturated fats, liquid at room temperature, are predominately vegetable in origin, including safflower, corn, sunflower, soybean, and cottonseed oils. The fat of fish is also polyunsaturated. Although studies suggested that the long-term consumption of polyunsaturated fat may present a potential risk for the development of cancer, this risk has not been substantiated. A high P/S ratio is recommended only for the dietary management of severe hypercholesterolemia and not for general use. Polyunsaturated oil or margarine is recommended for fat in food preparation. Table 10-6 shows the P/S ratio of some commonly used fat sources.

Monounsaturated fats.   Monounsaturated fats have a neutral effect on plasma cholesterol. Olives, olive oil, peanuts, peanut oil, peanut butter, and avocados contain monounsaturated fats.

Dairy Products Group (Appendix E, F)

Dairy products are a rich source of calcium. They also contribute a large amount of saturated fat to the diet unless skim or lowfat products are used. The daily calcium requirement for various ages (800 to 1,600 mg) can be met with lowfat dairy products, such as 2 to 4 cups of milk. Most cheeses provide a concentrated source of saturated fat. Cheese is made by decreasing the moisture content of milk or cream and allowing it to age, often in the presence of some type of bacteria to provide a characteristic flavor and texture. The percent of fat in natural cheese ranges from less than 1 percent (dry curd cottage cheese) to 34 percent (cream cheese and Roquefort). Some cheeses have been developed using skim milk and vegetable oil to replace the butterfat. These can be used on the Prudent Diet, although their fat content is greater than 12 percent.

Nondairy products or non-milk, fat-containing products that resemble or are used as dairy products can be high in saturated fat. Some are made with polyunsaturated oil; however, most products contain lauric oils, hydrogenated coconut oil, or palm kernel oil. The fat content of these products ranges from about 3 percent (for fluid filled milk) to 45 percent (for powdered nondairy toppings).[11]

Bread, Cereal, and Grain Products Group (Appendix G)

The bread, cereal, and grain products provide protein, vitamins, minerals, fiber, and energy. The protein provided by this group of products does not have the fat content of meats, eggs, and dairy products. Grain products contain no cholesterol.

Fiber, the fibrous material in the diet that is resistant to digestion, provides bulk, holds water and exchange ions, and binds small organic molecules. Fiber may play a role in reducing the risk of cardiovascular disease (see Chapter 6). *Bread products,* often thought to be high in calories, are excessive in calories because of the spread, such as margarine, butter, and gravy, that contributes more calories than the bread itself.

Alcoholic beverages are categorized with the bread, cereal, and grain group as a means of accounting for the calories. The Prudent Diet recommends no more than two servings of alcohol per day because of its tendency to increase weight and triglyceride levels. Alcohol consumption raises the level of HDL, but toxic effects of alcohol on the liver may be observed. Alcohol is not recommended as a means of raising HDL or preventing heart attacks because of the dangers associated with excessive alcohol consumption, including cirrhosis of the liver, hypertension, cardiomyopathy, psychosis, pancreatitis, and alcoholism itself (see Chapter 8).

Table 10-6.   Ratio of Polyunsaturated Fat to Saturated Fat[a]

Fat	P/S Ratio[b]
Animal Fats	
beef tallow	0.08
butter	0.06
chicken fat	0.70
lard (pork fat)	0.29
Margarine[c]	
corn oil (soft, tub)	2.21
corn oil (stick)	1.36
soybean and cottonseed (soft, tub)	1.76
soybean and cottonseed (stick)	0.97
Nuts	
almond	2.33
Brazil nut	1.47
cashew	0.81
coconut	0.02
Macadamia	0.21
peanut	1.58
pecan	2.94
pistachio	0.95
walnut, black	8.02
walnut, English	5.99
Shortening[c]	
soybean and cottonseed	1.04
lard and vegetable oil	0.27
Vegetable oils (nonhydrogenated)	
coconut oil	0.02
corn oil	4.62
cottonseed oil	2.00
olive oil	0.62
palm kernel oil	0.02
peanut oil	1.89
safflower oil	8.19
soybean oil	4.02
sunflower seed oil	6.37

[a]Data from Reeves JB: Composition of foods. Fats and oils. Raw, processed, prepared. Handbook 8-4. Washington, Science and Education Administration, US Department of Agriculture, 1979; and Fristrom GA: Comprehensive evaluation of fatty acids in foods. J Am Diet Assoc 66:482, 1975; 67:243, 351, 1975; 70:53, 111, 1977.
[b]Ratio of polyunsaturated fat to saturated fat
[c]May vary with hydrogenation in processing

Fruits Group (Appendix H)

Fruits are a source of simple carbohydrate and provide an excellent source of vitamins and minerals, especially vitamin C. Fruits and the amount considered as one serving are listed in the Appendix. Fruits rich in vitamins A and C are designated with an (A) or (C) beside them.

Vegetables (Appendix I)

Vegetables are divided into starchy or nonstarchy groups, depending on their carbohydrate content. Both are sources of complex carbohydrate and provide good sources of vitamins and minerals, especially vitamins A and C. The starchy vegetables are grouped with the bread, cereal, and grain products (Appendix G). The nonstarchy vegetables listed in Appendix I have been designated with an (A) or (C) if they are good sources of vitamins A or C.

Miscellaneous Foods (Appendix J)

Seasonings, herbs, spices, flavorings, and extracts can be used freely to complement the Prudent Diet. They can add creativity and interest to a variety of foods. A list of other foods that can also be used freely are listed in Appendix J.

Commercial Products

Many Americans are often interested in quick meals and do not want to spend time preparing foods "from scratch." Commercial products that have been partially or totally prepared can be great time savers. Nutrition labeling provides information that can be helpful in deciding if a specific food is low enough in total fat and calories to be included on the Prudent Diet. Unfortunately, at this time, information for cholesterol, saturated fat, and polyunsaturated fat is not required in nutrition labeling.

Eating Away From Home

Americans eat one of every three meals away from home. Most restaurants provide some food selections that are low in saturated fat and cholesterol; however, fast-food establishments and single-item specialty shops may only have fried or other high-fat foods available. General guidelines for selecting low-fat foods in a restaurant include:

1. Select seafood whenever possible, because it is naturally lower in fat; request that it be baked, broiled, or boiled without fat.
2. Eat bread, crackers and potatoes without butter or margarine, to help compensate for fat added to vegetables and other foods.
3. Trim fat off meat and remove skin from poultry.
4. Use lemon juice or vinegar on vegetable salads.

5. Remove the breading, batter, and skin from fried meat.
6. Push gravy and sauces aside.
7. Select a meatless entree, such as a fruit plate with cottage cheese or chef salad (without cheese).
8. Select hard rolls, bread sticks, English muffins, or French bread.
9. Use skim milk on cereal.
10. Request fresh fruit or sherbet, even though it may not appear on the menu.

When traveling by airplane, low-cholesterol or low-calorie meals can be requested at the time reservations are made.

Assessing Fat Intake in Food

For dietary management of hyperlipidemia and for control of plasma cholesterol for preventive reasons, it is important to assess food intake. The method should take into consideration both the cholesterol content and type of fat in each food. Anderson and coworkers[12] developed a means for identifying the cholesterol-raising or cholesterol-lowering effect of foods. Keys and coworkers[13,14] developed an equation for expressing the effect of dietary cholesterol and polyunsaturated fat on plasma lipids (see Chapters 3 and 5). The values for all the foods consumed during a day can be totaled according to food group and used to determine a food record rating. Nutrition counselors in the Multiple Risk Factor Intervention Trial 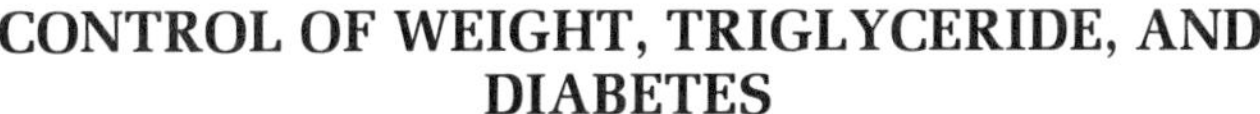 (MRFIT) described this technique and used it extensively.[15,16] They reported that the Food Record Rating (FRR) provides a mechanism for the acquisition and rapid analysis of food, which can systematically measure progressive diet changes. It is a valid and reliable means of monitoring dietary habits and has relevance in large-scale field trials and for individual nutrition counseling. The FRR is especially helpful for individuals who need to make dietary changes as a means of reducing their risk of heart disease.[17]

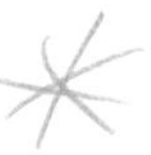

CONTROL OF WEIGHT, TRIGLYCERIDE, AND DIABETES

The Prudent Diet for control of cholesterol can be modified to control weight, triglyceride, and diabetes. The key factor in treatment is achieving and maintaining ideal body weight.

Obesity

Obesity, directly or indirectly, may affect cardiovascular risk. It tends to exacerbate hypertension, to elevate triglycerides, and to worsen glucose tolerance and diabetes. Increased calorie intake, decreased physical activity, or variations in energy metabolism may be causes of obesity (see Chapter 7). Excessive calories may be the result of a high-fat diet, which can lead to an increase in the serum cholesterol as well.

The goal in weight reduction is to achieve and maintain an ideal body weight. The most accurate way to determine ideal body weight is with the water submersion technique, which requires a large tank equipped to do water displacement. Without the use of body volume testing, an estimation of ideal body weight for women allows 100 lb for the first 5 ft of height, plus 5 lb for each additional inch of height. For men, 106 lb is allowed for the first 5 ft of height, plus 6 lb for each additional inch. Ten percent can be added or subtracted to the figure to adjust for small or large frame, respectively.

Obesity is inversely related to HDL cholesterol and directly related to VLDL cholesterol and triglyceride. Weight loss can decrease LDL cholesterol and raise HDL cholesterol. It is not clearly understood whether the drop in cholesterol results from the weight loss itself or from the change in sources of calories.

The first challenge in working with an obese patient is to determine caloric intake, which is often underestimated by the patient in terms of food consumption. It may be helpful to have the patient record food consumed for several days and total the calories prior to initiating treatment.

It is recommended that 1 to 2 lb per week be lost on a well-balanced diet. This can be achieved with the Prudent Diet for Control of Weight, Triglyceride, and Diabetes. A pound of body fat is equivalent to 3,500 kcal; in order to lose 2 pounds per week, daily calorie intake must be reduced by 1,000 kcal (1,000 kcal × 7 days = 7,000 kcal = 2 lb per week). Planning for adequate intake of the water-soluble vitamins and minerals is difficult with 1,200 kcal or less. This is especially true for iron and thiamine. It may be necessary to take a vitamin-mineral supplement if a restricted calorie diet is followed for a long period of time.

Diabetes Mellitus

Diabetes mellitus, characterized by an elevation of blood sugar, is one of the leading causes of death in the American population, and is a secondary risk factor for atherosclerosis. Diabetes, defined as a deficiency or inappropriate secretion of insulin by the pancreas in response to a particular amount of sugar, is classified into two major categories: Type I, which is insulin-dependent and often begins in childhood, and Type II, which is not insulin-dependent and usually affects adults. Type II diabetes comprises about 90 percent of all diabetes.

Diet, insulin (for Type I), and exercise are the cornerstones of treatment for diabetes. There is a high incidence of deaths among diabetics due to complications of the disease over a long period of time. Diabetics suffer from damage to the large and small arteries and capillaries. Diet plays a significant role in controlling blood sugar for insulin- and non-insulin-dependent diabetics. More than 80 percent of the Type II diabetics are overweight. The Prudent Diet for Control of Weight is recommended for use by diabetics because it controls carbohydrate and fat.

Controlling Calories

In order to limit calories, as a means of controlling body weight and/or triglycerides, the exchange system or calorie counting can be used. Either method provides a means for limiting calorie intake. Diabetics should use the exchange system, since it provides a means whereby carbohydrate and fat intake can be controlled. If the patient is counting calories, special emphasis needs to be placed on limiting saturated fat and cholesterol intake. The Food Record Rating System described may be beneficial (see p. 193).

A wide variety of nutritious and desirable foods are allowed, and they should be selected from all of the food groups (see Appendix). The exchange system serves as a guide and specifies the amount of food equivalent to one serving in each food group. The calories in each exchange are shown in Table 10-5. The number of servings from each food group to achieve various calorie levels is shown in Table 10-1.

CONTROL OF HYPERTENSION*

About one of every four persons between the ages of 18 and 79 years has hypertension, defined by the World Health Organization (WHO), and the American Heart Association as a blood pressure of 140/90 or greater. Hypertension, like elevated cholesterol and cigarette smoking, is an independent cardiovascular risk factor. The risk increases progressively as the systolic and diastolic pressures increase. Hypertension is a complex disorder affected by many factors, including sex, age, race, heredity, smoking, stress, obesity, and excessive dietary sodium intake. Treatment for mild to moderate hypertension begins with diet, which is important in all hypertensive patients, even those on medication. Control of sodium intake and maintenance of ideal body weight are the primary dietary goals for the control of hypertension.

Several studies[18,19] and reviews of the literature[20] provide good evidence that, throughout the world, populations with a higher sodium intake have a greater prevalence of hypertension. Parijs[21] investigated the relationship between blood pressure, sodium restricted diet, and 24-hour urinary sodium excretion, and developed the following equation:

$$y = -6.58 + 0.163x$$

(where y = reduction in systolic blood pressure [mm Hg], and
x = decrease in 24-hour urinary sodium excretion [mmol])

Parijs concluded that the average patient could expect a decrease in blood pressure of about 10/5 if daily salt consumption were reduced from 10 g (4 g sodium) to 5 g (2 g sodium). Stamler and coworkers[22] showed a positive relationship between the prevalence of hypertension and body weight. Stamler[23] and Dahl[24] demonstrated a significant correlation between weight reduction and decreases in blood pressure.

The first step in reducing sodium intake is to recognize sources of sodium in the diet. Almost half of the average sodium intake is from salt or sodium compounds added to foods during processing. The remaining sodium is approximately equally divided between salt added during home food preparation and from the natural sodium content of foods. All foods, whether of plant or animal origin, contain varying amounts of sodium. The average intake of sodium and potassium

---

* See also Chapter 9.

for infants, toddlers, and young adults living in the United States is presented in Table 10-7. The human subject needs only about 250 mg of sodium under normal conditions, or 400 mg when perspiring excessively. Since all food contains some sodium, an appropriate goal for sodium intake is 1,200 to 1,500 mg per 1,000 kcal energy intake per day.[25]

Sodium in Processed Foods

Sodium in processed foods accounts for a large portion of the total intake in the American diet. Salt has been a popular chemical preservative from the time of ancient man up to the present, since thousands of microbial species are unable to tolerate near-saturation levels of salt. Smaller amounts can be used to change flavor, texture, and overall characteristics of food. All fermented foods, whether vegetable, dairy, or meat, have salt added, generally amounting to 2 to 10 percent.[26] These foods include hundreds of varieties of cheese, milk drinks, sausages, and fermented vegetables such as sauerkraut, pickles, and olives. In canned foods, salt is used to effect stability and safety; however, in lower concentration it serves no function other than imparting a desirable flavor. Other sodium compounds used in canned foods include sodium salts of propionate, sorbate, bisulfite, and benzoate, used as preservatives; sodium ascorbate for curing or color preservation; monosodium glutamate as a flavor enhancer; sodium hydroxide as a lye peel; and sodium phosphate as a stabilizer or to improve texture.

Processed meats are another source of sodium in the diet. There are over 200 kinds of processed meats sold in the United States. Most types contain between 1.1 and 1.3 percent sodium. Salt is common not only to all processed meats, but also to all cured meats. Other types of protein added to processed meats increase their sodium content. Examples are milk-derived proteins, such as whey (1,250 mg sodium per 100 g) and calcium casinate whey blends (820 mg sodium per 100 g). Soy-derived products are increasingly popular because of their high protein content; textured soy flour has 50 percent protein. Textured soy flour has 10 to 30 mg sodium per 100 g; isolated soy protein (90 percent protein) can have up to 1,500 mg sodium per 100 g.[27]

Table 10-7.   Average Sodium and Potassium Contents* in Market Baskets

	Infant	Toddler	Adult
Sodium			
1977	885	1593	6697
1978	797	1685	6928
Potassium			
1977	1551	1714	4549
1978	1590	1846	4735

*Milligrams/Day

Reprinted with permission of the American Medical Association, "Sodium and Potassium in Foods and Drugs," 1982, copyright© American Medical Association.

Table 10-8. Conversions for Sodium and Salt

Conversions to mg of Sodium
  1 g salt = 400 mg of sodium (plus 600 mg chloride)
  1 g sodium = 1,000 mg sodium
  1mEq sodium = 23 mg sodium
  ¼ teaspoon salt = 533 mg sodium
Sodium to Salt
  .5 g sodium = 1.25 g salt
  2 g sodium = 5 g salt
  3 g sodium = 7.5 g salt
  5 g sodium = 12.5 g salt

Bakery products are a source of sodium in the American diet. Salt, some leavening acids, and sodium bicarbonate (baking soda) are the major sodium-containing ingredients present in most commercial bakery products.

Sodium-Potassium Ratio

Memelly and Battarbee[28] suggest that high sodium-low potassium diets perpetuate essential hypertension (see also Chapter 9). Studies have not yet examined the potassium intake of populations with regard to salt intake and hypertension, and the role of potassium in the etiology, prevention, and treatment of essential hypertension is undefined. Potassium is lost when diuretics are taken for the control of hypertension, unless a potassium-sparing diuretic is prescribed. It may be necessary to incorporate higher potassium foods into the diet or to take a potassium supplement when taking non-potassium-sparing diuretics. Hansen and Wyse[29] suggest that, for therapeutic reasons, sodium and potassium should be consumed in approximately equal molecular amounts. Shaw and Philips[30] suggest a sodium-potassium ratio of 0.5/0.25 as desirable, or 2,400 mg potassium per 1,000 kcal. The FDA Market Basket Survey[31] indicates intake of potassium is about one-half this amount (Table 10-7).

Limiting Sodium Intake

A specific level of sodium can be achieved by using either a point system[32] or by calculating milligrams of sodium. Generally, a "strict" sodium restricted diet has 200 to 500 mg sodium; "moderate" restriction, 800 to 1,200 mg; mild restriction, 2,000 to 3,000 mg, and a "no added salt" diet, 3,500 mg sodium.[33] Either system allows patients on low-sodium diets to know exactly what their intake is. Thus, it is possible to "personalize" the diet by occasionally eating a high-sodium food and then carefully selecting other low-sodium foods for that day.

Equations for converting sodium and salt values are shown in Table 10-8.

Low-Sodium Seasonings

Most spices, herbs, and extracts are low in sodium if "salt" is not specified as part of their name or as an ingredient. Garlic and celery salts and monosodium glutamate, for example, are high in sodium. Natural blends of herbs, spices, and dried vegetables that are available commercially are low in sodium. They can be used to add zest and flavor to low-sodium foods.

Salt Substitutes

Salt substitutes, low-sodium meat tenderizers, and seasoned salt substitutes usually contain potassium chloride, which may not be recommended for certain people.

Drugs

Some drugs have a relatively high sodium content. Generally, prescription drugs are not a hazard for patients on moderate sodium-restricted diets, even when used for long-term, chronic illness. However, certain nonprescription drugs can be potentially hazardous to persons following sodium-restricted diets. Certain antacids, analgesics, and laxatives have high sodium contents, ranging from 49 to 1,000 mg sodium per dose.[33]

Eating Out on the Sodium-controlled Diet

Foods prepared in restaurants may contain large amounts of sodium without tasting salty. Oriental and Mexican cuisines are usually high in sodium. The best choice of an entree in a restaurant is broiled or boiled meat, poultry, or seafood, prepared without salt or sauce. An inside cut of roast beef or poultry without skin or gravy can be a good selection. A plain vegetable, such as a baked potato or a tossed salad with oil and vinegar dressing, is also a good selection. Fruit and fruit juices add very little sodium. With advance notice, some restaurants and most airlines can provide low-sodium meals.

PREGNANCY AND LACTATION

It is recommended that a woman gain 22 to 27 lb during pregnancy regardless of her body weight before gestation. A thin woman may gain approximately 30 lb and retain some weight after the baby arrives. The overweight woman should keep her weight gain to 22 to 27 lbs. Pregnancy is not the time to undertake a strict weight reduction program. Insufficient weight gain may adversely affect fetal development.

The extra calories and nutrients required during pregnancy build new tissues and replenish nutrients used for growth of the baby. An increase of 300 kcal per day is usually recommended. Protein requirements increase by about 60 percent. Iron needs during pregnancy usually require an iron supplement. Iron is needed for the formation of hemoglobin and also for the fetus. A 3- to 4-month supply of iron is stored in the baby's liver, since the first food (milk) lacks iron. Folic acid, which regulates the formation of red blood cells in the bone marrow, should increase by 50 percent during pregnancy. Ascorbic acid facilitates the absorption of iron, and is required for production of collagen and for metabolism of folic acid. Sodium and potassium do not need to be increased or decreased during pregnancy and lactation.

Lipids During Pregnancy

During pregnancy, total cholesterol, LDL, VLDL, and triglycerides increase. Following delivery, the lipids return to prepregnancy levels by about 8 weeks postpartum. Hyperlipidemic women have even a greater increase in lipids during pregnancy than women with normal lipids. Cholesterol levels increase primarily during the third trimester; triglycerides steadily increase during all three trimesters.

Glueck and coworkers[34] observed the cholesterol level of a 28-year-old woman before, during, and after her pregnancy. She was following a diet containing 300 mg of cholesterol prior to the time she became pregnant; her plasma cholesterol and LDL cholesterol (C-LDL) were 352 and 286 mg/dl, respectively. At 8 weeks gestation, plasma cholesterol was 310 mg/dl, and C-LDL was 240 mg/dl. She was admitted to the hospital, and a cholesterol-free diet was given during the next 6 weeks. Her total serum cholesterol decreased by 25 percent, and C-LDL decreased by 33 percent. She returned to a 300 mg/day diet when she was discharged. During the remainder of her pregnancy, her serum cholesterol steadily increased to 420 mg/dl total cholesterol and 320 mg/dl of C-LDL. Two months postpartum, her lipids had decreased to prepregnancy levels. The results of this case study suggest that in hyperlipidemic women cholesterol-restricted diets could minimize the increase in serum lipids that occurs during pregnancy.

The Prudent Diet provides high quality food that is lower in total fat and calories than the average American diet. It is adequate for the pregnant woman except for milk, which needs to be increased to four cups of skim or low-fat milk daily. Diets lower in fat than 30 percent may need to be implemented if hyperlipidemia is severe. There are no known harmful effects of a low fat diet on the development of the fetus.

Lactating women need about 500 extra kcal per day. Lactation is not the time for a low-calorie diet. Requirements for all the nutrients are high, as during pregnancy. Fluid intake is essential to support the production of a quart of milk per day. The increased caloric requirements during lactation make it possible to lose extra pounds slowly and safely.

Lipids During Lactation

Lactation accentuates any preexisting hyperlipidemia, but to a lesser extent than does pregnancy. Severe fat restriction may make it difficult for a lactating woman to meet her energy requirements and may have a deleterious effect. Mellies and coworkers[35,36] investigated the effects of various types of vegetable fat on lipids of the mother and her breast-fed infant. In their study, fat made up 35 to 40 percent of the calories. On diets with a ratio of polyunsaturated fat to saturated fat (P/S) of 1.8, the proportion of linoleic acid in breast milk was doubled, and the stearic, palmitic, and myristic fatty acids were reduced. The infant's plasma linoleate increased on the high P/S diet. The long-term effect of rich polyunsaturated

Table 10-9.   Calorie Recommendation for Children and Adolescents[a]

Age (years)	Sex	Calories (kcal)
1 to 3	male and female	1,300
4 to 6	male and female	1,700
7 to 10	male and female	2,400
11 to 14	male	2,700
11 to 14	female	2,200
15 to 18	male	2,800
15 to 18	female	2,100

[a]Modified from Recommended Dietary Allowances, 9th ed. Washington, The National Research Council, National Academy of Sciences, 1980.

breast milk in growth and development is not known. The cholesterol content of breast milk is 2.4 mg/100 g and remains constant whether the mother eats a high or low-cholesterol diet.

CHILDREN AND ADOLESCENTS

Children develop eating habits early in life that affect their health as adults. These habits, if bad, can lead to the presence of cardiovascular risk factors in adult life, influencing elevated serum total cholesterol and LDL, hypertension, and obesity. Children whose parents have a history of hyperlipidemia or early cardiovascular disease have an increased risk of developing hyperlipidemia. Blackburn[37] suggests that mean serum cholesterol levels of 150 to 180 mg/dl in adults are consistently related to the lowest rates of coronary artery disease. To achieve these "lower" adult levels it may be necessary for children to have levels of serum cholesterol of 120 to 160 mg/dl.

The Eleventh Bethesda Conference on Prevention of Coronary Heart Disease[38] suggests that a preventive program for reducing risk factors would include identification and management of children with hypercholesterolemia, hypertension, and/or obesity. Diet plays a significant role in their treatment. The portion sizes of food to provide adequate calories varies with age and sex (Table 10-9). When children follow a restrictive diet, their nutrient intake should be carefully monitored by a dietitian. Iron may be low, especially if meat intake is limited, unless a supplement is prescribed.

In the Prudent Diet, it is recommended that healthy children beyond infancy consume no more than 300 mg of cholesterol, no more than 35 percent of calories as fat, less than 10 percent of fat calories as saturated fat, no more than 10 percent of fat calories as polyunsaturated fat, and the remainder of fat calories as monounsaturated fat.[38]

REFERENCES

1. Fredrickson DS, Goldstein JL, Brown MS: The familial hyperlipoproteinemias. In Stanbury JB, Wyngaarden JB, Fredrickson DS (eds): The Metabolic Basis of Inherited Disease. New York, McGraw-Hill, 1978.

2. U.S. Department of Agriculture: Food and nutrient intakes of individuals in 1 day in the United States, Spring 1977. Washington, U.S. Department of Agriculture, 1980.

3. Exler J, Weihrauch JL: Comprehensive evaluation of fatty acids in foods: XII. Shellfish. J Am Diet Assoc 71:518, 1977.

4. Exler J, Weihrauch, JL: Comprehensive evaluation of fatty acids in foods: VIII. Finfish. J Am Diet Assoc 69:243, 1976.

5. Anderson BA, Fristrom GA, Weihrauch JL: Comprehensive evaluation of fatty acids in foods: X. Lamb and veal. J Am Diet Assoc 70:53, 1977.

6. Anderson BA: Comprehensive evaluation of fatty acids in foods: XIII. Sausages and luncheon meats. J Am Diet Assoc 72:48, 1978.

7. Anderson, BA, Kinsella JA, Watt BK: Comprehensive evaluation of fatty acids in foods: II. Beef products. J Am Diet Assoc 67:35, 1975.

8. Fristrom GA, Weihrauch JL: Comprehensive evaluation of fatty acids in foods: IX. Fowl. J Am Diet Assoc 69:517, 1976.

9. Posati LP, Kinsella JE, Watt BK: Comprehensive evaluation of fatty acids in foods: III. Eggs and egg products. J Am Diet Assoc 67:111, 1975.

10. Rizek RL: Food supply studies and consumption survey statistics on fat in United States diets. Cancer Res 41:3729, 1981.

11. Posati LP, Kinsella JE, Watt BK: Comprehensive evaluation of fatty acids in foods: I. Dairy products. J Am Diet Assoc 66:482,1975.

12. Anderson JT, Jacobs DR, Foster N, Hall Y, Moss D, Mojonnier L, Blackburn H: Scoring systems for evaluating dietary pattern effect on serum cholesterol. Prev Med 8:525, 1979.

13. Keys A, Anderson JT, Grande F: Serum cholesterol response to changes in the diet. 1. Iodine value of dietary fat vs. 25-P. Metabolism 14:747, 1965.

14. Keys A, Anderson JT, Grande F: Serum cholesterol response to changes in the diet. 2. The effect of cholesterol in the diet. Metabolism 14:759, 1965.

15. Remmell PS, Gorder DD, Hall Y, Tillotson JL: Assessing dietary adherence in the Multiple Risk Factor Intervention Trial (MRFIT): I. Use of a dietary monitoring tool. J Am Diet Assoc 76:351, 1980.

16. The Multiple Risk Factor Intervention Trial (MRFIT): A national study of primary prevention of coronary heart disease. JAMA 235:825, 1976.

17. Remmel PS, Benfari RC: Assessing dietary adherence in the Multiple Risk Factor Intervention Trial (MRFIT): II. Food record rating as an indicator of compliance. J Am Diet Assoc 76:357, 1980.

18. Dahl LK, Love RA: Evidence for relationship between sodium (chloride) intake and human essential hypertension. Arch Intern Med 94:525, 1954.

19. Shaper AG, Leonard PJ, Jones KW, Jones M: Environmental effects on the body build, blood pressure and blood chemistry of nomadic warriors serving in the army in Kenya. East Afr Med J 46:282, 1969.

20. Page LB: Hypertension and atherosclerosis in primitive and acculturating societies. In: Hypertension Update, Vol 1. Cardiovascular Risk Factors and Consequences of Hypertension. Bloomington, NJ, Health Learning Systems Inc., 1979.

21. Parijs J, Joossens, JV, Linden LV, Verstreken G, Amery AKPC: Moderate sodium restriction and diuretics in the treatment of hypertension. Am Heart J 85:22, 1973.

22. Stamler R, Stamler J, Riedlinger WF: Weight and blood pressure: Findings in hypertension screenings of 1 million Americans. JAMA 240:1607, 1978.

23. Stamler J, Farinaro E, Mojonnier LM, Hall Y, Moss D, Stamler R: Prevention and control of hypertension by nutritional-hygienic means: Long-term experience of the Chicago Coronary Prevention Evaluation Program. JAMA 243:1819, 1980.

24. Dahl LK: Salt and hypertension. Am J Clin Nutr 25:231, 1972.

25. Filer LJ: Appropriate consumption of sodium and potassium. In White PL, Crocco SC (eds): Sodium and potassium in foods and drugs. Chicago, AMA, 1980.

26. Niven CF: Technology of sodium in processed foods: General bacteriological principles, with emphasis on canned fruits and vegetables, and dairy products. In White PL, Crocco SC (eds): Sodium and Potassium in Foods and Drugs. Chicago, AMA, 1981.

27. Marsden JL: Sodium containing additives in processed meats: A technological overview. In White PL, Crocco SC (eds): Sodium and Potassium in Foods and Drugs. Chicago, AMA, 1981.

28. Meneely GR, Battarbee HD: High sodium-low potassium environment and hypertension. Am J Cardiol 38:768, 1981.

29. Hansen RG, Wyse BW: Potassium and sodium compositions of food interpreted by nutrient density analysis. In White PW, Crocco Sc (eds): Sodium and Potassium in Foods and Drugs. Chicago, AMA, 1981.

30. Shaw RL, Phillips PM: The potassium and sodium requirements of certain mammals. Lancet 73:176, 1953.

31. Shank FR: Recent data on the amounts of sodium and potassium being consumed and future considerations for food labeling: In White PL, Crocco SC (eds): Sodium and Potassium in Foods and Drugs. Chicago, AMA, 1981.

32. Gotto AM, DeBakey ME, Scott LW, Foreyt JP: The Living Heart Diet. New York, Raven Press, (in press).

33. Bennett DR: Sodium content of prescription and nonprescription drugs. In White PL, Crocco SC (eds): Sodium and Potassium in Foods and Drugs. Chicago, AMA, 1981.

34. Glueck CJ, Christopher C, Tsang RC, Mellies MJ: Cholesterol-free diet and the physiologic hyperlipidemia of pregnancy in familial hypercholesterolemia. Metabolism 29: 949, 1980.

35. Mellies MJ, Ishikawa TT, Gartside PS, Burton K, MacGee J, Allen K, Steiner PM, Brady D, Glueck CJ: Effects of varying maternal dietary fatty acids in lactating women and their infants. Am J Clin Nutr 32:299, 1979.

36. Mellies MJ, Burton K, Larsen R, Fixler D, Glueck CJ: Cholesterol, phytosterols and polyunsaturated/saturated fatty acid ratios during the first 12 months of lactation. Am J Clin Nutr 32:2383, 1979.

37. Blackburn H, Berenson G, Christakis G: Conference on the health effects of blood lipids: Optimal distributions for populations. Workshop report: epidemiology section. Prev Med 8:612, 1979.

38. Jesse MJ, Cohen MM, Cunningham N, et al: The physician and children (pediatric and adolescent practice and the school): Task force I. Am J Cardiol 47:741, 1981.

Appendix

FOOD GROUP AND EXCHANGE SYSTEM TABLES

A. Meat, Poultry, and Seafood Guide
B. Estimating Portion Size of Meat, Poultry, and Seafood
C. Egg Guide
D. Fat Guide
E. Dairy Guide
F. Dairy Substitutes
G. Bread, Cereal, and Grain Products
H. Fruit Guide
I. Vegetable Guide
J. Miscellaneous Food Guide

HOW TO USE THE EXCHANGE SYSTEM TABLES

For *control of cholesterol,* choose foods from the "YES" list for each food group. The foods in this list are lower in total fat, saturated fat, and cholesterol than those in the "NO" list.

For *weight reduction* choose the desired calorie level (See Table 10-1). Then choose foods from the "YES" list that correspond to the food groups designated for the appropriate calorie level. Because the foods on the "YES" list are lower in fat and contain no sugar, they are lower in calories and higher in nutrient density than those on the "NO" list.

The *patient who is overweight, diabetic or hypertriglyceridemic* should follow the weight reduction plan.

Food items noted by (s) are high in sodium, and should be avoided by the *patient with hypertension.*

Fruit drinks and fruit juice with sugar added are high in simple sugar without being high in fat. They may be allowed on the diet of the patient with *elevated cholesterol* without obesity, diabetes, or endogenous hypertriglyceridemia, or the patient with chylomicronemia. Otherwise, these items should be avoided.

APPENDIX A   MEAT, POULTRY AND SEAFOOD GUIDE[a]

1 oz = 1 exchange
1 oz = 60 kcal, 8 g protein, 3 g fat

YES	NO
Fish and shellfish—all types except crayfish, eel, and fish roe	Fish and shellfish, crayfish, eel, fish roe, caviar
Chicken and turkey without skin	Poultry with skin, domesticated duck, goose
Lean, well-trimmed veal, beef, pork, and lamb	Beef, pork, lamb
Wild duck, pheasant, venison, and squirrel	all "prime" cuts
Liver—limit to 3 oz per month (very high in cholesterol)	bacon, brisket, sausage, corned beef, pastrami, ribs and spareribs, chili meat, regular ground meat
(s) Luncheon Meat	Organ meats
thinly sliced lean beef, chicken, turkey or ham	brains, chitterlings, gizzard, heart, kidney,
turkey franks	liver (more than 3 oz per month), pork maws,
turkey ham	sweetbreads
turkey pastrami	Game
Bean Products	venison sausage (if fat has been added)
soybean meat substitutes which have no saturated fat added	Luncheon Meat—all varieties of fresh or canned bologna, bratwurst, frankfurters, beef and
soybean meat extenders (textured vegetable protein)	pork, headcheese, liverwurst, pepperoni, salami
baked beans (without pork)—¼ cup	

[a](s) indicates high sodium content

APPENDIX B   ESTIMATING PORTION SIZE OF MEAT, POULTRY, AND SEAFOOD

Cooked weight = 3 oz

1 piece fish (3 × 2½ × ½ in)
½ large breast of chicken
1 leg and 1 thigh of chicken
½ rock Cornish hen
1 pound lean ground beef divided into 4 equal portions, one patty cooked
1 slice lean roast beef (3 × 3 × ¾ in)
1 medium pork chop (½ in thick)
Scallops, approximately 10 medium
Oysters, approximately 10 medium
Shrimp, 12 medium
1 slice beef, calf, pork, or lamb liver (3 × 2¼ × ⅜ in)
¾ cup chopped meat, fish or poultry

APPENDIX C   EGG GUIDE

1 whole egg = 1 oz lean meat
1 egg = 79 kcal, 6 g protein, 6 g fat

YES	NO
Egg yolks (2 per week) including those used in cooking Egg whites—free Egg substitutes—cholesterol free (1 egg equivalent = 1 oz meat)	Egg yolks—more than the 3 allowed per week Cakes, batters, sauces, rolls and other foods containing egg yolks Commercial cookies, cakes, mixes, and other commercial foods containing egg yolks Custard containing egg yolks (unless figured into weekly allowance) Egg substitutes that are not cholesterol free Eggnog and other beverages containing egg yolks

APPENDIX D   FAT GUIDE

1 exchange = 45 kcal, 5 g fat

YES	NO

Margarine—1 teaspoon tub or squeeze margarine listing either liquid safflower, sunflower, or corn oil as the first ingredient
Diet margarine—(same as the above)—2 teaspoons
Oil—1 teaspoon
  safflower
  walnut
  sunflower
  corn
  soybean
  cottonseed (or blends of soybean and cottonseed oils)
  sesame
Salad dressings—commercial or homemade
  salad dressings containing recommended ingredients—2 teaspoons
  mayonnaise—2 teaspoons
Nuts
  almonds — 7
  chestnuts — 5 small
  filberts — 5
  hazelnuts — 5
  hickory — 7 small
  mixed nuts — 4 to 6
  peanuts — 10
  pecans — 6 halves
  soynuts, toasted — 3 tablespoons
  walnuts[a] — 5 halves
Seeds
  pumpkin — 1 tablespoon
  sesame — 1 tablespoon
  sunflower — 1 tablespoon
Miscellaneous
  avocado (4 in diameter)—⅛
  olives—5 small
  peanut butter—2 teaspoons
	Margarine—any tub margarine not listing either safflower, sunflower, or corn oil as the first ingredient
	Saturated vegetable oils and shortening
	  coconut oil
	  palm kernel oil
	  partially hydrogenated vegetable oils
	  solid shortening
	Salad Dressings
	  blue cheese
	  green goddess
	  Roquefort
	  salad dressing made with sour cream or cheese
	Nuts
	  Brazil, cashew, macadamia, pistachio
	Food containing saturated fats
	  bacon
	  butter
	  chocolate
	  coconut
	  cream sauces
	  gravy made from meat drippings
	  ham hocks
	  lard
	  meat drippings
	  meat fat
	  salt pork

[a]Walnuts are highest in polyunsaturated fat of the nuts.

APPENDIX E   DAIRY GUIDE[a]

Amount listed is equal to 1 serving or 1 exchange
1 exchange = 80 kcal, 12 g carbohydrate, 8 g protein, less than 1 g fat

YES	NO
Milk	Milk
buttermilk made from skim milk—1 cup	buttermilk made from whole milk
buttermilk made from lowfat milk—1 cup + 1 fat exchange	chocolate milk
evaporated skim milk (undiluted)—½ cup or 1 cup diluted	condensed milk
evaporated lowfat milk (undiluted)—½ cup + 1 fat exchange or 1 cup diluted	evaporated milk
lowfat milk (1-2% butterfat)—1 cup + 1 fat exchange	whole milk
powdered skim milk—⅓ cup dry or 1 cup reconstituted	Cheese
powdered lowfat milk—⅓ cup dry or 1 cup reconstituted + 1 fat exchange	cheeses containing 12% butterfat or more
powdered buttermilk—⅓ cup dry or 1 cup reconstituted	Miscellaneous
skim milk (less than 1% butterfat)—1 cup	butter
Cheese	coffee cream
creamed cottage cheese—½ cup + 1 fat exchange	half and half
dry curd cottage cheese—½ cup	ice cream
lowfat cottage cheese—⅓ cup	mellorine
(s) skim milk cheese (1–5% butterfat)—2 oz	sour cream
(s) lowfat cheese (6–8% butterfat)—1½ oz	whipping cream
(s) vegetable oil cheeses—1 oz + 1 fat exchange	yogurt made from whole milk
Miscellaneous	yogurt with sweetened fruit
yogurt, plain, made from skim milk—1 cup	
yogurt, plain, made from lowfat milk—1 cup + 1 fat exchange	

[a](s) indicates high in sodium content

APPENDIX F   DAIRY SUBSTITUTES

1 exchange = 70 kcal, 15 g carbohydrate, 2 g protein

YES	NO
Products listing recommended oil as the predominant fat—1½ oz = 1 bread exchange	Imitation sour cream—tub, powdered, or canned
	Imitation whipped topping—tub, powdered, aerosol, or frozen
	Imitation coffee creamer—liquid, powdered, or frozen

APPENDIX G   BREAD, CEREAL, AND GRAIN PRODUCTS[a]

Any one of the following is a serving or exchange in the amount listed
1 exchange = 70 kcal, 15 g carbohydrate, 2 g protein

YES	NO
All whole grain and enriched bread products	Bread products
Bread, all varieties—1 slice	butter rolls
Cereal, cooked—½ cup	cheese breads
Cereal, dry, ready–to–eat—⅔ to ¾ cup	canned biscuits
[b]Cornbread, 2 inch cube—1 piece	commercial doughnuts
Hamburger bun, English muffin, bagel, or pita	muffins, sweet rolls
bread—½ each	waffles, and pancakes
[b]Muffin—1	croissants
[b]Pancake, 5 in diameter × ½ in thick—1	egg breads
Spaghetti, macaroni, lasagna, noodles—½ cup	Cereals
Tortilla, corn or flour—1	cereals containing coconut
	presweetened cereals
	Pastas
	egg noodles
	chow mein noodles
Low-fat crackers	Crackers
animal crackers—6	corn chips
Bread sticks (5 in × ½ in)—2	potato chips
flatbread or Finn crisp—4 to 6	tortilla chips
graham crackers (2½ in square)—2	commercial crackers
matzo (6 in square)—1	
melba toast (3½ × 1½ × ⅛ in)—4	
(s) oyster crackers—20	
(s) pretzels, large 3-ring (2½ in across)—4	
small 3-ring (1½ in across)—12	
rods (8 in)—3, sticks—20	
rye crackers (3½ × 1¾ in)—3	
(s) saltines (2 in square)—6	
(s) sesame wafers—3	
(s) soda crackers (2½ in square)—4	
zwiebach—2	
Desserts	Desserts
angel food cake (3 × 1 × ½ in)—1 slice	cheesecake pastries
sherbet or fruit ice—¼ cup	commercial cakes, pies, cookies, fried pies,
gelatin (regular)—⅓ cup	and cupcakes
ice milk or frozen yogurt—⅓ cup	commercial mixes containing dried eggs,
	whole milk, coconut oil, or
	hydrogenated shortening
	commercial sweet rolls
	ice cream
	mellorine
Starchy vegetables	
acorn squash—½ cup	
baked bean, canned or homemade (no pork)—	
¼ cup	
corn—⅓ cup or ½ large corn on the cob	
dried beans, peas, lentils, chick peas,	
garbanzos,soybeans, or lima beans—	
½ cup cooked	
green peas—½ cup cooked	
hominy—½ cup cooked	
parsnips—½ cup cooked	
popcorn (popped, no fat added)—1½ cups	
pumpkin—¾ cup	
[c]sweet potatoes, yams—¼ cup mashed	
[c]white potatoes—1 small or ½ cup mashed	

(continued)

APPENDIX G (continued)

YES	NO
Soup[d]	Soup
Soup such as broth, bouillon, and consomme may be included in the diet freely because they contain negligible calories.	Cream of potato, mushroom, chicken, celery and cheese soup, chunky type soups, vichyssoise
Vegetable soup—count soups made from starchy vegetables, such as corn, peas, beans, or potatoes as ½ cup = 1 bread exchange	
beef stew—count ounces of meat as meat exchanges and ½ cup starchy vegetable as 1 bread exchange	
mixed vegetable or tomato soup 1 cup = 1 bread exchange	
Alcohol	
The amount listed is 1 serving and may be exchanged for 1 serving from the Bread and Cereal Guide. Limit to 2 servings per day.	
bourbon, gin, rum, Scotch, tequila, vodka, whiskey—1 oz	
dessert or sweet wine—1½ oz	
dry table wine—2½ oz	
regular beer—5 oz	
light beer—check label for calorie and carbohydrate content	
Miscellaneous	
bread crumbs—3 tablespoons	
catsup—¼ cup	
chili sauce—¼ cup	
cocoa—5 tablespoons	
cornmeal—2 tablespoons	
cornstarch—2 tablespoons	
flour—2½ tablespoons	
tapioca—2 tablespoons	
tomato paste—6 tablespoons	
tomato sauce—1 cup	

[a](s) indicates high sodium content

[b]Recipe should be modified to contain ingredients from the ''Yes'' food lists, that is, lowfat or skim milk, margarine, and egg substitute.

[c]Without added fat. In preparation use ingredients from the ''Yes'' food lists and count added fat as part of daily allowance.

[d]Canned soup is high in sodium.

APPENDIX H   FRUIT GUIDE[a]

1 exchange = 40 kcal, 10 g carbohydrate
(A) (C) = good source of vitamins A and C

YES	NO
Apple (2″ in diameter)—1	Commercial fruit pie fillings
Apple juice (frozen or canned)—⅓ cup	Commercial fruit whips
Applesauce, unsweetened—½ cup	Fruits in sugar syrup
Apricots, fresh—2 medium	
Apricots, dried—4 halves	
Banana—½ small	
Blackberries—½ cup	
Blueberries—½ cup	
Cantaloupe (6 in diameter)—¼ (C) (A)	
Cherries—10 large	
Cranberry juice cocktail	
low-calorie—¾ cup	
regular—¼ cup	
Cranberry sauce—2 tablespoons	
Dates—2	
Dewberries—½ cup	
Figs, fresh—2 large	
Figs, dried—1 small	
Fruit cocktail, unsweetened—½ cup	
Grapefruit—½ small (C)	
Grapefruit juice (fresh, frozen, canned)—	
½ cup (C)	
Grapes, Tokay—12	
Grapes, green seedless—18	
Grape juice (frozen or canned)—¼ cup	
Honeydew melon (7 in diameter)—⅛	
Kumquats—4 medium	
Mandarin oranges—½ cup	
Mango—½ small (C)	
Mixed fruit (canned), unsweetened—½ cup	
Nectar—¼ cup	
Nectarine—1 medium	
Orange (2½ in diameter)—1 (C)	
Orange juice (fresh, frozen, canned)—½ cup (C)	
Papaya—⅓ medium (C)	
Peach—1 medium (A)	
Pear—1 small	
Pineapple, unsweetened	
chunk—½ cup	
slices—2 small	
juice (frozen or canned)—½ cup	
Plums—2 medium	
Prunes, dried—2 medium	
Prune juice—¼ cup	
Raisins—2 tablespoons	
Raspberries—½ cup	
Strawberries—1 cup (C)	
Tangerine—1 large (C)	
Tangerine juice—½ cup (C)	
(s) Tomato juice (up to 1 cup free)—1 cup (C)	
(s)Vegetable juice cocktail (up to 1 cup free)—1 cup	
Watermelon—1 cup	

[a](s) indicates high sodium content

APPENDIX I   VEGETABLE GUIDE

Vegetables may be fresh, frozen, or canned without sauce. Vegetables may be eaten as desired in moderate amounts either cooked or raw and not counted as part of the daily food exchanges. Starchy vegetables, such as potatoes and corn, are listed in the Bread Cereal and Grain Products Guide (Appendix G).

(A) (C) = good source of vitamins A and C.

YES	NO
Artichoke	Commercially fried vegetables such as fried potatoes, French fries, onion rings, okra, and eggplant
Asparagus (C)	
Bamboo shoots	
Beans, green and wax	Commercial vegetables, frozen or canned, packaged in a sauce or butter
Beets	
Broccoli (A) (C)	Dried beans or peas seasoned with bacon fat, salt pork, or ham hocks
Brussels sprouts	
Cabbage, any variety (C)	Frozen French fries and fried onion rings
Carrots (A)	
Cauliflower	
Celery	
Chicory (A)	
Cucumbers, escarole (A)	
Eggplant, ginger root	
Greens (A) (C)	
beet kale	
chard mustard	
collard spinach	
dandelion turnip	
Kohlrabi	
Leeks	
Lettuce	
Mushrooms	
Okra	
Onions	
Parsley	
Pepper (green and red) (C)	
Pimento	
Radishes	
Rutabagas	
Sauerkraut	
Shallots	
Spinach (C)	
Sprouts (alfalfa and bean)	
Summer squash (zucchini, yellow, etc.)	
Tomatoes (C)	
Turnips	
Watercress (A)	
Water chestnuts	

APPENDIX J   MISCELLANEOUS FOOD GUIDE[a]

Some foods are low enough in calories that it is not necessary to consider their total calories. Spices and herbs add flavor without adding calories. Many beverages such as coffee, tea, and diet carbonated drinks also add variety.

YES	NO
These foods are *very low* in calories and may be eaten freely:	These foods are *high* in calories and may lead to weight gain and/or an elevation in triglycerides:
Bitters	Alcoholic beverages—beer, wine, whiskey, etc. (except as exchanged for bread in Appendix G)
Bouillon (fat free)	Candy
Clear broth (fat free)	Cakes
Club soda	Cookies
Cocoa (limit 1 tablespoon free)	Fruit flavored drinks, punches, ades
Coffee, black	Fruit whips
Consomme (fat free)	Gum
Cranberries (unsweetened)	Honey
Decaffeinated coffee	Jelly, jam, marmalade, preserves
Diet salad dressing (limit to 1 tablespoon per meal)	Molasses
Diet gelatin	Pastries
Diet soft drinks	Pies
Dietetic jelly, jam, preserves, syrup	Puddings
Flavoring essence (maple, butter, etc.)	Regular carbonated beverages
Gelatin, unflavored	Sugar
Horseradish, hot sauce	Syrup
Lemon, lime	
Liquid smoke, mustard	
Picante sauce	
(s)Pickles (unsweetened)	
Rennet tablets	
Rhubarb (unsweetened)	
(s)Soy sauce	
Spices and herbs	
Sugar substitute	
Sugarless gum	
Tea, no sugar	
Vinegar	
(s)Worcestershire sauce	

[a](s) indicates high sodium content

Index